AIDS
SOURCEBOOK

Seventh Edition

Health Reference Series

Seventh Edition

AIDS
SOURCEBOOK

Basic Consumer Health Information about the Human Immunodeficiency Virus (HIV) and Acquired Immunodeficiency Syndrome (AIDS), Including Facts about Its Origins, Stages, Types, Transmission, Risk Factors, and Prevention, and Featuring Details about Diagnostic Testing, Antiretroviral Treatments, and Co-Occurring Infections, Such as Cytomegalovirus, Mycobacterium avium *Complex,* Pneumocystis carinii *Pneumonia, and Toxoplasmosis*

Along with Tips for Living with HIV/AIDS, Updated Statistics, Reports on Current Research Initiatives, a Glossary of Related Terms, and a List of Resources for Additional Help and Information

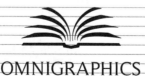

OMNIGRAPHICS
615 Griswold, Ste. 901, Detroit, MI 48226

Bibliographic Note
Because this page cannot legibly accommodate all the copyright notices, the Bibliographic Note portion of the Preface constitutes an extension of the copyright notice.

* * *

OMNIGRAPHICS
Angela L. Williams, *Managing Editor*
***

Copyright © 2018 Omnigraphics

ISBN 978-0-7808-1636-7
E-ISBN 978-0-7808-1637-4

Library of Congress Cataloging-in-Publication Data

Names: Omnigraphics, Inc., issuing body.

Title: AIDS sourcebook: basic consumer health information about the human immunodeficiency virus (HIV) and acquired immunodeficiency syndrome (AIDS), including facts about its origins, stages, types, transmission, risk factors, and prevention, and featuring details about diagnostic testing, antiretroviral treatments, and co-occurring infections, such as Cytomegalovirus, Mycobacterium Avium Complex, Pneumocystis Carinii Pneumonia, and Toxoplasmosis; along with tips for living with HIV/AIDS, updated statistics, reports on current research initiatives, a glossary of related terms, and a list of resources for additional help and information.

Description: Seventh edition. | Detroit, MI: Omnigraphics, [2018] | Series: Health reference series | Includes bibliographical references and index.

Identifiers: LCCN 2018019925 (print) | LCCN 2018020119 (ebook) | ISBN 9780780816374 (eBook) | ISBN 9780780816367 (hardcover: alk. paper)

Subjects: LCSH: AIDS (Disease)--Popular works.

Classification: LCC RC606.64 (ebook) | LCC RC606.64.A337 2018 (print) | DDC 362.19697/92--dc23

LC record available at https://lccn.loc.gov/2018019925

Table of Contents

Part II: HIV/AIDS Transmission, Risk Factors, and Prevention

Part III: Receiving an HIV/AIDS Diagnosis

Part IV: Treatments and Therapies for HIV/AIDS

Part V: Common Co-Occurring Infections and Complications of HIV/AIDS

Part VI: Living with HIV Infection

Part VII: Additional Help and Information

Preface

About This Book

According to the Centers for Disease Control and Prevention (CDC), more than 1.1 million Americans are living with human immunodeficiency virus (HIV) infection. Nearly 40,000 people in the United States were diagnosed with HIV in 2016, the most recent year for which statistics are available. This devastating disease attacks the immune system and affects all parts of the body, eventually leading to acquired immunodeficiency syndrome (AIDS), its most deadly and advanced stage, for which there is currently no cure. Yet there is hope for the many Americans living with HIV infection or AIDS. Researchers are developing new and more effective drug combinations, and scientists are growing ever closer to a vaccine. Improvements in medications and earlier diagnosis mean that those infected with HIV are living longer, healthier, and more productive lives. Still, many Americans are unaware of even the basic facts about HIV—how it is transmitted, how HIV progresses to AIDS, and how HIV and AIDS are treated.

AIDS Sourcebook, Seventh Edition provides basic consumer information about the HIV and AIDS, including information about the stages and types of the disease and about how it is transmitted. It includes guidelines for preventing disease transmission and details about how it is diagnosed and the various drug regimens used in its treatment. Information on co-occurring infections, complications, and tips for living with HIV infection are also included. The book concludes with a glossary of related terms and a list of resources for additional help and information.

How to Use This Book

This book is divided into parts and chapters. Parts focus on broad areas of interest. Chapters are devoted to single topics within a part.

Part I: Basic Information about Human Immunodeficiency Virus/ Acquired Immunodeficiency Syndrome (HIV/AIDS) defines HIV and AIDS, briefs up about what is known regarding the origin of the virus, symptoms, and facts. It describes the life cycle, stages, and types of HIV infection, and explains how HIV causes AIDS. It also includes a brief discussion of the prevalence and incidence of HIV and AIDS in the United States and especially among specific populations.

Part II: HIV/AIDS Transmission, Risk Factors, and Prevention presents the facts about the transmission of the human immunodeficiency virus and debunks some of the rumors about how this infection is transmitted. It explains the factors that put people at risk for HIV, provides tips for avoiding these risks, and answers questions related to transmission, risk, PrEP, and prevention.

Part III: Receiving an HIV/AIDS Diagnosis describes the different types of HIV testing and explains consumer rights regarding confidentiality and counseling. It provides a detailed explanation of what the test results mean and how to determine if you have AIDS. It provides tips for choosing a provider and navigating the healthcare system and concludes with answers to frequently asked questions on testing and window period.

Part IV: Treatment and Therapies for HIV/AIDS gives an overview of treatment options, details the antiretroviral treatment process, describes the common side effects and complications of this treatment, and explains how the effectiveness of treatment is monitored and what to do in the event of treatment failure. It also discusses complementary and alternative HIV/AIDS treatments, other treatments currently being developed including the ones which are being researched, and how treatment varies in the special cases of children and pregnant women. It also offers information regarding paying for HIV care and provides answer to questions pertaining to treatment.

Part V: Common Co-Occurring Infections and Complications of HIV / AIDS describes the bacterial, fungal, parasitic, and viral infections that often accompany HIV and AIDS. It also offers tips on how to avoid these infections and explains how they are treated when they do occur. In addition, AIDS-related cancer, wasting syndrome, HIV-associated neurocognitive disorders, and other AIDS-related health concerns are discussed.

Part VI: Living with HIV Infection offers advice on coping with an HIV/ AIDS diagnosis and explains how diet and exercise can help maintain health. It discusses legal responsibility for disclosure and provides tips for telling a spouse or sexual partners, family and friends, co-workers, and healthcare providers about HIV status. The part concludes with a discussion about laws that apply to people with HIV and a description of the public benefits, insurance, and housing options available, including information about providing home care for someone with AIDS.

Part VII: Additional Help and Information includes a glossary of terms related to AIDS and HIV and a directory of resources for additional help and support.

Bibliographic Note

This volume contains documents and excerpts from publications issued by the following government agencies: Centers for Disease Control and Prevention (CDC); Centers for Medicare and Medicaid Services (CMS); *Eunice Kennedy Shriver* National Institute of Child Health and Human Development (NICHD); Genetic and Rare Diseases Information Center (GARD); Health Resources and Services Administration (HRSA); National Cancer Institute (NCI); National Heart, Lung, and Blood Institute (NHLBI); National Institute of Allergy and Infectious Diseases (NIAID); National Institute of Dental and Craniofacial Research (NIDCR); National Institute of Diabetes and Digestive and Kidney Diseases (NIDDK); National Institute of Mental Health (NIMH); National Institute of Neurological Disorders and Stroke (NINDS); National Institute on Drug Abuse (NIDA); National Institutes of Health (NIH); Office on Women's Health (OWH); U.S. Department of Health and Human Services (HHS); U.S. Department of Justice (DOJ); U.S. Department of Labor (DOL); U.S. Department of Veterans Affairs (VA); U.S. Food and Drug Administration (FDA); U.S. National Library of Medicine (NLM); and U.S. Social Security Administration (SSA).

About the Health Reference Series

The *Health Reference Series* is designed to provide basic medical information for patients, families, caregivers, and the general public. Each volume takes a particular topic and provides comprehensive coverage. This is especially important for people who may be dealing with a newly diagnosed disease or a chronic disorder in themselves or in a family member. People looking for preventive guidance, information about disease warning signs, medical statistics, and risk factors for health problems will also find answers to their questions in the *Health Reference Series*. The *Series*, however, is not intended to serve as a tool for diagnosing illness, in prescribing treatments, or as a substitute for the physician/patient relationship. All people concerned about medical symptoms or the possibility of disease are encouraged to seek professional care from an appropriate healthcare provider.

A Note about Spelling and Style

Health Reference Series editors use *Stedman's Medical Dictionary* as an authority for questions related to the spelling of medical terms and the *Chicago Manual of Style* for questions related to grammatical structures, punctuation, and other editorial concerns. Consistent adherence is not always possible, however, because the individual volumes within the *Series* include many documents from a wide variety of different producers, and the editor's primary goal is to present material from each source as accurately as is possible. This sometimes means that information in different chapters or sections may follow other guidelines and alternate spelling authorities.

Medical Review

Omnigraphics contracts with a team of qualified, senior medical professionals who serve as medical consultants for the *Health Reference Series*. As necessary, medical consultants review reprinted and originally written material for currency and accuracy. Citations including the phrase, "Reviewed (month, year)" indicate material reviewed by this team. Medical consultation services are provided to the *Health Reference Series* editors by:

Dr. Vijayalakshmi, MBBS, DGO, MD
Dr. Senthil Selvan, MBBS, DCH, MD
Dr. K. Sivanandham, MBBS, DCH, MS (Research), PhD

Our Advisory Board

We would like to thank the following board members for providing initial guidance on the development of this series:

- Dr. Lynda Baker, Associate Professor of Library and Information Science, Wayne State University, Detroit, MI

- Nancy Bulgarelli, William Beaumont Hospital Library, Royal Oak, MI

- Karen Imarisio, Bloomfield Township Public Library, Bloomfield Township, MI

- Karen Morgan, Mardigian Library, University of Michigan-Dearborn, Dearborn, MI

- Rosemary Orlando, St. Clair Shores Public Library, St. Clair Shores, MI

Health Reference Series *Update Policy*

The inaugural book in the *Health Reference Series* was the first edition of *Cancer Sourcebook* published in 1989. Since then, the *Series* has been enthusiastically received by librarians and in the medical community. In order to maintain the standard of providing high-quality health information for the layperson the editorial staff at Omnigraphics felt it was necessary to implement a policy of updating volumes when warranted.

Medical researchers have been making tremendous strides, and it is the purpose of the *Health Reference Series* to stay current with the most recent advances. Each decision to update a volume is made on an individual basis. Some of the considerations include how much new information is available and the feedback we receive from people who use the books. If there is a topic you would like to see added to the update list, or an area of medical concern you feel has not been adequately addressed, please write to:

Managing Editor
Health Reference Series
Omnigraphics
615 Griswold, Ste. 901
Detroit, MI 48226

Part One

Basic Information about Human Immunodeficiency Virus / Acquired Immunodeficiency Syndrome (HIV/AIDS)

Chapter 1

Definition and Origin of HIV and AIDS

Human immunodeficiency virus (HIV) is a virus spread through certain body fluids that attacks the body's immune system, specifically the CD4 cells, often called T cells. Over time, HIV can destroy so many of these cells that the body can't fight off infections and disease. These special cells help the immune system fight off infections. Untreated, HIV reduces the number of CD4 cells (T cells) in the body. This damage to the immune system makes it harder and harder for the body to fight off infections and some other diseases. Opportunistic infections or cancers take advantage of a very weak immune system and signal that the person has acquired immunodeficiency syndrome (AIDS). Learn more about the stages of HIV and how to know whether you're infected.

What Is Human Immunodeficiency Virus (HIV)?

HIV stands for human immunodeficiency virus. It is the virus that can lead to acquired immunodeficiency syndrome, or AIDS, if not treated.

This chapter contains text excerpted from the following sources: Text in this chapter begins with text excerpted from "What Are HIV and AIDS?" HIV.gov, U.S. Department of Health and Human Services (HHS), May 15, 2017; Text under the heading "Where Did HIV Come From?" is excerpted from "Origins of HIV and the AIDS Pandemic," U.S. National Library of Medicine (NLM), September 1, 2011. Reviewed June 2018. Text under the heading "How Do I Know If I Have HIV?" is excerpted from "About HIV/AIDS—HIV Basics," Centers for Disease Control and Prevention (CDC), March 16, 2018.

Unlike some other viruses, the human body can't get rid of HIV completely, even with treatment. So once you get HIV, you have it for life.

HIV attacks the body's immune system, specifically the CD4 cells (T cells), which help the immune system fight off infections. Untreated, HIV reduces the number of CD4 cells (T cells) in the body, making the person more likely to get other infections or infection-related cancers. Over time, HIV can destroy so many of these cells that the body can't fight off infections and disease. These opportunistic infections or cancers take advantage of a very weak immune system and signal that the person has AIDS, the last stage of HIV infection.

No effective cure currently exists, but with proper medical care, HIV can be controlled. The medicine used to treat HIV is called antiretroviral therapy or ART. If taken the right way, every day, this medicine can dramatically prolong the lives of many people infected with HIV, keep them healthy, and greatly lower their chance of infecting others. Before the introduction of ART in the mid-1990s, people with HIV could progress to AIDS in just a few years. Today, someone diagnosed with HIV and treated before the disease is far advanced can live nearly as long as someone who does not have HIV.

What Is Acquired Immunodeficiency Syndrome (AIDS)?

AIDS is the most severe phase of HIV infection. People with AIDS have such badly damaged immune systems that they get an increasing number of severe illnesses, called opportunistic infections.

What Are the Stages of HIV Infection?

Without treatment, HIV advances in stages, overwhelming your immune system and getting worse over time. The three stages of HIV infection are (1) acute HIV infection, (2) clinical latency, and (3) AIDS (acquired immunodeficiency syndrome).

However, there's good news: by using HIV medicines (called antiretroviral therapy or ART) consistently, you can prevent HIV from progressing to AIDS. ART helps control the virus so that you can live a longer, healthier life and greatly reduces the risk of transmitting HIV to others.

These are the three stages of HIV infection:

Acute HIV Infection Stage

Within 2 to 4 weeks after infection, many, but not all, people develop flu-like symptoms, often described as "the worst flu ever." Symptoms can include fever, swollen glands, sore throat, rash, muscle and joint aches and pains, and headache. This is called "acute retroviral syndrome" (ARS) or "primary HIV infection," and it's the body's natural response to the HIV infection. People who think that they may have been infected recently and are in the acute stage of HIV infection should seek medical care right away. Starting treatment at this stage can have significant benefits to your health.

During this early period of infection, large amounts of virus are being produced in your body. The virus uses CD4 cells to replicate and destroys them in the process. Because of this, your CD4 cells can fall rapidly. Eventually, your immune response will begin to bring the level of virus in your body back down to a level called a viral set point, which is a relatively stable level of virus in your body. At this point, your CD4 count begins to increase, but it may not return to preinfection levels. It may be particularly beneficial to your health to begin ART during this stage.

During the acute HIV infection stage, you are at very high risk of transmitting HIV to your sexual or needle-sharing partners because the levels of HIV in your bloodstream are extremely high. For this reason, it is very important to take steps to reduce your risk of transmission.

Clinical Latency Stage

After the acute stage of HIV infection, the disease moves into a stage called the "clinical latency" stage. "Latency" means a period where a virus is living or developing in a person without producing symptoms. During the clinical latency stage, people who are infected with HIV experience no symptoms, or only mild ones. (This stage is sometimes called "asymptomatic HIV infection" or "chronic HIV infection.")

During the clinical latency stage, the HIV virus continues to reproduce at very low levels, even if it cannot be detected with standard laboratory tests. If you take ART, you may live with clinical latency for decades and never progress to AIDS because treatment helps keep the virus in check.

People in this symptom-free stage are still able to transmit HIV to others. The risk of transmission is greatly reduced by HIV treatment. In studies looking at the effects of HIV treatment on transmission, no new HIV infections have been linked to someone with very low or undetectable (suppressed) viral load.

For people who are not on ART, the clinical latency stage lasts an average of 10 years, but some people may progress through this stage faster. As the disease progressions, eventually your viral load will begin to rise and your CD4 count will begin to decline. As this happens, you may begin to have constitutional symptoms of HIV as the virus levels increase in your body before you develop AIDS.

AIDS

This is the stage of HIV infection that occurs when your immune system is badly damaged and you become vulnerable to opportunistic infections. When the number of your CD4 cells falls below 200 cells per cubic millimeter of blood (200 cells/mm^3), you are considered to have progressed to AIDS. (In someone with a healthy immune system, CD4 counts are between 500 and 1,600 cells/mm^3.) You are also considered to have progressed to AIDS if you develop one or more opportunistic illnesses, regardless of your CD4 count.

Without treatment, people who progress to AIDS typically survive about 3 years. Once you have a dangerous opportunistic illness, life-expectancy without treatment falls to about 1 year. ART can be helpful for people who have AIDS when diagnosed and can be lifesaving. Treatment is likely to benefit people with HIV no matter when it is started, but people who start ART soon after they get HIV experience more benefits from treatment than do people who start treatment after they have developed AIDS.

In the United States, most people with HIV do not develop AIDS because effective ART stops disease progression. People with HIV who are diagnosed early can have a lifespan that is about the same as someone like them who does not HIV.

People living with HIV may progress through these stages at different rates, depending on a variety of factors, including their genetic makeup, how healthy they were before they were infected, how much virus they were exposed to and its genetic characteristics, how soon after infection they are diagnosed and linked to care and treatment, whether they see their healthcare provider regularly and take their HIV medications as directed, and different health-related choices they make, such as decisions to eat a healthful diet, exercise, and not smoke.

Is There a Cure for HIV?

No effective cure currently exists for HIV. But with proper medical care, HIV can be controlled. Treatment for HIV is called antiretroviral therapy or ART. If taken the right way, every day, ART can dramatically prolong the lives of many people infected with HIV, keep them healthy, and greatly lower their chance of infecting others. Before the introduction of ART in the mid-1990s, people with HIV could progress to AIDS (the last stage of HIV infection) in a few years. Today, someone diagnosed with HIV and treated before the disease is far advanced can live nearly as long as someone who does not have HIV.

Where Did HIV Come From?

Acquired immunodeficiency syndrome (AIDS) was first recognized as a new disease in 1981 when increasing numbers of young homosexual men succumbed to unusual opportunistic infections and rare malignancies. A retrovirus, now termed human immunodeficiency virus type 1 (HIV-1), was subsequently identified as the causative agent of what has since become one of the most devastating infectious diseases to have emerged in recent history. HIV-1 spreads by sexual, percutaneous, and perinatal routes; however, 80 percent of adults acquire HIV-1 following exposure at mucosal surfaces, and AIDS is thus primarily a sexually transmitted disease. Since its first identification almost three decades ago, the pandemic form of HIV-1, also called the main (M) group, has infected at least 60 million people and caused more than 25 million deaths. Developing countries have experienced the greatest HIV/AIDS morbidity and mortality, with the highest prevalence rates recorded in young adults in sub-Saharan Africa. Although antiretroviral treatment has reduced the toll of AIDS-related deaths, access to therapy is not universal, and the prospects of curative treatments and an effective vaccine are uncertain. Thus, AIDS will continue to pose a significant public health threat for decades to come.

Ever since HIV-1 was first discovered, the reasons for its sudden emergence, epidemic spread, and unique pathogenicity have been a subject of intense study. A first clue came in 1986 when a morphologically similar but antigenically distinct virus was found to cause AIDS in patients in western Africa. Curiously, this new virus, termed human immunodeficiency virus type 2 (HIV-2), was only distantly related to HIV-1 but was closely related to a simian virus that caused immunodeficiency in captive macaques. Soon thereafter, additional viruses, collectively termed simian immunodeficiency viruses (SIVs) with a suffix to denote their species of origin, were found in various different primates from sub-Saharan Africa, including African green monkeys, sooty mangabeys, mandrills, chimpanzees, and others. Surprisingly, these viruses appeared to be largely nonpathogenic in their natural hosts, despite clustering together with the human and simian AIDS viruses in a single phylogenetic lineage within the radiation of lentiviruses. Interestingly, close simian relatives of HIV-1 and HIV-2 were found in chimpanzees and sooty mangabeys, respectively. These relationships provided the first evidence that AIDS had emerged in both humans and macaques as a consequence of cross-species infections with lentiviruses from different primate species. Indeed, subsequent studies confirmed that SIVmac was not a natural pathogen of macaques (which are Asian primates), but had been generated inadvertently in U.S. primate centers by inoculating various species of macaques with blood and/or tissues from naturally infected sooty mangabeys. Similarly, it became clear that HIV-1 and HIV-2 were the result of zoonotic transfers of viruses infecting primates in Africa.

How Do I Know If I Have HIV?

The only way to know for sure whether you have HIV is to get tested. Knowing your status is important because it helps you make healthy decisions to prevent getting or transmitting HIV.

Some people may experience a flu-like illness within 2–4 weeks after infection (stage 1 HIV infection). But some people may not feel sick during this stage. Flu-like symptoms include fever, chills, rash, night sweats, muscle aches, sore throat, fatigue, swollen lymph nodes, or mouth ulcers. These symptoms can last anywhere from a few days to several weeks. During this time, HIV infection may not show up on an HIV test, but people who have it are highly infectious and can spread the infection to others.

If you have these symptoms, that doesn't mean you have HIV. Each of these symptoms can be caused by other illnesses. But if you have these symptoms after a potential exposure to HIV, see a healthcare provider and tell them about your risk. The only way to determine whether you are infected is to be tested for HIV infection.

To find places near you that offer confidential HIV testing,

- Visit gettested.cdc.gov,

- Text your ZIP code to KNOW IT (566948), or

- Call 800-CDC-INFO (800-232-4636).

You can also use a home testing kit, available for purchase in most pharmacies and online.

After you get tested, it's important to find out the result of your test so you can talk to your healthcare provider about treatment options if you're HIV-positive or learn ways to prevent getting HIV if you're HIV-negative.

Chapter 2

HIV Stages and Types

Chapter Contents

Section 2.1

The HIV Life Cycle

This section includes content from "The HIV Life Cycle,"
AIDS*info*, U.S. Department of Health and Human
Services (HHS), August 18, 2017.

Human immunodeficiency virus (HIV) infection attacks and destroys the cluster of differentiation 4 (CD4) cells of the immune system. CD4 cells are a type of white blood cell (WBC) that play a major role in protecting the body from infection. HIV uses the machinery of the CD4 cells to multiply (make copies of itself) and spread throughout the body. This process, which is carried out in seven steps or stages, is called the HIV life cycle.

The Seven Stages of the HIV Life Cycle

The seven stages of the HIV life cycle are:

1. **Binding** (also called attachment). HIV binds (attaches itself) to receptors on the surface of a CD4 cell.

2. **Fusion.** The HIV envelope and the CD4 cell membrane fuse (join together), which allows HIV to enter the CD4 cell.

3. **Reverse transcription.** Inside the CD4 cell, HIV releases and uses reverse transcriptase (an HIV enzyme) to convert its genetic material—HIV ribonucleic acid (RNA)—into HIV deoxyribonucleic acid (DNA). The conversion of HIV RNA to HIV DNA allows HIV to enter the CD4 cell nucleus and combine with the cell's genetic material—cell DNA.

4. **Integration.** Inside the CD4 cell nucleus. HIV releases integrase (an HIV enzyme). HIV uses integrase to insert (integrate) its viral DNA into the DNA of the CD4 cell.

5. **Replication.** Once integrated into the CD4 cell DNA, HIV begins to use the machinery of the CD4 cell to make long chains of HIV proteins. The protein chains are the building blocks for more HIV.

6. **Assembly.** Now HIV proteins and HIV RNA move to the surface of the cell and assemble into immature (noninfectious) HIV.

7. **Budding.** Newly formed immature (noninfectious) HIV pushes itself out of the host CD4 cell. The new HIV releases protease (an HIV enzyme). Protease acts to break up the long protein chains that form the immature virus. The smaller HIV proteins combine to form mature (infectious) HIV.

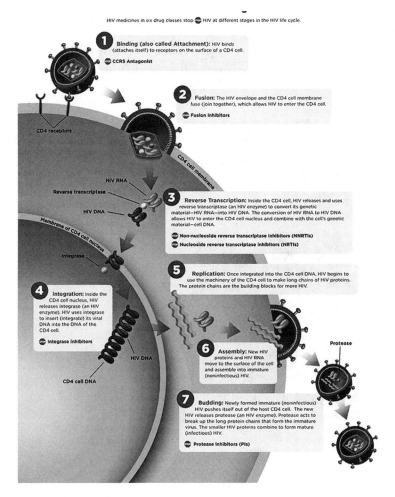

Figure 2.1. *HIV Life Cycle*

Connection between the HIV Life Cycle and HIV Medicines

Antiretroviral therapy (ART) is the use of HIV medicines to treat HIV infection. HIV medicines protect the immune system by blocking

HIV at different stages of the HIV life cycle. HIV medicines are grouped into different drug classes according to how they fight HIV. Each class of drugs is designed to target a specific step in the HIV life cycle. ART combines HIV medicines from at least two different HIV drug classes, making it very effective at preventing HIV from multiplying. Having less HIV in the body protects the immune system and prevents HIV from advancing to acquired immunodeficiency syndrome (AIDS). ART also reduces the risk of HIV drug resistance.

ART can't cure HIV, but HIV medicines help people with HIV live longer, healthier lives. HIV medicines also reduce the risk of HIV transmission (the spread of HIV to others).

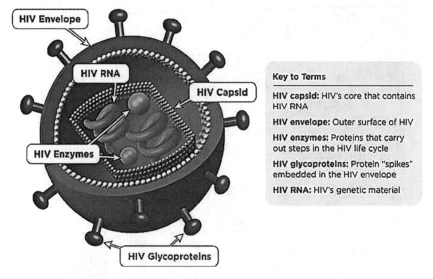

Figure 2.2. *Human Immunodeficiency Virus*

Section 2.2

Stages of HIV Infection

This section includes content from "About HIV/AIDS,"
Centers for Disease Control and Prevention (CDC), March 16, 2018.

When people get human immunodeficiency virus (HIV) and don't receive treatment, they will typically progress through three stages of disease. Medicine to treat HIV, known as antiretroviral therapy (ART), helps people at all stages of the disease if taken the right way, every day. Treatment can slow or prevent progression from one stage to the next. It can also dramatically reduce the chance of transmitting HIV to someone else.

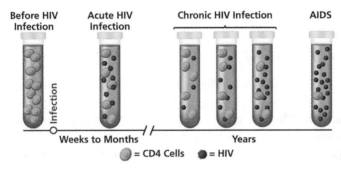

Figure 2.3. *Stages of HIV*

Three Stages of Human Immunodeficiency Virus (HIV) Infection

Stage 1. Acute HIV Infection

Within 2–4 weeks after infection with HIV, people may experience a flu-like illness, which may last for a few weeks. This is the body's natural response to infection. When people have acute HIV infection, they have a large amount of virus in their blood and are very contagious. But people with acute infection are often unaware that they're infected because they may not feel sick right away or at all. To know whether someone has an acute infection, either a fourth-generation antibody/antigen test or a nucleic acid (NAT) test is necessary. If you think you have been exposed to HIV through sex or drug use and you have flu-like symptoms, seek medical care and ask for a test to diagnose acute infection.

Stage 2. Clinical Latency (HIV Inactivity or Dormancy)

This period is sometimes called asymptomatic HIV infection or chronic HIV infection. During this phase, HIV is still active but reproduces at very low levels. People may not have any symptoms or get sick during this time. For people who aren't taking medicine to treat HIV, this period can last a decade or longer, but some may progress through this phase faster. People who are taking medicine to treat HIV (ART) the right way, every day may be in this stage for several decades. It's important to remember that people can still transmit HIV to others during this phase, although people who are on ART and stay virally suppressed (having a very low level of virus in their blood) are much less likely to transmit HIV than those who are not virally suppressed. At the end of this phase, a person's viral load starts to go up and the CD4 cell count begins to go down. As this happens, the person may begin to have symptoms as the virus levels increase in the body, and the person moves into stage 3.

Stage 3. Acquired Immunodeficiency Syndrome (AIDS)

Acquired immunodeficiency syndrome (AIDS) is the most severe phase of HIV infection. People with AIDS have such badly damaged immune systems that they get an increasing number of severe illnesses, called opportunistic illnesses.

Without treatment, people with AIDS typically survive about 3 years. Common symptoms of AIDS include:

- Chills
- Fever
- Sweats
- Swollen lymph glands
- Weakness
- Weight loss

People are diagnosed with AIDS when their CD4 cell count drops below 200 cells/mm or if they develop certain opportunistic illnesses. People with AIDS can have a high viral load and be very infectious.

Section 2.3

Acute HIV Infection

This section includes content from "Patient Information Sheet—Acute HIV Infection," Centers for Disease Control and Prevention (CDC), May 14, 2014. Reviewed June 2018.

HIV stands for human immunodeficiency virus. This is the virus that causes acquired immunodeficiency syndrome (AIDS). Acute HIV infection is a name for the earliest stage of HIV infection when you first get infected with the HIV virus. It is sometimes also called primary HIV infection. Many people with acute HIV infection have the following:

- A fever

- A tired feeling

- Swollen lymph nodes (also called lymph glands)

- Swollen tonsils (also called tonsillitis)

- A sore throat

- Joint and muscle aches

- Diarrhea

- A rash

These signs and symptoms of acute HIV infection can begin a few days after you are exposed to HIV and usually last for about 14 days. They could last for just a few days, or they could last for several months.

You might not realize your illness is acute HIV infection. For one thing, you may not have known that the person you had sex with had HIV infection. And the signs and symptoms of HIV infection may feel just like other common viral infections like flu, a cold, sore throat, or mononucleosis (mono).

Diagnostic Tests for Acute Human Immunodeficiency Virus (HIV) Infection

When HIV enters your body, it moves inside white blood cells called CD4 lymphocytes. HIV takes over the CD4 cells and makes billions of copies of the virus each day. The virus spread through your body.

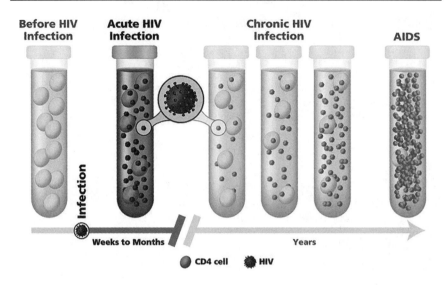

Figure 2.4. *HIV Progression*

Your body tries to defend itself against HIV by making antibodies (these antibodies try to block the virus from spreading in your body). Most HIV tests check to see if antibodies against HIV are in your blood. But it takes a few weeks before your body makes enough antibodies for the usual HIV tests to see them.

However, when you have acute HIV infection, you have a high amount of the HIV virus in your blood. Special tests can measure the amount of HIV in your blood. At the time you have acute HIV infection, you probably won't have enough HIV antibodies in your blood to measure, but you will have enough virus to measure. So if the blood tests do not find any antibody but do see the virus, your doctor will know that you're feeling sick because you have acute HIV infection.

Diagnosing HIV at an Early Stage

First, preexposure prophylaxis (PrEP) is used to help lower your chances of getting HIV infection. If you already have acute HIV infection you should not take PrEP. Second, while PrEP helps protect people, especially when they take their doses every day, it is still possible to get HIV infection. So if you are taking PrEP and have the signs and symptoms mentioned above, it is important to see your doctor to be checked. If you have some other infection, like the flu, you should continue your PrEP medicines but if it is discovered that you have acute HIV infection, you should stop taking PrEP as soon as your tests show that you have HIV infection.

Third, people who take PrEP for more than a couple of weeks while they have HIV infection can easily develop the virus that can't be treated with those same drugs (resistant virus). So finding out quickly that you have HIV infection and stopping PrEP can protect your long-term health and keep your treatment options open.

And fourth, when people have lots of virus in their body during acute HIV infection, they are more likely to pass the virus on to people they have sex with, especially since they may not know yet that they have gotten infected. For example, if your last HIV test result was negative and your partner also had a recent negative HIV test result, you might choose to have sex without a condom just at the time when it's very likely you would pass the virus on. So the sooner you know you have become infected, the more careful you can be to protect others from getting HIV infection.

HIV Treatment

People who have HIV infection are treated with combinations of 3 or more medicines that fight HIV. Some doctors start people on treatment medications as soon as they become infected; other doctors wait for a while because the greatest benefits to a person's health are seen after they have been infected a while. Early treatment also reduces the chances that a person with HIV infection will pass the virus on to their sex partners.

Having Suspicion of Being Infected with Acute HIV

First, contact your doctor's office and arrange to be examined and have the right blood tests. Second, discuss with your doctor whether to stop your PrEP medications or continue them until your test results are back. Third, be especially careful to use condoms and take other safer sex measures to protect your partner(s).

Section 2.4

HIV Drug Resistance

This section includes content from "HIV Treatment,"
AIDS*info*, U.S. Department of Health and Human
Services (HHS), June 7, 2018.

What Is Human Immunodeficiency Virus (HIV) Drug Resistance?

Once a person has HIV, the virus begins to multiply (make copies of itself) in the body. As HIV multiplies, it sometimes mutates (changes form) and produces variations of itself. Variations of HIV that develop while a person is taking HIV medicines can lead to drug-resistant strains of HIV.

With drug resistance, HIV medicines that previously controlled the person's HIV are not effective against the new, drug-resistant HIV. In other words, the HIV medicines can't prevent the drug-resistant HIV from multiplying. Drug resistance can cause HIV treatment to fail.

Drug-resistant HIV can spread from person to person. People initially infected with drug-resistant HIV have drug resistance to one or more HIV medicines even before they start taking HIV medicines.

How Does Poor Medication Adherence Increase the Risk of Drug Resistance?

Medication adherence means taking HIV medicines every day and exactly as prescribed. HIV medicines prevent HIV from multiplying. Skipping HIV medicines allows HIV to multiply, which increases the risk that the virus will mutate and produce drug-resistant HIV.

As a result of drug resistance, one or more HIV medicines in a person's HIV regimen may no longer be effective.

What Is Drug-Resistance Testing?

Cross-resistance is when resistance to one HIV medicine causes resistance to other medicines in the same HIV drug class. (HIV medicines are grouped into drug classes according to how they fight HIV.) As a result of cross-resistance, a person's HIV may be resistant even to HIV medicines that the person has never taken. Cross-resistance limits the number of HIV medicines available to include in an HIV regimen.

What Is Cross Resistance?

Drug-resistance testing is done to identify which, if any, HIV medicines won't be effective against a person's strain of HIV. Drug-resistance testing is done using a sample of blood.

Drug-resistance testing is done when a person first begins receiving care for HIV infection. Resistance testing should be done whether the person decides to start taking HIV medicines immediately or to delay treatment. If treatment is delayed, resistance testing may be repeated when HIV medicines are started.

Drug-resistance testing done before a person starts HIV medicines for the first time can show whether the person was initially infected with a drug-resistant strain of HIV. Drug-resistance testing results are used to decide which HIV medicines to include in a person's first HIV regimen.

After treatment is started, drug-resistance testing is repeated if viral load testing indicates that a person's HIV regimen isn't controlling the virus. If drug-resistance testing shows that the HIV regimen isn't effective because of drug resistance, the test results can be used to select a new HIV regimen.

Drug-resistance testing is also recommended for all pregnant women with HIV before starting HIV medicines and also in some pregnant women already taking HIV medicines. Pregnant women will work with their healthcare providers to decide if drug-resistance testing is needed.

How Can a Person Taking HIV Medicines Reduce the Risk of Drug Resistance?

Adherence to an effective HIV treatment regimen reduces the risk of drug resistance.

Here are some tips on medication adherence for people living with HIV:

- Once you decide to start treatment, work closely with your healthcare provider to choose an HIV regimen that suits your needs. A regimen that meets your needs will make adherence easier. Tell your healthcare provider about any issues that can make adherence difficult. For example, tell your healthcare provider if you have a busy schedule that makes it hard to take medicines on time or lack health insurance to cover the cost of HIV medicines. Your healthcare provider can recommend resources to help you address any issues before you start taking HIV medicines.

- When you start treatment, closely follow your HIV regimen. Take your HIV medicines every day and exactly as prescribed. Use medication aids such as a 7-day pill box or pill diary to stay on track. Download the AIDS*info* Drug Database app to set daily pill reminders.

- Keep your medical appointments so that your healthcare provider can monitor your HIV treatment. Appointments are a good time to ask questions and ask for help to manage problems that make it hard to follow an HIV regimen.

Chapter 3

Symptoms of HIV

The symptoms of human immunodeficiency virus (HIV) vary, depending on the individual and what stage of the disease you are in: the early stage, the clinical latency stage, or acquired immunodeficiency syndrome (AIDS) (the late stage of HIV infection). Below are the symptoms that some individuals may experience in these three stages. Not all individuals will experience these symptoms.

Early Stage Human Immunodeficiency Virus (HIV)

About 40–90 percent of people have flu-like symptoms within 2–4 weeks after HIV infection. Other people do not feel sick at all during this stage, which is also known as acute HIV infection. Early infection is defined as HIV infection in the past six months (recent) and includes acute (very recent) infections. Flu-like symptoms can include:

- Fever
- Chills
- Rash
- Night sweats
- Muscle aches

This chapter includes text excerpted from "About HIV and AIDS: Symptoms of HIV," HIV.gov, U.S. Department of Health and Human Services (HHS), May 2017.

- A sore throat
- Fatigue
- Swollen lymph nodes
- Mouth ulcers

These symptoms can last anywhere from a few days to several weeks. During this time, HIV infection may not show up on some types of HIV tests, but people who have it are highly infectious and can spread the infection to others.

You should not assume you have HIV just because you have any of these symptoms. Each of these symptoms can be caused by other illnesses. And some people who have HIV do not show any symptoms at all for 10 years or more.

However, if you think you may have been exposed to HIV and could be in the early stage of HIV infection, get an HIV test. Most HIV tests detect antibodies (proteins your body makes as a reaction against the presence of HIV), not HIV itself. But it can take a few weeks or longer for your body to produce these antibodies.

Some places use HIV tests that can detect acute and recent infections, but others do not. So be sure to let your testing site know if you think you may have been recently infected with HIV. Tests that can detect acute infection look for HIV ribonucleic acid (RNA) or p24 antigen (a viral protein). Most doctors and clinics that provide a full range of healthcare services can do this test, but some places that only do HIV testing may not have it. So you may want to contact the site before you go to ask if they can test you for acute HIV infection.

After you get tested, it's important to find out the result of your test. If you're HIV-positive, you should see a doctor and start HIV treatment as soon as possible. You are at high risk of transmitting HIV to others during the early stage of HIV infection, even if you have no symptoms. For this reason, it is very important to take steps to reduce your risk of transmission. If you're HIV-negative, explore HIV-prevention options, like preexposure prophylaxis (PrEP), that can help you stay negative.

Clinical Latency Stage

After the early stage of HIV infection, the disease moves into a stage called the clinical latency stage (also called chronic HIV infection). During this stage, HIV is still active but reproduces at very low levels. People with chronic HIV infection may not have any HIV-related symptoms or only mild ones.

For people who aren't taking medicine to treat HIV (called antiretroviral therapy or ART), this period can last a decade or longer, but some may progress through this phase faster. People who are taking medicine to treat HIV, and who take their medications the right way, every day, maybe in this stage for several decades because treatment helps keep the virus in check.

It's important to remember that people can still transmit HIV to others during this phase even if they have no symptoms, although people who are on ART and stay virally suppressed (having a very low level of virus in their blood) are much less likely to transmit HIV than those who are not virally suppressed.

Progression to Acquired Immunodeficiency Syndrome (AIDS)

If you have HIV and you are not on ART, eventually the virus will weaken your body's immune system and you will progress to acquired immunodeficiency syndrome (AIDS), the late stage of HIV infection. Symptoms can include:

- Rapid weight loss
- Recurring fever or profuse night sweats
- Extreme and unexplained tiredness
- Prolonged swelling of the lymph glands in the armpits, groin, or neck
- Diarrhea that lasts for more than a week
- Sores of the mouth, anus, or genitals
- Pneumonia
- Red, brown, pink, or purplish blotches on or under the skin or inside the mouth, nose, or eyelids
- Memory loss, depression, and other neurologic disorders

Each of these symptoms can also be related to other illnesses. So the only way to know for sure if you have HIV is to get tested.

Many of the severe symptoms and illnesses of HIV disease come from the opportunistic infections that occur because your body's immune system has been damaged.

You can't rely **ON SYMPTOMS**
to tell if you have **HIV.**

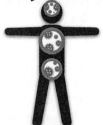

The only way to know for sure is to

GET TESTED

Figure 3.1. *Get Tested for AIDS*

How Can I Tell If I Have Human Immunodeficiency Virus (HIV)?

You cannot rely on symptoms to tell whether you have HIV. The only way to know for sure if you have HIV is to get tested. Knowing your status is important because it helps you make healthy decisions to prevent getting or transmitting HIV.

Use HIV.gov's HIV Testing Sites and Care Services Locator (locator. hiv.gov) to find a testing site near you.

Knowing your HIV status helps you
make **healthy decisions** to prevent
getting or transmitting HIV.

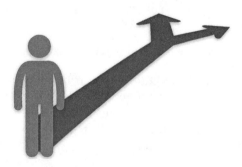

Figure 3.2. *Know Your HIV Status*

Chapter 4

How HIV Causes AIDS

A significant component of the research effort of the National Institute of Allergy and Infectious Diseases (NIAID) is devoted to the pathogenesis of human immunodeficiency virus (HIV) disease. Studies on pathogenesis address the complex mechanisms that result in the destruction of the immune system of an HIV-infected person. A detailed understanding of HIV and how it establishes infection and causes the acquired immunodeficiency syndrome (AIDS) is crucial to identifying and developing effective drugs and vaccines to fight HIV and AIDS. This chapter summarizes the state of knowledge in this area and provides a brief glossary of terms.

Overview

HIV disease is characterized by a gradual deterioration of immune function. Most notably, crucial immune cells called CD4+ T cells are disabled and killed during the typical course of infection. These cells sometimes called "T-helper cells," play a central role in the immune response, signaling other cells in the immune system to perform their special functions.

A healthy, uninfected person usually has 800–1,200 CD4+ T cells per cubic millimeter (mm^3) of blood. During HIV infection, the number

This chapter includes text excerpted from "How HIV Causes AIDS," AIDS*info*, U.S. Department of Health and Human Services (HHS), October 2001. Reviewed June 2018.

of these cells in a person's blood progressively declines. When a person's CD4+ T cell count falls below 200/mm^3, he or she becomes particularly vulnerable to the opportunistic infections and cancers that typify AIDS, the end stage of HIV disease. People with AIDS often suffer infections of the lungs, intestinal tract, brain, eyes and other organs, as well as debilitating weight loss, diarrhea, neurologic conditions and cancers such as Kaposi's sarcoma and certain types of lymphomas.

Most scientists think that HIV causes AIDS by directly inducing the death of CD4+ T cells or interfering with their normal function, and by triggering other events that weaken a person's immune function. For example, the network of signaling molecules that normally regulates a person's immune response is disrupted during HIV disease, impairing a person's ability to fight other infections. The HIV-mediated destruction of the lymph nodes and related immunologic organs also plays a major role in causing the immunosuppression seen in people with AIDS.

Scope of the HIV Epidemic

Although HIV was first identified in 1983, studies of previously stored blood samples indicate that the virus entered the U.S. population sometime in the late 1970s. In the United States, 774,467 cases of AIDS, and 448,060 deaths among people with AIDS had been reported to the Centers for Disease Control and Prevention (CDC) as of the end of 2000. Approximately 40,000 new HIV infections occur each year in the United States, 70 percent of them among men and 30 percent among women. Minority groups in the United States have been disproportionately affected by the epidemic.

Worldwide, an estimated 36.1 million people (47 percent of whom are female) were living with HIV/AIDS as of December 2000, according to the Joint United Nations Programme on HIV/AIDS (UNAIDS). Through 2000, cumulative HIV/AIDS-associated deaths worldwide numbered approximately 21.8 million: 17.5 million adults and 4.3 million children younger than 15 years. Globally, approximately 5.3 million new HIV infections and 3.0 million HIV/AIDS-related deaths occurred in the year 2000 alone.

HIV is a Retrovirus

HIV belongs to a class of viruses called retroviruses. Retroviruses are ribonucleic acid (RNA) viruses, and in order to replicate, they must make a deoxyribonucleic acid (DNA) copy of their RNA. It is the DNA genes that allow the virus to replicate.

Like all viruses, HIV can replicate only inside cells, commandeering the cell's machinery to reproduce. However, only HIV and other retroviruses, once inside a cell, use an enzyme called reverse transcriptase to convert their RNA into DNA, which can be incorporated into the host cell's genes.

Slow Viruses

HIV belongs to a subgroup of retroviruses known as lentiviruses or "slow" viruses. The course of infection with these viruses is characterized by a long interval between initial infection and the onset of serious symptoms.

Other lentiviruses infect nonhuman species. For example, the feline immunodeficiency virus (FIV) infects cats and the simian immunodeficiency virus (SIV) infects monkeys and other nonhuman primates. Like HIV in humans, these animal viruses primarily infect immune system cells, often causing immunodeficiency and AIDS-like symptoms. These viruses and their hosts have provided researchers with useful, albeit imperfect, models of the HIV disease process in people.

Structure of HIV

The viral envelope. HIV has a diameter of 1/10,000 of a millimeter and is spherical in shape. The outer coat of the virus, known as the viral envelope, is composed of two layers of fatty molecules called lipids, taken from the membrane of a human cell when a newly formed virus particle buds from the cell. Recent evidence from NIAID-supported researchers indicates that HIV may enter and exit cells through special areas of the cell membrane known as "lipid rafts." These rafts are high in cholesterol and glycolipids and may provide a new target for blocking HIV.

Embedded in the viral envelope are proteins from the host cell, as well as 72 copies (on average) of a complex HIV protein (frequently called "spikes") that protrudes through the surface of the virus particle (virion). This protein, known as Env, consists of a cap made of three molecules called glycoprotein (gp) 120, and a stem consisting of three gp41 molecules that anchor the structure in the viral envelope. Much of the research to develop a vaccine against HIV has focused on these envelope proteins.

The viral core. Within the envelope of a mature HIV, particle is a bullet-shaped core or capsid, made of 2000 copies of another viral protein, p24. The capsid surrounds two single strands of HIV RNA, each of which has a copy of the virus's nine genes. Three of these, gag, pol and env, contain information needed to make structural proteins for new virus particles. The env gene, for example, codes for a protein called gp160 that is broken down by a viral enzyme to form gp120 and gp41, the components of Env.

Six regulatory genes, tat, rev, nef, vif, vpr, and vpu, contain information necessary for the production of proteins that control the ability of HIV to infect a cell, produce new copies of virus or cause disease. The protein encoded by nef, for instance, appears necessary for the virus to replicate efficiently, and the vpu-encoded protein influences the release of new virus particles from infected cells.

The ends of each strand of HIV RNA contain an RNA sequence called the long terminal repeat (LTR). Regions in the LTR act as switches to control production of new viruses and can be triggered by proteins from either HIV or the host cell.

The core of HIV also includes a protein called p7, the HIV nucleocapsid protein; and three enzymes that carry out later steps in the virus's life cycle: reverse transcriptase, integrase, and protease. Another HIV protein called p17, or the HIV matrix protein, lies between the viral core and the viral envelope.

Replication Cycle of HIV

Entry of HIV into cells. Infection typically begins when an HIV particle, which contains two copies of the HIV RNA, encounters a cell with a surface molecule called cluster designation 4 (CD4). Cells carrying this molecule are known as CD4 positive (CD4+) cells.

One or more of the virus's gp120 molecules binds tightly to CD4 molecule(s) on the cell's surface. The binding of gp120 to CD4 results in a conformational change in the gp120 molecule allowing it to bind to a second molecule on the cell surface known as a coreceptor. The envelope of the virus and the cell membrane then fuse, leading to entry of the virus into the cell. The gp41 of the envelope is critical to the fusion process. Drugs that block either the binding or the fusion process are being developed and tested in clinical trials.

Studies have identified multiple coreceptors for different types of HIV strains; these coreceptors are promising targets for new anti-HIV drugs, some of which are now being tested in preclinical and clinical studies. In the early stage of HIV disease, most people harbor viruses that use, in addition to CD4, a receptor called CCR5 to enter their target cells. With disease progression, the spectrum of coreceptor usage expands in approximately 50 percent of patients to include other receptors, notably a molecule called CXCR4. Virus that utilizes CCR5 is called R5 HIV and virus that utilizes CXCR4 is called X4 HIV.

Although CD4+ T cells appear to be the main targets of HIV, other immune system cells with and without CD4 molecules on their surfaces are infected as well. Among these are long-lived cells called monocytes and macrophages, which apparently can harbor large quantities of the virus without being killed, thus acting as reservoirs of HIV. CD4+ T cells also serve as important reservoirs of HIV: a small proportion of these cells harbor HIV in a stable, inactive form. Normal immune processes may activate these cells, resulting in the production of new HIV virions

Cell-to-cell spread of HIV also can occur through the CD4-mediated fusion of an infected cell with an uninfected cell.

Reverse transcription. In the cytoplasm of the cell, HIV reverse transcriptase converts viral RNA into DNA, the nucleic acid form in which the cell carries its genes. Nine of the 15 antiviral drugs approved in the United States for the treatment of people with HIV infection— AZT, ddC, ddI, d4T, 3TC, nevirapine, delavirdine, abacavir and efavirenz—work by interfering with this stage of the viral life cycle.

Integration. The newly made HIV DNA moves to the cell's nucleus, where it is spliced into the host's DNA with the help of HIV integrase. HIV DNA that enters the DNA of the cell is called a "provirus." Integrase is an important target for the development of new drugs.

Transcription. For a provirus to produce new viruses, RNA copies must be made that can be read by the host cell's protein-making machinery. These copies are called messenger RNA (mRNA), and production of mRNA is called transcription, a process that involves the host cell's own enzymes. Viral genes in concert with the cellular machinery control this process: the tat gene, for example, encodes a protein that accelerates transcription. Genomic RNA is also transcribed for later incorporation in the budding virion.

Cytokines, proteins involved in the normal regulation of the immune response, also may regulate transcription. Molecules such as tumor necrosis factor (TNF)-alpha and interleukin (IL)-6, secreted in elevated levels by the cells of HIV-infected people, may help to activate HIV proviruses. Other infections, by organisms such as *Mycobacterium tuberculosis*, may also enhance transcription by inducing the secretion of cytokines.

Translation. After HIV mRNA is processed in the cell's nucleus, it is transported to the cytoplasm. HIV proteins are critical to this process: for example, a protein encoded by the rev gene allows mRNA encoding HIV structural proteins to be transferred from the nucleus to the cytoplasm. Without the rev protein, structural proteins are not made.

In the cytoplasm, the virus co-opts the cell's protein-making machinery—including structures called ribosomes—to make long chains of viral proteins and enzymes, using HIV mRNA as a template. This process is called translation.

Assembly and budding. Newly made HIV core proteins, enzymes and genomic RNA gather just inside the cell's membrane, while the viral envelope proteins aggregate within the membrane. An immature viral particle forms and buds off from the cell, acquiring an envelope that includes both cellular and HIV proteins from the cell membrane. During this part of the viral life cycle, the core of the virus is immature and the virus is not yet infectious. The long chains of proteins and enzymes that make up the immature viral core are now cleaved into smaller pieces by a viral enzyme called protease. This step results in infectious viral particles.

Drugs called protease inhibitors interfere with this step of the viral life cycle. Six such drugs—saquinavir, ritonavir, indinavir, amprenavir, nelfinavir, and lopinavir—have been approved for marketing in the United States.

Transmission of HIV

Among adults, HIV is spread most commonly during sexual intercourse with an infected partner. During sex, the virus can enter the body through the mucosal linings of the vagina, vulva, penis, or rectum after intercourse or, rarely, via the mouth and possibly the upper gastrointestinal tract after oral sex. The likelihood of transmission is increased by factors that may damage these linings, especially other sexually transmitted diseases that cause ulcers or inflammation.

Research suggests that immune system cells of the dendritic cell type, which reside in the mucosa, may begin the infection process after sexual exposure by binding to and carrying the virus from the site of infection to the lymph nodes where other immune system cells become infected.

HIV also can be transmitted by contact with infected blood, most often by the sharing of needles or syringes contaminated with minute quantities of blood containing the virus. The risk of acquiring HIV from blood transfusions is now extremely small in the United States, as all blood products in this country are screened routinely for evidence of the virus.

Almost all HIV-infected children acquire the virus from their mothers before or during birth. In the United States, approximately 25 percent of pregnant HIV-infected women not receiving antiretroviral therapy have passed on the virus to their babies. In 1994, researchers demonstrated that a specific regimen of the drug zidovudine (AZT) can reduce the risk of transmission of HIV from mother to baby by two-thirds. The use of combinations of antiretroviral drugs has further reduced the rate of mother-to-child HIV transmission in the United States. In developing countries, cheap and simple antiviral drug regimens have been proven to significantly reduce mother-to-child transmission in resource-poor settings.

The virus also may be transmitted from an HIV-infected mother to her infant via breastfeeding.

Early Events in HIV Infection

Once it enters the body, HIV infects a large number of CD4+ cells and replicates rapidly. During this acute or primary phase of infection, the blood contains many viral particles that spread throughout the body, seeding various organs, particularly the lymphoid organs. Lymphoid organs include the lymph nodes, spleen, tonsils, and adenoids.

Two to four weeks after exposure to the virus, up to 70 percent of HIV-infected persons suffer flu-like symptoms related to the acute infection. The patient's immune system fights back with killer T cells (CD8+ T cells) and B-cell-produced antibodies, which dramatically reduce HIV levels. A patient's CD4+ T cell count may rebound somewhat and even approach its original level. A person may then remain free of HIV-related symptoms for years despite continuous replication of HIV in the lymphoid organs that had been seeded during the acute phase of infection.

One reason that HIV is unique is the fact that despite the body's aggressive immune responses, which are sufficient to clear most viral infections, some HIV invariably escapes. This is due in large part to the high rate of mutations that occur during the process of HIV replication. Even when the virus does not avoid the immune system by mutating, the body's best soldiers in the fight against HIV - certain subsets of killer T cells that recognize HIV may be depleted or become dysfunctional.

In addition, early in the course of HIV infection, patients may lose HIV-specific CD4+ T cell responses that normally slow the replication of viruses. Such responses include the secretion of interferons and other antiviral factors, and the orchestration of CD8+ T cells.

Finally, the virus may hide within the chromosomes of an infected cell and be shielded from surveillance by the immune system. Such cells can be considered as a latent reservoir of the virus.

Course of HIV Infection

Among patients enrolled in large epidemiologic studies in western countries, the median time from infection with HIV to the development of AIDS-related symptoms has been approximately 10–12 years in the absence of antiretroviral therapy. However, researchers have observed a wide variation in disease progression. Approximately 10 percent of HIV-infected people in these studies have progressed to AIDS within the first two to three years following infection, while up to 5 percent of individuals in the studies have stable CD4+ T cell counts and no symptoms even after 12 or more years.

Factors such as age or genetic differences among individuals, the level of virulence of an individual strain of virus, and coinfection with other microbes may influence the rate and severity of disease progression. Drugs that fight the infections associated with AIDS have improved and prolonged the lives of HIV-infected people by preventing or treating conditions such as *Pneumocystis carinii* pneumonia, cytomegalovirus disease, and diseases caused by a number of fungi.

HIV co-receptors and disease progression. Recent research has shown that most infecting strains of HIV use a co-receptor molecule called CCR5, in addition to the CD4 molecule, to enter certain of its target cells. HIV-infected people with a specific mutation in one of their two copies of the gene for this receptor may have a slower disease course than people with two normal copies of the gene. Rare individuals with two mutant copies of the CCR5 gene appear - in most cases - to be completely protected from HIV infection. Mutations in the gene for other HIV co-receptors also may influence the rate of disease progression.

Viral burden predicts disease progression. Numerous studies show that people with high levels of HIV in their bloodstream are more likely to develop new AIDS-related symptoms or die than individuals with lower levels of virus. For instance, in the Multicenter AIDS

Cohort Study (MACS), investigators demonstrated that the level of HIV in an untreated individual's plasma 6 months to a year after infection - the so-called viral "set point"—is highly predictive of the rate of disease progression; that is, patients with high levels of virus are much more likely to get sicker, faster, than those with low levels of virus. The MACS and other studies have provided the rationale for providing aggressive antiretroviral therapy to HIV-infected people, as well as for routinely using newly available blood tests to measure viral load when initiating, monitoring and modifying anti-HIV therapy.

Potent combinations of three or more anti-HIV drugs known as highly active antiretroviral therapy or HAART can reduce a person's "viral burden" to very low levels and in many cases delay the progression of HIV disease for prolonged periods. However, antiretroviral regimens have yet to completely and permanently suppress the virus in HIV-infected people. Recent studies have shown that HIV persists in a replication-competent form in resting CD4+ T cells even in patients receiving aggressive antiretroviral therapy who have no readily detectable HIV in their blood. Investigators around the world are working to develop the next generation of anti-HIV drugs.

HIV is Active in the Lymph Nodes

Although HIV-infected individuals often exhibit an extended period of clinical latency with little evidence of disease, the virus is never truly completely latent although individual cells may be latently infected. Researchers have shown that even early in disease, HIV actively replicates within the lymph nodes and related organs, where large amounts of virus become trapped in networks of specialized cells with long, tentacle-like extensions. These cells are called follicular dendritic cells (FDCs).

FDCs are located in hot spots of immune activity in lymphoid tissue called germinal centers. They act like flypaper, trapping invading pathogens (including HIV) and holding them until B cells come along to initiate an immune response.

Close on the heels of B cells are CD4+ T cells, which rush into the germinal centers to help B cells fight the invaders. CD4+ T cells, the primary targets of HIV, may become infected as they encounter HIV trapped on FDCs. Research suggests that HIV trapped on FDCs remains infectious, even when coated with antibodies. Thus, FDCs are an important reservoir of HIV, and the large quantity of infectious HIV trapped on FDCs may explain in part how the momentum of HIV infection is maintained

Once infected, CD4+ T cells may infect other CD4+ cells that congregate in the region of the lymph node surrounding the germinal center.

Over a period of years, even when little virus is readily detectable in the blood, significant amounts of virus accumulate in the lymphoid tissue, both within infected cells and bound to FDCs. In and around the germinal centers, numerous CD4+ T cells are probably activated by the increased production of cytokines such as TNF-alpha and IL-6 by immune system cells within the lymphoid tissue. Activation allows uninfected cells to be more easily infected and increases replication of HIV in already infected cells.

While greater quantities of certain cytokines such as TNF-alpha and IL-6 are secreted during HIV infection, other cytokines with key roles in the regulation of normal immune function may be secreted in decreased amounts. For example, CD4+ T cells may lose their capacity to produce interleukin 2 (IL-2), a cytokine that enhances the growth of other T cells and helps to stimulate other cells' response to invaders. Infected cells also have low levels of receptors for IL-2, which may reduce their ability to respond to signals from other cells.

Breakdown of FDC networks. Ultimately, accumulated HIV overwhelms the FDC networks. As these networks break down, their trapping capacity is impaired, and large quantities of virus enter the bloodstream.

Although it remains unclear why FDCs die and the FDC networks dissolve, some scientists think that this process may be as important in HIV pathogenesis as the loss of CD4+ T cells. The destruction of the lymphoid tissue structure seen late in HIV disease may preclude a successful immune response against not only HIV but other pathogens as well. This devastation heralds the onset of the opportunistic infections and cancers that characterize AIDS.

Role of CD8+ T Cells

Rapid Replication and Mutation of HIV

HIV replicates rapidly; several billion new virus particles may be produced every day. In addition, the HIV reverse transcriptase enzyme makes many mistakes while making DNA copies from HIV RNA. As a consequence, many variants of HIV develop in an individual, some of which may escape destruction by antibodies or killer T cells. Additionally, different strains of HIV can recombine to produce a wide range of variants or strains.

During the course of HIV disease, viral strains emerge in an infected individual that differ widely in their ability to infect and kill different cell types, as well as in their rate of replication. Scientists are investigating why strains of HIV from patients with advanced disease appear to be more virulent and infect more cell types than strains obtained earlier from the same individual.

Theories of Immune System Cell Loss in HIV Infection

Researchers around the world are studying how HIV destroys or disables CD4+ T cells, and many think that a number of mechanisms may occur simultaneously in an HIV-infected individual. Recent data suggest that billions of CD4+ T cells may be destroyed every day, eventually overwhelming the immune system's regenerative capacity.

Direct cell killing. Infected CD4+ T cells may be killed directly when large amounts of virus are produced and bud off from the cell surface, disrupting the cell membrane, or when viral proteins and nucleic acids collect inside the cell, interfering with cellular machinery.

Apoptosis. Infected CD4+ T cells may be killed when the regulation of cell function is distorted by HIV proteins, probably leading to cell suicide by a process known as programmed cell death or apoptosis. Recent reports indicate that apoptosis occurs to a greater extent in HIV-infected individuals, both in the bloodstream and lymph nodes. Apoptosis is closely correlated with the aberrant cellular activation seen in HIV disease.

Uninfected cells also may undergo apoptosis. Investigators have shown in cell cultures that the HIV envelope alone or bound to antibodies sends an inappropriate signal to CD4+ T cells causing them to undergo apoptosis, even if not infected by HIV.

Innocent bystanders. Uninfected cells may die in an innocent bystander scenario: HIV particles may bind to the cell surface, giving them the appearance of an infected cell and marking them for destruction by killer T cells after antibody attaches to the viral particle on the cell. This process is called antibody-dependent cellular cytotoxicity.

Killer T cells also may mistakenly destroy uninfected cells that have consumed HIV particles and that display HIV fragments on their surfaces. Alternatively, because HIV envelope proteins bear some resemblance to certain molecules that may appear on CD4+ T cells, the body's immune responses may mistakenly damage such cells as well.

Anergy. Researchers have shown in cell cultures that CD4+ T cells can be turned off by activation signals from HIV that leaves them unable to respond to further immune stimulation. This inactivated state is known as anergy.

Damage to precursor cells. Studies suggest that HIV also destroys precursor cells that mature to have special immune functions, as well as the microenvironment of the bone marrow and the thymus needed for the development of such cells. These organs probably lose the ability to regenerate, further compounding the suppression of the immune system.

Central Nervous System Damage

Although monocytes and macrophages can be infected by HIV, they appear to be relatively resistant to killing by the virus. However, these cells travel throughout the body and carry HIV to various organs, including the brain, which may serve as a hiding place or "reservoir" for the virus that may be relatively impervious to most anti-HIV drugs.

Neurologic manifestations of HIV disease are seen in up to 50 percent of HIV-infected people, to varying degrees of severity People infected with HIV often experience cognitive symptoms, including impaired short-term memory, reduced concentration, and mental slowing; motor symptoms such as fine motor clumsiness or slowness, tremor, and leg weakness; and behavioral symptoms including apathy, social withdrawal, irritability, depression, and personality change. More serious neurologic manifestations in HIV disease typically occur in patients with high viral loads, generally when an individual has advanced HIV disease or AIDS.

Neurologic manifestations of HIV disease are the subject of many research projects. Current evidence suggests that although nerve cells do not become infected with HIV, supportive cells within the brain, such as astrocytes and microglia (as well as monocyte/macrophages that have migrated to the brain) can be infected with the virus. Researchers postulate that infection of these cells can cause a disruption of normal neurologic functions by altering cytokine levels, by delivering aberrant signals, and by causing the release of toxic products in the brain. The use of anti-HIV drugs frequently reduces the severity of neurologic symptoms, but in many cases does not, for reasons that are unclear.

Role of Immune Activation in HIV Disease

During a normal immune response, many components of the immune system are mobilized to fight an invader. CD4+ T cells, for instance, may quickly proliferate and increase their cytokine secretion, thereby signaling other cells to perform their special functions. Scavenger cells called macrophages may double in size and develop numerous organelles, including lysosomes that contain digestive enzymes used to process ingested pathogens. Once the immune system clears the foreign antigen, it returns to a relative state of quiescence.

Paradoxically, although it ultimately causes immune deficiency, HIV disease for most of its course is characterized by immune system hyperactivation, which has negative consequences. As noted above, HIV replication and spread are much more efficient in activated CD4+ cells. Chronic immune system activation during HIV disease may also result in a massive stimulation of B cells, impairing the ability of these cells to make antibodies against other pathogens.

Chronic immune activation also can result in apoptosis, and an increased production of cytokines that may not only increase HIV replication but also have other deleterious effects. Increased levels of TNF-alpha, for example, may be at least partly responsible for the severe weight loss or wasting syndrome seen in many HIV-infected individuals.

The persistence of HIV and HIV replication plays an important role in the chronic state of immune activation seen in HIV-infected people. In addition, researchers have shown that infections with other organisms activate immune system cells and increase production of the virus in HIV-infected people. Chronic immune activation due to persistent infections, or the cumulative effects of multiple episodes of immune activation and bursts of virus production, likely contribute to the progression of HIV disease.

NIAID Research on the Pathogenesis of AIDS

National Institute of Allergy and Infectious Diseases (NIAID)-supported scientists conduct research on HIV pathogenesis in laboratories on the campus of the National Institutes of Health (NIH) in Bethesda, Md., at the Institute's Rocky Mountain Laboratories in Hamilton, Montana, and at universities and medical centers in the United States and abroad.

An NIAID-supported resource, the NIH AIDS Research and Reference Reagent Program, in collaboration with the World Health Organization, provides critically needed AIDS-related research materials free to qualified researchers around the world.

In addition, the Institute convenes groups of investigators and advisory committees to exchange scientific information, clarify research priorities and bring research needs and opportunities to the attention of the scientific community.

Chapter 5

HIV/AIDS: A Statistical Overview

Annual human immunodeficiency virus (HIV) infections and diagnoses are declining in the United States. The declines may be due to targeted HIV prevention efforts. However, progress has been uneven, and annual infections and diagnoses have increased among some groups.

Human Immunodeficiency Virus (HIV) Infections

There were an estimated 37,600 addition of HIV infections in 2014. Among all populations in the United States, the estimated number of annual infections declined 10 percent from 2010 (41,900) to 2014 (37,600).

HIV Diagnoses

In 2016, 39,782 people received an HIV diagnosis. The annual number of HIV diagnoses declined 5 percent between 2011–2015.

This chapter includes text excerpted from "HIV in the United States: At a Glance," Centers for Disease Control and Prevention (CDC), November 29, 2017.

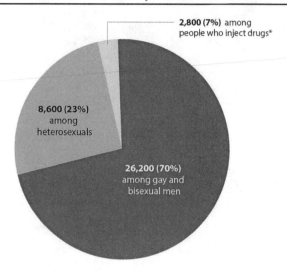

Figure 5.1. *Estimated New HIV Infections in the United States by Transmission Category, 2014.*

*Includes infections attributed to male-to-male sexual contact and injection drug use.

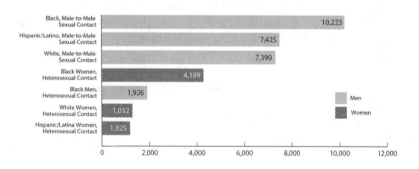

Figure 5.2. *HIV Diagnoses in the United States for the Most-Affected Subpopulations, 2016.*

Subpopulations representing 2 percent or less of HIV diagnoses are not reflected in this chart.

Gay and Bisexual Men

Gay and bisexual men are the population most affected by HIV. In 2016:

- Gay and bisexual men accounted for 67 percent (26,570) of all HIV diagnoses and 83 percent of diagnoses among males.

- Black/African American gay and bisexual men accounted for the largest number of HIV diagnoses (10,223), followed by Hispanic/Latino (7,425) and white (7,390) gay and bisexual men.

Trends among gay and bisexual men have varied by race. From 2011–2015:

- Among white gay and bisexual men, diagnoses decreased by 10 percent.

- Among African American gay and bisexual men, diagnoses increased by 4 percent.

- After years of sharp increases, diagnoses among young African American gay and bisexual men (aged 13–24) stayed about the same.

- Among Hispanic/Latino gay and bisexual men, diagnoses increased by 14 percent.

Heterosexuals and People Who Inject Drugs (PWID)

Heterosexuals and people who inject drugs (PWID) also continue to be affected by HIV. In 2016:

- Heterosexual contact accounted for 24 percent (9,578) of HIV diagnoses.

- Women accounted for 19 percent (7,529) of HIV diagnoses (primarily attributed to heterosexual contact (87%, or 6,541) or injection drug use (12%, or 939).

- PWID accounted for 9 percent (3,425) of HIV diagnoses (includes 1,201 diagnoses among gay and bisexual men who inject drugs).

From 2011–2015:

- Diagnoses among all women declined by 16 percent.

- Among all heterosexuals, diagnoses declined 15 percent, and among PWID, diagnoses declined by 17 percent.

By Race / Ethnicity

By race/ethnicity, African Americans and Hispanics/Latinos are disproportionately affected by HIV. In 2016:

- African Americans represented 12 percent of the population but accounted for 44 percent (17,528) of HIV diagnoses. African

Americans have the highest rate of HIV diagnoses compared to other races and ethnicities.

- Hispanics/Latinos represented 18 percent of the population but accounted for 25 percent (9,766) of HIV diagnoses.

By Location

HIV diagnoses are not evenly distributed geographically. The population rates (per 100,000 people) of people who received an HIV diagnosis were highest in the South (16.8), followed by the Northeast (11.2), the West (10.2), and the Midwest (7.5).

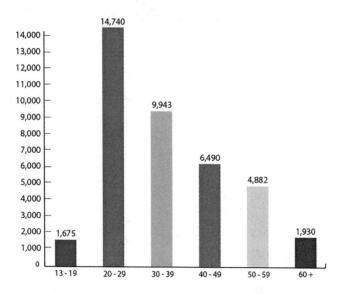

Figure 5.3. *HIV Diagnoses in the United States by Age, 2016*

Living with HIV

An estimated 1,122,900 adults and adolescents were living with HIV at the end of 2015. Of those, 162,500 (15%) had not received a diagnosis. Young people were the most likely to be unaware of their infection. Among people aged 13–24 who were living with HIV, an estimated 44 percent didn't know.

In 2014, among all adults and adolescents living with HIV (diagnosed or undiagnosed):

- 62 percent received some HIV medical care,

- 48 percent were retained in continuous HIV care, and

- 49 percent had achieved viral suppression (having a very low level of the virus).

A person living with HIV who takes HIV medicine as prescribed and gets and stays virally suppressed can stay healthy and has effectively no risk of sexually transmitting HIV to HIV-negative partners.

AIDS Diagnoses and Deaths

In 2016, 18,160 people received an acquired immunodeficiency syndrome (AIDS) diagnosis. Since the epidemic began in the early 1980s, 1,232,346 people have received an AIDS diagnosis. In 2014, 6,721 deaths were attributed directly to HIV.

Chapter 6

Impact of HIV on Racial and Ethnic Minorities in the United States

Chapter Contents

Section 6.1

HIV among African Americans

This section includes text excerpted from "HIV among
African Americans," Centers for Disease Control and
Prevention (CDC), May 15, 2018.

Blacks/African Americans account for a higher proportion of new
human immunodeficiency virus (HIV) diagnoses, those living with
HIV, and those who have ever received an acquired immunodeficiency
syndrome (AIDS) diagnosis, compared to other races/ethnicities. In
2016, African Americans accounted for 44 percent of HIV diagnoses,
though they comprise 12 percent of the U.S. population.

The Numbers

Human immunodeficiency virus (HIV) and Acquired Immunodeficiency Syndrome (AIDS) Diagnoses
In 2016:

- 17,528 African Americans received an HIV diagnosis in the
  United States (12,890 men and 4,560 women).

- More than half (58 percent, 10,223) of African Americans with
  diagnosed HIV were gay or bisexual men.

- Among African American gay and bisexual men who received an
  HIV diagnosis, 39 percent (3,993) were young men aged 25–34.

- Forty-seven percent (8,501) of those who received an AIDS
  diagnosis in the United States were African American.

From 2011–2015:

- HIV diagnoses decreased by 8 percent among African Americans
  overall.

- HIV diagnoses decreased by 16 percent among African American
  heterosexual men.

- The number of HIV diagnoses among African American women
  fell 20 percent, though it is still high compared to women of
  other races/ethnicities. In 2016, 4,560 African American women
  received an HIV diagnosis, compared with 1,450 white women
  and 1,168 Hispanic/Latina women.

- HIV diagnoses decreased by 39 percent among African Americans who inject drugs.

- HIV diagnoses among African American gay and bisexual men remained stable.

- HIV diagnoses among young African American gay and bisexual men aged 13–24 remained stable.

- HIV diagnoses among African American gay and bisexual men aged 25–34 increased by 30 percent.

Living with HIV and Deaths

At the end of 2014, an estimated 471,500 African Americans were living with HIV (43 percent of everyone living with HIV in the United States), and 16 percent were unaware of their infection.

Among all African Americans living with HIV in 2014, 84 percent had received a diagnosis, 59 percent received HIV medical care in 2014, 46 percent were retained in HIV care, and 43 percent had a suppressed viral load.

In 2015, 3,379 African Americans died from HIV disease, accounting for 52 percent of total deaths attributed to the disease that year.

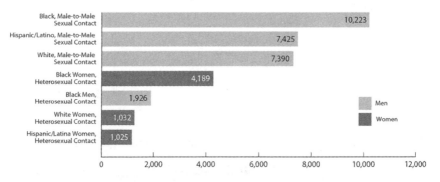

Figure 6.1. *HIV Diagnoses in the United States for the Most-Affected Subpopulations, 2016*

Subpopulations representing 2 percent or less of HIV diagnoses are not reflected in this chart.

Prevention Challenges

In all communities, lack of awareness of HIV status contributes to HIV risk. People who do not know they have HIV cannot take advantage of HIV care and treatment and may unknowingly pass HIV to others.

A number of challenges contribute to the higher rates of HIV infection among African Americans. The greater number of people living with HIV (prevalence) in African American communities and the tendency for African Americans to have sex with partners of the same race/ethnicity means that African Americans face a greater risk of HIV infection. Some African American communities also experience higher rates of other sexually transmitted diseases (STDs) than other racial/ ethnic communities in the United States. Having another STD can significantly increase a person's chance of getting or transmitting HIV.

Stigma, fear, discrimination, and homophobia may place many African Americans at higher risk for HIV. Also, the poverty rate is higher among African Americans than other racial/ethnic groups. The socioeconomic issues associated with poverty—including limited access to high-quality healthcare, housing, and HIV prevention education— directly and indirectly, increase the risk for HIV infection and affect the health of people living with and at risk for HIV. These factors may explain why African Americans have worse outcomes on the HIV continuum of care, including lower rates of linkage to care and viral suppression.

Section 6.2

HIV among American Indians and Alaska Natives

This section includes text excerpted from "HIV among American Indians and Alaska Natives in the United States," Centers for Disease Control and Prevention (CDC), April 3, 2018.

Human immunodeficiency virus (HIV) is a public health issue among American Indians and Alaska Natives (AI/AN), who represent about 1.3 percent of the U.S. population. Overall, diagnosed HIV infections among AI/AN are proportional to their population size. Compared with other racial/ethnic groups, AI/AN ranked fourth in rates of HIV diagnoses in 2016, with a lower rate than blacks/African Americans, Hispanics/Latinos, and people reporting multiple races, but a higher rate than Native Hawaiians/other Pacific Islanders, Asians, and whites.

The Numbers

Human Immunodeficiency Virus (HIV) and Acquired Immunodeficiency Syndrome (AIDS) Diagnoses

Of the 39,782 HIV diagnoses in the United States in 2016, 1 percent (243) were among AI/AN. Of those, 81 percent (198) were men, and 19 percent (45) were women. Of the 198 HIV diagnoses among AI/AN men in 2016, most (77%; 152) were attributed to male-to-male sexual contact. Most of the 45 HIV diagnoses among AI/AN women in 2016 were attributed to heterosexual contact (69%; 31).

From 2011–2015, the annual number of HIV diagnoses increased 38 percent (from 143 to 197) among AIs/ANs overall and 54 percent (from 74–114) among AI/AN gay and bisexual men. In 2016, 102 AIs/ANs were diagnosed with AIDS. Of them, 75 percent (77) were men and 24 percent (24) were women.

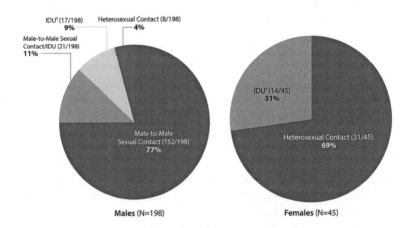

Figure 6.2. *HIV Diagnoses among American Indians/Alaska Natives in the United States by Transmission Category and Sex, 2016*

†Injection Drug Use
The terms male-to-male sexual contact and male-to-male sexual contact and injection drug use are used in the Centers for Disease Control and Prevention (CDC) surveillance systems. They indicate the behaviors that transmit HIV infection, not how individuals self-identify in terms of their sexuality.

Living with HIV and Deaths

An estimated 3,500 AI/AN were living with HIV in 2015, and 81 percent of them had received a diagnosis. Of AI/AN who were living with HIV in 2014, 58 percent received HIV care during 2014, 45 percent were retained in care, and 47 percent had achieved viral suppression. During 2015, 53 AI/AN died from HIV disease.

Prevention Challenges

Sexually transmitted diseases (STDs). From 2012–2016, AI/AN had the second highest rates of chlamydia and gonorrhea among all racial/ethnic groups. Having another STD increases a person's risk for getting or transmitting HIV.

Awareness of HIV status. An estimated 81 percent of AI/AN living with HIV in 2015 had received a diagnosis. It is important for everyone to know their HIV status. People who do not know they have HIV cannot take advantage of HIV care and treatment and may unknowingly pass HIV to others.

Stigma. AI/AN gay and bisexual men may face culturally based stigma and confidentiality concerns that could limit opportunities for education and HIV testing, especially among those who live in rural communities or on reservations.

Cultural diversity. There are over 560 federally recognized AI/AN tribes, whose members speak over 170 languages. Because each tribe has its own culture, beliefs, and practices, creating culturally appropriate prevention programs for each group can be challenging.

Socioeconomic issues. Poverty, including limited access to high-quality housing, directly and indirectly, increases the risk for HIV infection and affects the health of people living with and at risk for HIV infection. Compared with other racial/ethnic groups, AI/AN have higher poverty rates, have completed fewer years of education, are younger, are less likely to be employed, and have lower rates of health insurance coverage.

Alcohol and illicit drug use. Alcohol and substance use can impair judgment and lead to behaviors that increase the risk of HIV. Injection drug use can directly increase the risk of HIV through sharing contaminated needles, syringes, and other equipment. Compared with other racial/ethnic groups, AI/AN tend to use alcohol and drugs at a younger age and use them more often and in higher quantities.

Data limitations. Racial misidentification of AI/AN may lead to the undercounting of this population in HIV surveillance systems and may contribute to the underfunding of targeted services for AI/AN.

Section 6.3

HIV among Asians

This section includes text excerpted from "HIV among Asians in the United States," Centers for Disease Control and Prevention (CDC), May 23, 2018.

Between 2011–2015, the Asian population in the United States grew around 12 percent, four times as fast as the total U.S. population. During the same period, the number of Asians receiving a human immunodeficiency virus (HIV) diagnosis increased by 28 percent, driven primarily by an increase in HIV diagnoses among Asian gay and bisexual men. Asians, who make up 6 percent of the population, continue to account for only a small percentage of new HIV diagnoses in the United States and 6 dependent areas.

The Numbers

Human Immunodeficiency Virus (HIV) Infections

From 2010–2015, estimated annual HIV infections, both diagnosed and undiagnosed, remained stable among Asians in the United States.

HIV and Acquired Immunodeficiency Syndrome (AIDS) Diagnosis

Adult and adolescent Asians accounted for 2 percent (970) of the 40,324 new HIV diagnoses in the United States and 6 dependent areas in 2016. Of Asians who received an HIV diagnosis in 2016, 84 percent (825) were men and 15 percent (145) were women. Infections attributed to male-to-male sexual contact accounted for 90 percent (740) of all HIV diagnoses among Asian men in 2016. Among Asian women who received an HIV diagnosis, 94 percent (136) of infections were attributed to heterosexual contact.

From 2011–2015, annual HIV diagnoses increased by 35 percent among Asian gay and bisexual men in the United States and 6 dependent areas. In 2016, 336 Asians received a diagnosis of acquired immunodeficiency syndrome (AIDS), representing 2 percent of the 18,409 AIDS diagnoses in the United States and 6 dependent areas.

Living with HIV

Of the 15,800 Asians estimated to be living with HIV in the United States in 2015, 80 percent had received a diagnosis, a lower percentage than for any other race/ethnicity. Of Asians living with HIV in 2014, 57 percent received HIV medical care, 46 percent were retained in HIV care, and 51 percent had achieved viral suppression. A person living with HIV who takes HIV medicine as prescribed and gets and stays virally suppressed can stay healthy and has effectively no risk of sexually transmitting HIV to HIV-negative partners.

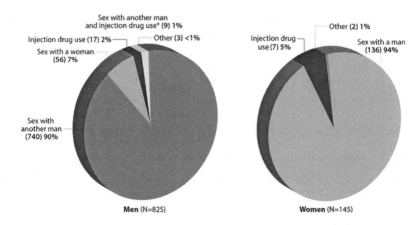

Figure 6.3. *HIV Diagnoses among Adult and Adolescent Asians in the United States and 6 Dependent Areas by Transmission Category and Sex, 2016*

*Had both risk factors.

Prevention Challenges

There are some behaviors that put everyone at risk for HIV. These include having vaginal or anal sex without a condom or without being on medicines that prevent HIV or sharing injection drug equipment with someone who has HIV. Other factors that affect Asians particularly include:

- **Undiagnosed HIV.** People living with undiagnosed HIV cannot obtain the care they need to stay healthy and may unknowingly transmit HIV to others.

- **Cultural factors.** Some Asians may avoid seeking testing, counseling, or treatment because of language barriers or fear of discrimination, the stigma of homosexuality, immigration issues, or fear of bringing shame to their families.

- **Limited research.** Limited research about Asian health and HIV infection has resulted in few targeted prevention programs and behavioral interventions in this population.

- **Data limitations.** The reported number of HIV cases among Asians may not reflect the true HIV diagnoses in this population because of race/ethnicity misidentification. This could lead to the underestimation of HIV infection in this population.

Section 6.4

HIV among Hispanics/Latinos

This section includes text excerpted from "HIV among Hispanics/Latinos," Centers for Disease Control and Prevention (CDC), February 12, 2018.

Human immunodeficiency virus (HIV) continues to be a serious threat to the health of the Hispanic/Latino community. In 2015, Hispanics/Latinos accounted for about one-quarter of all new diagnoses of HIV in the United States, despite representing about 18 percent of the total U.S. population.

The Numbers

Increase in Human Immunodeficiency Virus (HIV) Infections

From 2010–2014, estimated annual HIV infections increased 14 percent (from 6,400–7,300) among Hispanic/Latino gay, bisexual, and other men who have sex with men.

HIV and Acquired Immunodeficiency Syndrome (AIDS) Diagnoses

In 2015, Hispanics/Latinos accounted for 24 percent (9,798) of the 40,040 new diagnoses of HIV infection in the United States and 6 dependent areas. Of those, 87 percent (8,563) were in men, and 12 percent (1,223) were in women. Gay and bisexual men accounted for 85 percent (7,271) of the HIV diagnoses among Hispanic/Latino men in 2015. Among Hispanic women/Latinas, 90 percent (1,096) of the diagnosed HIV infections were attributed to heterosexual contact.

From 2010–2014, HIV diagnoses increased 2 percent among all Hispanics/Latinos, but trends varied among subgroups.

- Diagnoses among Hispanic women/Latinas declined steadily (16 percent).

- Diagnoses among all Hispanic/Latino gay and bisexual men increased (13 percent).

- Diagnoses among young Hispanic/Latino gay and bisexual men (aged 13–24) increased 16 percent, a slower increase than in previous years.

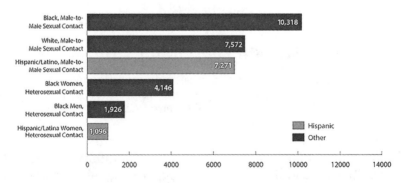

Figure 6.4. *HIV Diagnoses in the United States and 6 Dependent Areas for the Most-Affected Subpopulations, 2015*

Living with HIV and Deaths

At the end of 2014, an estimated 235,600 Hispanics/Latinos were living with HIV in the United States. Of these, an estimated 17 percent were living with undiagnosed HIV. Among all Hispanics/Latinos living with HIV in 2014, 83 percent had received a diagnosis, 58 percent received HIV medical care in 2014, 48 percent were retained in HIV care, and 48 percent had a suppressed viral load. In 2014, 916 deaths among Hispanics/Latinos were attributed directly to HIV.

Prevention Challenges

Hispanics / Latinos Are at Higher Risk

In all communities, lack of awareness of HIV status contributes to HIV transmission. People who do not know they have HIV cannot take advantage of HIV care and treatment and may unknowingly pass HIV to others. A number of challenges contribute to the higher rates of HIV infection among Hispanics/Latinos:

- More Hispanics/Latinos are living with HIV than some other races/ethnicities.

- Hispanics/Latinos have higher rates of some STDs than some other races/ethnicities. Having another STD can increase a person's chance of getting or transmitting HIV.

- Though not unique to Hispanics/Latinos, stigma, fear, discrimination, and homophobia impact Hispanic/Latino lives. These issues may put many Hispanics/Latinos at higher risk for HIV infection.

- Poverty, migration patterns, lower educational level, and language barriers may make it harder for Hispanics/Latinos to get HIV testing and care.

- Undocumented Hispanics/Latinos may be less likely to use HIV prevention services, get an HIV test, or get treatment if HIV-positive because of concerns about being arrested and deported.

Section 6.5

HIV among Native Hawaiians and Other Pacific Islanders

This section includes text excerpted from "HIV among
Native Hawaiians and Other Pacific Islanders in the
United States and 6 Dependent Areas," Centers for
Disease Control and Prevention (CDC), May 7, 2017.

Although Native Hawaiians and Other Pacific Islanders (NHOPI)
account for a very small percentage of new human immunodeficiency
virus (HIV) diagnoses, HIV affects NHOPI in ways that are not always
apparent because of their small population sizes. In 2016, NHOPI
made up 0.2 percent of the U.S. population.

The Numbers

Human Immunodeficiency Virus (HIV) and Acquired Immunodeficiency Syndrome (AIDS) Diagnoses

In 2016:

- Fifty-four NHOPI received an HIV diagnosis (45 men and 9
  women), representing less than 1 percent of new HIV diagnoses
  in the United States and 6 dependent areas.

- Gay and bisexual men accounted for 65 percent (35) of HIV
  diagnoses among NHOPI.

- Twenty NHOPI received an acquired immunodeficiency
  syndrome (AIDS) diagnosis.

HIV and Native Hawaiians and Other Pacific Islanders

From 2011–2015, HIV diagnoses:

- Increased 51 percent (from 55–83) among NHOPI overall

- Increased 50 percent (from 42–63) among NHOPI gay and
  bisexual men

Living with HIV

In 2015, an estimated 1,100 NHOPI were living with HIV in the
United States. Of those, 82 percent had received a diagnosis. Among

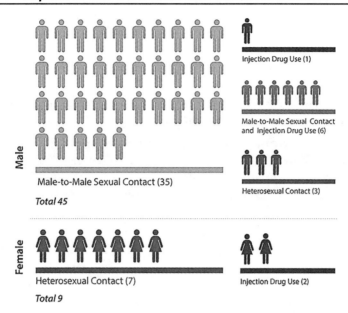

Figure 6.5. *Diagnoses of HIV Infection among Adult and Adolescent Native Hawaiians and Other Pacific Islanders*

NHOPI living with HIV in 2014, 60 percent received HIV medical care, 43 percent were retained in HIV care, and 50 percent had a suppressed viral load.

Prevention Challenges

Some behaviors put everyone at risk for HIV, including NHOPI. These behaviors include having vaginal or anal sex without a condom or without medicines to prevent or treat HIV, sharing injection drug equipment with someone who has HIV, or lack of awareness of HIV status. People who do not know they have HIV cannot take advantage of HIV care and treatment and may unknowingly pass HIV to others. Factors that particularly affect NHOPI include:

- **Socioeconomic factors.** Poverty, inadequate or no healthcare coverage, language barriers, and lower educational attainment among NHOPI may contribute to lack of awareness about HIV risk and higher-risk behaviors.

- **Cultural factors.** NHOPI cultural customs, such as not talking about sex across generations, may stigmatize sexuality in general, and homosexuality specifically, as well as interferes with HIV risk-reduction strategies, such as condom use.

- **Limited research.** Limited research about NHOPI health and HIV infection and small population numbers have resulted in a lack of targeted prevention programs and behavioral interventions for this population.

- **Data limitations.** The low reported number of HIV cases among NHOPI may not reflect the true burden of HIV in this population because of race/ethnicity misidentification. This could lead to an underestimation of HIV infection in this population.

Chapter 7

HIV/AIDS among Specific Populations

Chapter Contents

Section 7.1

HIV among Children and Adolescents

This section includes text excerpted from "HIV and Children and Adolescents," AIDS*info*, U.S. Department of Health and Human Services (HHS), April 17, 2018.

Does Human Immunodeficiency Virus (HIV) Affect Children and Adolescents?

Yes, children and adolescents are among the people living with human immunodeficiency virus (HIV) in the United States. According to the Centers for Disease Control and Prevention (CDC), 122 cases of HIV were diagnosed in children younger than 13 years of age in the United States and 6 dependent areas in 2016.

CDC reports that youth 13–24 years of age accounted for more than 1 in 5 new HIV diagnoses in the United States in 2015. Most of the HIV infections among youth occur among gay and bisexual males, with young black/African American and Hispanic/Latino gay and bisexual males especially affected.

How Do Most Children Become Infected with HIV?

HIV can pass from a mother with HIV to her child during pregnancy, childbirth, or breastfeeding (called mother-to-child transmission of HIV). In the United States, most cases of HIV diagnosed in children under 13 years of age are due to mother-to-child transmission of HIV.

Fortunately, women with HIV can take HIV medicines during pregnancy and childbirth to prevent mother-to-child transmission of HIV. In addition, babies born to women with HIV receive HIV medicine for 4–6 weeks after birth. The HIV medicine protects the babies from any HIV that may have passed from mother to child during childbirth. A mother can also prevent transmitting HIV to her baby by not breastfeeding and by not feeding her baby prechewed food.

How Do Adolescents Become Infected with HIV?

Most people in the United States who acquired HIV infection through mother-to-child transmission are now adolescents or young adults. However, most youth who get HIV during adolescence are infected through sex. Many adolescents with HIV are recently infected and don't know that they are HIV positive.

What Factors Increase the Risk of HIV Infection in Adolescents?

Several factors make it challenging to prevent HIV in adolescents. Many adolescents lack basic information about HIV and how to prevent becoming infected with HIV. The following are some factors that put adolescents at risk of HIV infection:

- **Low rates of condom use.** Always using a condom correctly during vaginal, anal, or oral sex reduces the risk of HIV infection.

- **High rates of sexually transmitted diseases (STDs) among youth.** An STD increases the risk of getting or spreading HIV.

- **Alcohol or drug use.** Adolescents under the influence of alcohol or drugs are more likely to engage in risky behaviors, such as having sex without a condom.

Is HIV Treatment the Same for Children and Adolescents Living with HIV as It Is for Adults?

The use of HIV medicines to treat HIV infection is called antiretroviral therapy (ART). ART is recommended for everyone with HIV, including children and adolescents. Children and adolescents with HIV are living longer, healthier lives because of HIV medicines.

When to start ART and what HIV medicines to take depends on many factors. Growth and development and medication adherence are issues that affect HIV treatment in children and adolescents.

How Does Growth and Development Affect the Use of Antiretroviral Therapy (ART)?

Because children and adolescents with HIV are still growing, dosing of HIV medicines is not always based on age. Instead, weight or stage of development is usually used to determine the appropriate dose of an HIV medicine.

The form of an HIV medicine to use can depend on a child's age. For example, some HIV medicines come in a liquid form, which can make it easier for infants and young children to take their medicines.

Why Can Medication Adherence Be Difficult for Children and Adolescents?

Medication adherence means taking HIV medicines every day and exactly as prescribed. Effective ART depends on good adherence. Several factors can make adherence difficult for children and adolescents with HIV. For example, a child may refuse to take an HIV medicine because it tastes unpleasant.

Negative beliefs and attitudes about HIV (stigma) can make adherence especially difficult for adolescents living with HIV. They may skip medicine doses to hide their HIV-positive status from others.

The following factors can also affect medication adherence in children and adolescents:

- A busy schedule that makes it hard to take HIV medicines on time every day

- Side effects from HIV medicines

- Issues within a family, such as physical or mental illness, an unstable housing situation, or alcohol or drug abuse

- Lack of health insurance to cover the cost of HIV medicines

Section 7.2

HIV among Women

This section includes text excerpted from "Women and HIV," Office on Women's Health (OWH), U.S. Department of Health and Human Services (HHS), March 2, 2018.

One in four people living with human immunodeficiency virus (HIV) in the United States is a woman. Women of all ages, races, and ethnicities can get HIV, but some women are more at risk than others.

Who Is at Risk for Human Immunodeficiency Virus (HIV)?

All women can get HIV, but your risk for getting HIV is higher if you:

- Have unprotected sex
- Have injected illegal drugs, either now or in the past
- Had sex with someone to get money or drugs in return or with someone who has traded sex for money or drugs
- Had sex with someone who:
  - Has HIV
  - Has sex with both men and women
  - Injects drugs
- Have another sexually transmitted infection (STI)
- Had a blood transfusion between 1978–1985

Women Who Have Sex with Men

In the United States, most women get HIV from having sex with a man. Women are more likely than men to get HIV during vaginal sex because:

- The vagina has a larger surface area (compared with the penis) that can be exposed to HIV-infected semen.

- Semen can stay in your vagina for several days after sex. This means you are exposed to the virus longer.

- Having a vaginal yeast infection, bacterial vaginosis, or an untreated STI makes HIV transmission more likely. This is because the yeast or bacterial infection or STI brings white blood cells (and therefore, cluster of differentiation 4 (CD4) cells that can be infected with HIV) into the vaginal area. Small cuts on the skin of your vagina (common with genital ulcers from herpes or syphilis) are hard to notice but may allow HIV to pass into your body.

As a woman, you are more likely to get HIV during vaginal sex when:

- You are unaware of your partner's risk factors for HIV. Some men, for example, have sex with men as well as women but do not tell their female partners.

- Your male partner was recently infected. During this time, the amount of HIV in his semen is higher. Exposure during early infection may cause up to half of all HIV transmissions in the United States.

- Your partners do not use male latex condoms or you do not use female condoms correctly every time you have sex

- You have a history of sexual abuse, which can lead to riskier future behavior

- You have sex with multiple partners or have sex with someone who is having sex with multiple partners

- You have sex in exchange for money or drugs

- You misuse drugs or alcohol before or during sex

Women Who Inject Drugs or Share Needles

Women who use injection drugs or share needles or syringes and other injection equipment are at high risk for HIV. In fact, sharing needles is the second most common way that HIV is spread. (Sex is the most common way that HIV is spread.) Use of injected drugs also raises your risk for risky behaviors, such as not using a condom during sex. In a study of U.S. cities with high levels of HIV, 72 percent of women who injected drugs reported having sex without a condom in the past year.

If you use injection drugs, talk to your doctor about medicine, called preexposure prophylaxis (PrEP), to prevent getting HIV.

Women Who Have Sex with Women

Women who have sex only with women might think they are safe from HIV. This type of HIV transmission is rare. If you are a woman and your female partner has HIV, you can get it if you have cuts, bleeding gums, or sores in your mouth and you give oral sex. It is also possible to spread HIV through menstrual blood and shared sex toys.

As a woman who has sex with women, it is also possible to get HIV if:

- You inject or your partner injects drugs with someone who has HIV

- You have or your partner has sex with a man who has HIV

- You are trying to get pregnant and use semen that has not been tested for HIV or STIs

Lower your risk of getting HIV or passing it to your partner:

- Know your HIV status and your partner's HIV status.

- Take steps to protect yourself and others from HIV.

- Use latex condoms correctly and every time if you have sex with men.

- Use dental dams correctly.

- Never share sex toys.

Younger Women

Young women are at risk for HIV:

- According to a 2013 survey, only half of the female high school students used a condom the last time they had sex. Only one in eight female high school students in the study had ever been tested for HIV.

- Younger women are more likely to have an STI. Having an untreated STI makes HIV transmission more likely. An untreated vaginal yeast or bacterial infection can also increase the risk of transmission. This is because the infection brings white blood cells (and therefore, CD4 cells that can be infected with HIV) into the area. This is especially true for women because small cuts on the skin of the vagina are hard to notice but may allow HIV to pass into your body.

- Teen girls and younger women are at higher risk for HIV infection than adult women because their reproductive tract is still developing.

Older Women

Women over 50 are still at risk for HIV. Older women are more likely than younger women to be diagnosed with HIV much later after they are first infected.

This may be because older women may think they do not need condoms because they do not worry about getting pregnant. They may not talk about safe sex with their doctors or partner or get tested regularly for HIV and other STIs. Their doctors may also not suspect their symptoms could be caused by HIV. A later diagnosis can mean a later start to treatment and possibly more damage to your immune system. It can also raise the risk of spreading HIV to other people.

You can get HIV at any age. In fact, the decrease in hormone levels during and after menopause means your vagina will probably not be as lubricated (wet) as it used to be. This means that you have a greater risk for tiny cuts in your vagina during sex that can make it easier for HIV to get in.

Other Health Concerns

Older women with HIV also need to think about other health problems, such as heart disease and osteoporosis. If you have HIV, talk to your doctor about steps you can take to lower your risk of these problems. Ask about screening tests you might need as you age.

African-American and Hispanic Women

Women of color, especially African-American and Hispanic women, are disproportionately affected by HIV.

- African-American women made up more than 61 percent of new HIV infections among women in 2015 but are only 14 percent of the female population in the United States. African-American women face the highest risk of HIV and other STIs compared with women of other groups. However, many African-American women do not know their HIV status. Poverty, stigma, and fear of discrimination may prevent women from getting tested or seeking care if infected.

- Hispanic women made up 15 percent of new HIV infections among women in 2015. Cultural challenges may raise Hispanic women's risk for HIV. Hispanic women may avoid seeking testing, counseling, or treatment if infected because of their immigration status, stigma, or fear of discrimination. Poverty may also prevent Hispanic women from getting care.

Act against AIDS: Take Charge. Take the Test.

Take Charge. Take the Test.™ urges African-American women to get tested for HIV. The program is part of the Act Against AIDS campaign by the Centers for Disease Control and Prevention (CDC). The effort helps you recognize your risk of getting HIV and the need for HIV testing. It provides you with the information and helps you need to take charge of your life—whatever your HIV test result.

Section 7.3

HIV among Older Adults

This section includes text excerpted from "HIV and
Older Adults," AIDS*info*, U.S. Department of Health
and Human Services (HHS), April 2, 2018.

Does Human Immunodeficiency Virus (HIV) Affect Older Adults?

Yes, anyone—including older adults—can get human immunodeficiency virus (HIV). According to the Centers for Disease Control and Prevention (CDC), in 2014, an estimated 45 percent of Americans living with diagnosed HIV were aged 50 and older.

The population of older adults living with HIV is increasing for the following reasons:

- Many people who received an HIV diagnosis at a younger age are growing older. Life-long treatment with HIV medicines (called antiretroviral therapy or ART) is helping these people live longer, healthier lives.

- Thousands of older people become infected with HIV every year.

For these reasons, the population of people living with HIV will increasingly include older adults.

Are the Risk Factors for HIV the Same for Older Adults?

Many risk factors for HIV are the same for adults of any age. But like many younger people, older adults may not be aware of their HIV risk factors. HIV is most commonly spread by:

- having sex without using a condom with someone who is HIV positive or whose HIV status you don't know; or

- injecting drugs and sharing needles, syringes, or other drug equipment.

Some age-related factors also put older adults at risk for HIV infection. For example, older adults who begin dating again after a divorce or the death of a partner may not use condoms if they are unaware of the risk of HIV.

Age-related thinning and dryness of the vagina may increase the risk of HIV infection in older women. In addition, women who are no longer concerned about pregnancy may not use a female condom or ask their partners to use a male condom during sex.

Talk to your healthcare provider about your risk of HIV infection and ways to reduce your risk.

Should Older Adults Get Tested for HIV?

The CDC recommends that everyone 13–64 years old get tested for HIV at least once and that people at high risk of infection get tested more often. Your healthcare provider may recommend HIV testing if you are over 64 and at risk for HIV infection.

For several reasons, older people are less likely to get tested for HIV:

- Healthcare providers may not think to ask older adults about their HIV risk factors, including sexual activity, and may not recommend HIV testing.

- Some older people may be embarrassed to discuss HIV testing with their healthcare providers.

- In older adults, signs of HIV infection may be mistaken for symptoms of aging or of age-related conditions. Consequently, HIV testing is often not offered to older adults.

For these reasons, HIV is more likely to be diagnosed at an advanced stage in many older adults. When diagnosed late, HIV is more likely to advance to acquired immunodeficiency syndrome (AIDS).

Ask your healthcare provider whether HIV testing is right for you.

Is HIV Treatment the Same for Older Adults?

Treatment with HIV medicines is recommended for everyone with HIV, and HIV treatment recommendations are the same for older and younger adults. However, age-related factors can complicate HIV treatment in older adults.

- Liver and kidney functions decline with age. This decline may make it harder for the body to process HIV medicines and increase the risk of side effects.

- Older adults with HIV may have other conditions, like diabetes and heart disease, that can make it more difficult to manage

HIV infection. In addition, HIV may affect the aging process and increase the risk of age-related conditions such as dementia, bone loss, and some cancers. Taking HIV medicines and medicines for other conditions at the same time may increase the risk of drug-drug interactions and side effects.

• The immune system may not recover as well or as quickly in older adults taking HIV medicines as it does in younger people.

Despite these age-related factors, some studies have shown that older adults are more adherent to their HIV medicine regimens— meaning they take their HIV medicines every day and exactly as pre-scribed—than younger adults.

Section 7.4

HIV among Gay and Bisexual Men

This section includes text excerpted from "HIV among Gay and Bisexual Men," Centers for Disease Control and Prevention (CDC), February 27, 2018.

In 2014, gay and bisexual men made up an estimated 2 percent of the U.S. population but accounted for 70 percent of new human immu-nodeficiency virus (HIV) infections. Approximately 492,000 sexually active gay and bisexual men are at high risk for HIV; however, we have more tools to prevent HIV than ever before.

The Numbers

Human Immunodeficiency Virus (HIV) Infections

In 2014, gay and bisexual men accounted for an estimated 70 percent (26,200) of new HIV infections in the United States. From 2010–2014, estimated annual HIV infections remained stable at about 26,000 per year among all gay and bisexual men. However, trends varied by age and race/ethnicity. Estimated HIV infections

- Declined 16 percent among gay and bisexual men aged 13–24

- Increased 23 percent among gay and bisexual men aged 25–34

- Declined 16 percent among gay and bisexual men aged 35– 44

- Declined 11 percent among white gay and bisexual men

- Increased 14 percent among Hispanic/Latino gay and bisexual men

- Remained stable among black or African American gay and bisexual men, at about 10,000 per year

HIV and Acquired Immunodeficiency Syndrome (AIDS) Diagnoses

In 2015:

- Gay and bisexual men accounted for 82 percent (26,376) of new HIV diagnoses among all males aged 13 and older and 67 percent of the total new diagnoses in the United States.

- Gay and bisexual men aged 13–24 accounted for 92 percent of new HIV diagnoses among all men in their age group and 27 percent of new diagnoses among all gay and bisexual men.

- Gay and bisexual men accounted for 55 percent (10,047) of people who received an AIDS diagnosis. Of those men, 39 percent were African American, 31 percent were white, and 24 percent were Hispanic/Latino.

From 2010–2014:

- HIV diagnoses remained stable at about 26,000 per year among all gay and bisexual men.

- After years of increases, diagnoses stabilized among young (aged 13–24) African American and white gay and bisexual men. Diagnoses increased 14 percent among young Hispanic/Latino gay and bisexual men.

Living with HIV and Deaths

At the end of 2014, an estimated 615,400 gay and bisexual men were living with HIV. Of those, 17.3 percent were unaware of their infection. Among all gay and bisexual men living with HIV in 2014, 83 percent had received a diagnosis, 61 percent received HIV medical

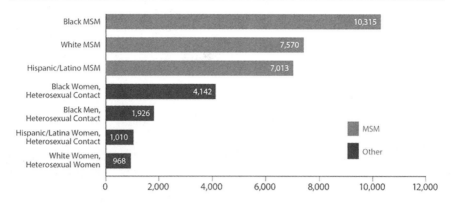

Figure 7.1. *HIV Diagnoses among the Most-Affected Subpopulations, 2015—United States*

Subpopulations representing 2 percent or less of HIV diagnoses are not reflected in this chart. Abbreviation: MSM=men who have sex with men.

care in 2014, 48 percent were receiving continuous HIV care, and a person living with HIV who gets and stays virally suppressed can stay healthy and has effectively no risk of sexually transmitting HIV to HIV-negative partners. In 2014, there were 6,110 deaths among gay and bisexual men living with diagnosed HIV infection.

Prevention Challenges

A much higher proportion of gay and bisexual men are living with HIV compared to any other group in the United States. Therefore, gay and bisexual men have an increased chance of having an HIV-positive partner.

One in six gay and bisexual men living with HIV are unaware they have it. People who don't know they have HIV cannot get the medicines they need to stay healthy and prevent transmitting HIV to their partners. Therefore, they may transmit the infection to others without knowing it.

Most gay and bisexual men get HIV through having anal sex without condoms or medicines to prevent or treat HIV. Anal sex is the riskiest type of sex for getting or transmitting HIV. Receptive anal sex is 13 times as risky for getting HIV as insertive anal sex.

Gay and bisexual men are also at increased risk for other sexually transmitted diseases (STDs), like syphilis, gonorrhea, and chlamydia. Condoms can protect from some STDs, including HIV.

Homophobia, stigma, and discrimination may place gay and bisexual men at risk for multiple physical and mental health problems and affect whether they take protective actions with their partners or seek and are able to obtain high-quality health services.

Section 7.5

HIV among Transgender People

This section includes text excerpted from "HIV among Transgender People," Centers for Disease Control and Prevention (CDC), April 23, 2018.

Transgender is a term for people whose gender identity or expression is different from their sex assigned at birth. Gender identity refers to a person's internal understanding of their own gender. Gender expression describes a person's outward presentation of their gender (for example, how they dress). Transgender women describe people who were assigned the male sex at birth but identify as women. Transgender men describes people who were assigned the female sex at birth but identify as men.

The Numbers

A 2017 paper used meta-analysis and synthesized national surveys to estimate that 1 million adults in the United States are transgender. From 2009–2014, 2,351 transgender people were diagnosed with human immunodeficiency virus (HIV) in the United States. Eighty-four percent (1,974) were transgender women, 15 percent (361) were transgender men, and less than 1 percent (16) had another gender identity. Around half of the transgender people (43 percent (844) of transgender women; 54 percent (193) of transgender men) who received an HIV diagnosis from 2009–2014 lived in the South.

According to estimates, around a quarter (22–28 percent) of transgender women are living with HIV, and more than half (an estimated 56 percent) of black/African American transgender women are living with HIV.

Among the 3 million HIV testing events reported to CDC in 2015, the percentage of transgender people who received a new HIV diagnosis was more than 3 times the national average.

Nearly two-thirds of transgender women and men surveyed by the Behavioral Risk Factor Surveillance System (BRFSS) in 2014 and 2015 from 28 jurisdictions reported never testing for HIV.

Prevention Challenges

Multiple factors have put transgender people at risk for HIV infection and transmission, including multiple sexual partners, anal or vaginal sex without condoms or medicines to prevent HIV, injecting hormones or drugs with shared syringes and other drug paraphernalia, commercial sex work, mental health issues, incarceration, homelessness, unemployment, and high levels of substance misuse compared to the general population, as well as violence and lack of family support.

HIV behavioral interventions developed for other at-risk groups have been adapted for use with transgender people. However, the effectiveness of these interventions is understudied. According to a 2017 study, most existing interventions target behavior change among transgender women, with only one HIV prevention program evaluated for transgender men. Evidence-based multilevel interventions that address the structural, biomedical, and behavioral risks for HIV among transgender populations, including transgender men, are needed to address disparities in HIV prevalence.

Many transgender people face stigma, discrimination, social rejection, and exclusion that prevent them from fully participating in society, including accessing healthcare, education, employment, and housing. These factors affect the health and well-being of transgender people, placing them at increased risk for HIV.

Transgender women and men might not be sufficiently reached by current HIV testing measures. Tailoring HIV testing activities to overcome the unique barriers faced by transgender women and men might increase rates of testing among these populations.

Transgender men's sexual health has not been well studied. Transgender men, particularly those who have sex with cisgender (persons whose sex assigned at birth is the same as their gender identity or expression) men, are at high risk for infection. Over half of transgender men with diagnosed HIV infection had no identified or reported risk. Additional research is needed to understand HIV risk behavior among transgender men, especially those who have sex with other men.

Insensitivity to transgender issues by healthcare providers can be a barrier for transgender people diagnosed with HIV and seeking quality treatment and care services. Few healthcare providers receive proper training or are knowledgeable about transgender health issues and their unique needs. This can lead to limited healthcare access and negative healthcare encounters.

Transgender women and men might not fully engage in medical care. In the United States, transgender and other gender minority youth are an at-risk group understudied in HIV prevention (e.g., preexposure prophylaxis or PrEP) and HIV treatment. In one study, medical gender affirmation and stigma in HIV care were each independently associated with elevated odds of having missed HIV care appointments. In a study of transgender men living with HIV who were receiving medical care, 60 percent had maintained an undetectable viral load over the previous 12 months. A 2015 study found that 50.8 percent of transgender women who were receiving medical care had maintained an undetectable viral load over the previous 12 months. Sustaining an undetectable viral load through effective treatment is the best thing people living with HIV can do to stay healthy and protect their sexual partners. People living with HIV who sustain an undetectable viral load have effectively no risk of sexually transmitting HIV to an HIV-negative partner.

Transgender-specific data are limited. Some federal, state and local agencies do not collect or have complete data on transgender individuals. Using the two-step data collection method of asking for sex assigned at birth and current gender identity can help increase the likelihood that transgender people are correctly identified in HIV surveillance programs. Accurate data on transgender status can lead to more effective public health actions.

Section 7.6

HIV among Incarcerated Populations

This section includes text excerpted from "HIV among
Incarcerated Populations," Centers for Disease Control and
Prevention (CDC), February 12, 2018.

More than 2 million people in the United States are incarcerated
in federal, state, and local correctional facilities on any given day.
In 2010, the rate of diagnosed human immunodeficiency virus (HIV)
infection among inmates in state and federal prisons was more than
five times greater than the rate among people who were not incarcerated. Most inmates with HIV acquire it in their communities, before
they are incarcerated.

The Numbers

In 2012, 1.57 million people were incarcerated in state and federal
prisons and at midyear 2013 there were 731,208 people detained in
local jails. In 2010, there were 20,093 inmates with HIV/acquired
immunodeficiency syndrome (AIDS) in state and federal prisons with
91 percent being men. Among state and federal jurisdictions reporting
in 2010, there were 3,913 inmates living with an AIDS diagnosis.

Rates of AIDS-related deaths among state and federal prisoners
declined an average of 16 percent per year between 2001–2010, from
24 deaths/100,000 in 2001 to 5/100,000 in 2010.

Among jail populations, African American men are 5 times as likely
as white men, and twice as likely as Hispanic/Latino men, to be diagnosed with HIV. Among jail populations, African American women
are more than twice as likely to be diagnosed with HIV as white or
Hispanic/Latino women.

Prevention Challenges

**Lack of awareness about HIV and lack of resources for HIV
testing and treatment in inmates' home communities.** Most
inmates with HIV become infected in their communities, where they
may engage in high-risk behaviors or be unaware of available prevention and treatment resources.

**Lack of resources for HIV testing and treatment in correc-
tional facilities.** Prison and jail administrators must weigh the costs

of HIV testing and treatment against other needs, and some correctional systems may not provide such services. HIV testing can identify inmates with HIV before they are released. Early diagnosis and treatment can potentially reduce the level of HIV in communities to which inmates return.

Rapid turnover among jail populations. While most HIV programs in correctional facilities are in prisons, most incarcerated people are detained in jails. Nine out of ten jail inmates are released in under 72 hours, which makes it hard to test them for HIV and help them find treatment.

Inmate concerns about privacy and fear of stigma. Many inmates do not disclose their high-risk behaviors, such as anal sex or injection drug use, because they fear being stigmatized. Healthcare providers should keep inmate's healthcare information confidential, know the public health confidentiality and reporting laws, and inform inmates about them.

Section 7.7

HIV among Sex Workers

This section includes text excerpted from "HIV Risk among Persons Who Exchange Sex for Money or Nonmonetary Items," Centers for Disease Control and Prevention (CDC), September 26, 2016.

The phrase "people who exchange sex for money or nonmonetary items" (hereinafter referred to as "people who exchange sex") includes a broad range of persons who trade sex for income or other items including food, drugs, medicine, and shelter. Persons who exchange sex are at increased risk of getting or transmitting human immunodeficiency virus (HIV) and other sexually transmitted diseases (STDs) because they are more likely to engage in risky sexual behaviors (e.g., sex without a condom, sex with multiple partners) and substance use. Those who exchange sex more regularly as a source of ongoing income are at higher risk for HIV than those who do so infrequently. Persons who engage in such activities include escorts; people who work in massage parlors, brothels, and the adult film industry; exotic dancers; state-regulated prostitutes (in Nevada); and men, women, and transgender persons who participate in survival sex, i.e., trading sex to meet basic needs of daily life. For any of the above, sex can be consensual or nonconsensual.

It is important for people who exchange sex to get tested for HIV regularly and know their status. Knowing one's status helps determine the best prevention or care options:

- Condoms are highly effective in preventing a person from getting or transmitting HIV infection if used the right way every time during sex.

- For persons who are HIV-negative, prevention options like preexposure prophylaxis (PrEP), taking HIV medicines daily to prevent getting HIV, may be beneficial.

- For people who are living with HIV, taking medicines to treat HIV (called antiretroviral therapy or ART) the right way every day can help keep them healthy and greatly reduce their chance of transmitting HIV to others.

Prevention Challenges

Lack of Data

There is a lack of population-based studies on persons who exchange sex, although some studies have been done in singular settings such as prisons and exotic dance clubs. However, the illegal—and often criminalized—nature of exchange sex makes it difficult to gather population-level data on HIV risk among this population. This lack of data creates significant barriers to developing targeted HIV prevention efforts.

Socioeconomic Factors

Many persons who exchange sex face stigma, poverty, and lack of access to healthcare and other social services—all of which pose challenges to HIV prevention efforts. Existing research shows that:

- Many persons who exchange sex may have a history of homelessness, unemployment, incarceration, mental health issues, violence, emotional/physical/sexual abuse, and drug use.

- Some transgender persons may turn to exchange sex because of discrimination and lack of economic opportunities. They may exchange sex to generate income for rent, drugs, medicines, hormones, and gender-related surgeries.

Sexual Risk Factors

Persons who exchange sex may not use condoms consistently. Several factors may contribute to this behavior, including:

- **Economics.** Persons who exchange sex may receive more money for sex without a condom.

- **Partner type.** Persons who exchange sex may use condoms less often with regular clients than with one-time clients and even less frequently with intimate partners.

- **Power dynamics.** Unequal power in a relationship with clients may make it difficult for persons who exchange sex to negotiate condom use.

Other risk factors for this population include:

- Multiple high-risk sex partners, e.g., partners who do not know they are living with HIV or other STDs.

- More money for sex with partners known to be HIV positive.

Drug and Alcohol Use

There is a strong link between exchange sex and drug and alcohol use. Persons who exchange sex, if under the influence of drugs or alcohol, may have impaired judgment, engage in riskier forms of sex such as anal sex, and have difficulty negotiating safer sex (condom use, for example) with their customers. People who trade sex for drugs tend to have more clients, use condoms less often, and are more likely to share needles and other drug works.

Knowledge of HIV Status

Many persons who exchange sex may not know their HIV status because they:

- Do not know where to access available services

- Are uncomfortable sharing information about sexual and substance use histories as part of HIV testing protocol

Some persons who know their HIV status may be reluctant to seek or stay in care because of:

- Mistrust of the healthcare system

- Concern that they may lose income if identified as being HIV-positive

- Financial circumstances and other barriers (e.g., health insurance) that affect healthcare access

Part Two

HIV/AIDS Transmission, Risk Factors, and Prevention

Chapter 8

HIV Transmission: Questions and Answers

Myths persist about how human immunodeficiency virus (HIV) is transmitted. This chapter provides the facts about HIV risk from different types of sex, injection drug use, and other activities.

Frequently Asked Questions about Human Immunodeficiency Virus (HIV) Transmission

How Is HIV Passed from One Person to Another?

You can get or transmit HIV only through specific activities. Most commonly, people get or transmit HIV through sexual behaviors and needle or syringe use.

Only certain body fluids—blood, semen (cum), preseminal fluid (precum), rectal fluids, vaginal fluids, and breast milk—from a person who has HIV can transmit HIV. These fluids must come in contact with a mucous membrane or damaged tissue or be directly injected into the bloodstream (from a needle or syringe) for transmission to occur. Mucous membranes are found inside the rectum, vagina, penis, and mouth.

This chapter contains text excerpted from "HIV Transmission," Centers for Disease Control and Prevention (CDC), March 16, 2018.

In the United States HIV is spread mainly by:

- Having anal or vaginal sex with someone who has HIV without using a condom or taking medicines to prevent or treat HIV.

- For the HIV-negative partner, receptive anal sex (bottoming) is the highest-risk sexual behavior, but you can also get HIV from insertive anal sex (topping).

- Either partner can get HIV through vaginal sex, though it is less risky for getting HIV than receptive anal sex.

- Sharing needles or syringes. Rinse water, or other equipment (works) used to prepare drugs for injection with someone who has HIV. HIV can live in a used needle up to 42 days depending on temperature and other factors.

Less commonly, HIV may be spread:

- From mother to child during pregnancy, birth, or breastfeeding. Although the risk can be high if a mother is living with HIV and not taking medicine, recommendations to test all pregnant women for HIV and start HIV treatment immediately have lowered the number of babies who are born with HIV.

- By being stuck with an HIV-contaminated needle or other sharp object. This is a risk mainly for healthcare workers.

In extremely rare cases, HIV has been transmitted by:

- Oral sex—putting the mouth on the penis (fellatio), vagina (cunnilingus), or anus (rimming). In general, there's little to no risk of getting HIV from oral sex. But transmission of HIV, though extremely rare, is theoretically possible if an HIV-positive man ejaculates in his partner's mouth during oral sex.

- Receiving blood transfusions, blood products, or organ/tissue transplants that are contaminated with HIV. This was more common in the early years of HIV, but now the risk is extremely small because of rigorous testing of the U.S. blood supply and donated organs and tissues.

- Eating food that has been prechewed by an HIV-infected person. The contamination occurs when infected blood from a caregiver's mouth mixes with food while chewing. The only known cases are among infants.

- Being bitten by a person with HIV. Each of the very small number of documented cases has involved severe trauma with extensive tissue damage and the presence of blood. There is no risk of transmission if the skin is not broken.

- Contact between broken skin, wounds, or mucous membranes and HIV-infected blood or blood-contaminated body fluids

- Deep, open-mouth kissing if both partners have sores or bleeding gums and blood from the HIV-positive partner gets into the bloodstream of the HIV-negative partner. HIV is not spread through saliva.

How Well Does HIV Survive outside the Body?

HIV does not survive long outside the human body (such as on surfaces), and it cannot reproduce outside a human host. It is not spread by:

- Mosquitoes, ticks, or other insects

- Saliva, tears, or sweat that is not mixed with the blood of an HIV-positive person

- Hugging, shaking hands, sharing toilets, sharing dishes, or closed-mouth or "social" kissing with someone who is HIV-positive

- Other sexual activities that don't involve the exchange of body fluids (for example, touching)

Can I Get HIV from Anal Sex?

Yes. In fact, anal sex is the riskiest type of sex for getting or trans-mitting HIV. HIV can be found in certain body fluids—blood, semen (cum), preseminal fluid (precum), or rectal fluids—of a person who has HIV. Although receptive anal sex (bottoming) is much riskier for getting HIV than insertive anal sex (topping), it's possible for either partner—the top or the bottom—to get HIV. The bottom's risk is very high because the lining of the rectum is thin and may allow HIV to enter the body during anal sex. The top is also at risk because HIV can enter the body through the opening at the tip of the penis (or urethra); the foreskin if the penis isn't circumcised; or small cuts, scratches, or open sores anywhere on the penis.

Can I Get HIV from Vaginal Sex?

Yes. Either partner can get HIV through vaginal sex, though it is less risky for getting HIV than receptive anal sex. When a woman has vaginal sex with a partner who's HIV-positive, HIV can enter her body through the mucous membranes that line the vagina and cervix. Most women who get HIV get it from vaginal sex.

Men can also get HIV from having vaginal sex with a woman who's HIV-positive. This is because vaginal fluid and blood can carry HIV. Men get HIV through the opening at the tip of the penis (or urethra); the foreskin if they're not circumcised; or small cuts, scratches, or open sores anywhere on the penis.

Can I Get HIV from Oral Sex?

The chance that an HIV-negative person will get HIV from oral sex with an HIV-positive partner is extremely low. Oral sex involves putting the mouth on the penis (fellatio), vagina (cunnilingus), or anus (anilingus). In general, there's little to no risk of getting or transmitting HIV through oral sex.

Factors that may increase the risk of transmitting HIV through oral sex are ejaculation in the mouth with oral ulcers, bleeding gums, genital sores, and the presence of other sexually transmitted diseases (STDs), which may or may not be visible.

You can get other STDs from oral sex. And, if you get feces in your mouth during anilingus, you can get hepatitis A and B, parasites like *Giardia*, and bacteria like *Shigella*, *Salmonella*, *Campylobacter*, and *E. coli*.

Is There a Connection between HIV and Other Sexually Transmitted Infections (STIs)?

Yes. Having another sexually transmitted disease (STD) can increase the risk of getting or transmitting HIV. If you have another STD, you're more likely to get or transmit HIV to others. Some of the most common STDs include gonorrhea, chlamydia, syphilis, trichomoniasis, human papillomavirus (HPV), genital herpes, and hepatitis. The only way to know for sure if you have an STD is to get tested. If you're sexually active, you and your partners should get tested for STDs (including HIV if you're HIV-negative) regularly, even if you don't have symptoms.

If you are HIV-negative but have an STD, you are about 3 times as likely to get HIV if you have unprotected sex with someone who has HIV. There are two ways that having an STD can increase the likelihood of getting HIV. If the STD causes irritation of the skin (for example, from syphilis, herpes, or human papillomavirus), breaks or sores may make it easier for HIV to enter the body during sexual contact. Even STDs that cause no breaks or open sores (for example, chlamydia, gonorrhea, trichomoniasis) can increase your risk by causing inflammation that increases the number of cells that can serve as targets for HIV.

If you are HIV-positive and also infected with another STD, you are about 3 times as likely as other HIV-infected people to spread HIV through sexual contact. This appears to happen because there is an increased concentration of HIV in the semen and genital fluids of HIV-positive people who also are infected with another STD.

Does My HIV-Positive Partner's Viral Load Affect My Risk of Getting HIV?

Yes, as an HIV-positive person's viral load goes down, the chance of transmitting HIV goes down. Viral load is the amount of HIV in the blood of someone who is HIV-positive. When the viral load is very low, it is called viral suppression. Undetectable viral load is when the amount of HIV in the blood is so low that it can't be measured.

In general, the higher someone's viral load, the more likely that person is to transmit HIV. People who have HIV but are in care, taking HIV medicines, and have a very low or undetectable viral load are much less likely to transmit HIV than people who have HIV and do not have a low viral load.

However, a person with HIV can still potentially transmit HIV to a partner even if they have an undetectable viral load, because:

- HIV may still be found in genital fluids (semen, vaginal fluids). The viral load test only measures virus in blood.

- A person's viral load may go up between tests. When this happens, they may be more likely to transmit HIV to partners.

Sexually transmitted diseases increase viral load in genital fluids.

If you're HIV-positive, getting into care and taking HIV medicines (called antiretroviral therapy or ART) the right way, every day will give you the greatest chance to get and stay virally suppressed, live a longer, healthier life, and reduce the chance of transmitting HIV to your partners.

If you're HIV-negative and have an HIV-positive partner, encourage your partner to get into care and take HIV treatment medicines.

Taking other actions, like using a condom the right way every time you have sex or taking daily medicine to prevent HIV (called preexposure prophylaxis or PrEP) if you're HIV-negative, can lower your chances of transmitting or getting HIV even more.

Can I Get HIV from Injecting Drugs?

Yes. Your risk for getting HIV is very high if you use needles or works (such as cookers, cotton, or water) after someone with HIV has used them. People who inject drugs, hormones, steroids, or silicone can get HIV by sharing needles or syringes and other injection equipment. The needles and equipment may have someone else's blood in them, and blood can transmit HIV. Likewise, you're at risk for getting hepatitis B and C if you share needles and works because these infections are also transmitted through blood.

Another reason people who inject drugs can get HIV (and other sexually transmitted diseases) is that when people are high, they're more likely to have risky sex.

Stopping injection and other drug use can lower your chances of getting HIV a lot. You may need help to stop or cut down using drugs, but many resources are available. To find a substance abuse treatment center near you, check out the locator tools on SAMHSA.gov or HIV.gov, or call 800-662-4357.

If you keep injecting drugs, you can lower your risk for getting HIV by using only new, sterile needles and works each time you inject. Never share needles or works.

Can I Get HIV from Using Other Kinds of Drugs?

When you're drunk or high, you're more likely to make decisions that put you at risk for HIV, such as having sex without a condom.

Drinking alcohol, particularly binge drinking, and using "club drugs" like Ecstasy, ketamine, gamma-hydroxybutyrate (GHB), and poppers can alter your judgment, lower your inhibitions, and impair your decisions about sex or other drug use. You may be more likely to have unplanned and unprotected sex, have a harder time using a condom the right way every time you have sex, have more sexual partners or use other drugs, including injection drugs or meth. Those behaviors can increase your risk of exposure to HIV. If you have HIV, they can also increase your risk of spreading HIV to others. Being drunk or high affects your ability to make safe choices.

If you're going to a party or another place where you know you'll be drinking or using drugs, you can bring a condom so that you can reduce your risk if you have vaginal or anal sex.

Therapy, medicines, and other methods are available to help you stop or cut down on drinking or using drugs. Talk with a counselor, doctor, or other healthcare provider about options that might be right for you.

If I Am Living with HIV, How Can I Prevent Passing It to Others*

There are many actions you can take to lower your risk of transmitting HIV to a partner. The more actions you take, the safer you can be.

- The most important thing you can do is to take medicines to treat HIV infection (ART) the right way, every day. These medicines reduce the amount of virus (viral load) in your blood and body fluids. They can keep you healthy for many years and greatly reduce your chance of transmitting HIV to your partners if you have a very low or undetectable viral load.

- If you're taking medicines to treat HIV (ART), follow your healthcare provider's advice. Visit your healthcare provider regularly and always take your medicines as directed.

- Use condoms the right way every time you have sex.

- Choose less risky sexual behaviors. Anal sex is the highest-risk sexual activity for HIV transmission. If your partner is HIV-negative, it's less risky if they're the insertive partner (top) and you're the receptive partner (bottom) during anal sex. Oral sex is much less risky than anal or vaginal sex. Sexual activities that don't involve contact with body fluids (semen, vaginal fluid, or blood) carry no risk of HIV transmission. If you inject drugs, never share your needles or works with anyone.

- Talk to your partners about PrEP, taking HIV medicines the right way, every day to prevent HIV infection.

- Talk to your partners about postexposure prophylaxis (pep. html) (PEP) if you think they've recently had a possible exposure to HIV (for example, if they had anal or vaginal sex without a condom or if the condom broke during sex). Your partners should talk to a healthcare provider right away (within 72 hours) after a possible exposure. Starting PEP immediately and taking it daily for 28 days will reduce their chance of getting HIV.

- Get tested and treated for other STDs and encourage your partners to do the same. If you are sexually active, get tested at least once a year. STDs can have long-term health consequences. They can also increase the risk of getting or transmitting HIV. Find an STD testing site.

Also, encourage your partners who are HIV-negative to get tested for HIV so they are sure about their status and can take action to keep themselves healthy.

*Source: "HIV Transmission," Centers for Disease Control and Prevention (CDC), March 16, 2018.

If I Already Have HIV, Can I Get Another Kind of HIV?

Yes. This is called HIV superinfection. HIV superinfection is when a person with HIV gets infected with another strain of the virus. The new strain of HIV can replace the original strain or remain along with the original strain.

The effects of superinfection differ from person to person. Superinfection may cause some people to get sicker faster because they become infected with a new strain of the virus that is resistant to the medicine (ART) they're taking to treat their original infection.

Research suggests that a hard-to-treat superinfection is rare. Taking medicine to treat HIV (ART) may reduce someone's chance of getting a superinfection.

Are Healthcare Workers at Risk of Getting HIV on the Job?

The risk of healthcare workers being exposed to HIV on the job (occupational exposure) is very low, especially if they use protective practices and personal protective equipment to prevent HIV and other blood-borne infections. For healthcare workers on the job, the main risk of HIV transmission is from being stuck with an HIV-contaminated needle or other sharp object. However, even this risk is small. Scientists estimate that the risk of HIV infection from being stuck with a needle used on an HIV-infected person is less than 1 percent.

Can I Get HIV from Receiving Medical Care?

Although HIV transmission is possible in healthcare settings, it is extremely rare.

Careful practice of infection control, including universal precautions (using protective practices and personal protective equipment to prevent HIV and other blood-borne infections), protects patients as well as healthcare providers from possible HIV transmission in medical and dental offices and hospitals.

The risk of getting HIV from receiving blood transfusions, blood products, or organ/tissue transplants that are contaminated with HIV is extremely small because of rigorous testing of the U.S. blood supply and donated organs and tissues.

It is important to know that you cannot get HIV from donating blood. Blood collection procedures are highly regulated and safe.

Can I Get HIV from Casual Contact ("Social Kissing," Shaking Hands, Hugging, Using a Toilet, Drinking from the Same Glass, or the Sneezing and Coughing of an Infected Person)?

No. HIV isn't transmitted:

- By hugging, shaking hands, sharing toilets, sharing dishes, or closed-mouth or "social" kissing with someone who is HIV-positive

- Through saliva, tears, or sweat that is not mixed with the blood of an HIV-positive person

- By mosquitoes, ticks or other blood-sucking insects

- Through the air

Only certain body fluids—blood, semen (cum), preseminal fluid (precum), rectal fluids, vaginal fluids, and breast milk—from an HIV-infected person can transmit HIV. Most commonly, people get or transmit HIV through sexual behaviors and needle or syringe use. Babies can also get HIV from an HIV-positive mother during pregnancy, birth, or breastfeeding.

Can I Get HIV from a Tattoo or a Body Piercing?

There are no known cases in the United States of anyone getting HIV this way. However, it is possible to get HIV from a reused or not properly sterilized tattoo or piercing needle or other equipment, or from contaminated ink.

It's possible to get HIV from tattooing or body piercing if the equipment used for these procedures has someone else's blood in it or if the ink is shared. The risk of getting HIV this way is very low, but the risk increases when the person doing the procedure is unlicensed, because of the potential for unsanitary practices such as sharing needles or ink. If you get a tattoo or a body piercing, be sure that the person doing the procedure is properly licensed and that they use only new or sterilized needles, ink, and other supplies.

Can I Get HIV from Being Spit on or Scratched by an HIV-Infected Person?

No. HIV isn't spread through saliva, and there is no risk of transmission from scratching because no body fluids are transferred between people.

Can I Get HIV from Mosquitoes?

No. HIV is not transmitted by mosquitoes, ticks, or any other insects.

Can I Get HIV from Food?

You can't get HIV from consuming food handled by an HIV-infected person. Even if the food contained small amounts of HIV-infected blood or semen, exposure to the air, heat from cooking, and stomach acid would destroy the virus.

Though it is very rare, HIV can be spread by eating food that has been prechewed by an HIV-infected person. The contamination occurs when infected blood from a caregiver's mouth mixes with food while chewing. The only known cases are among infants.

Are Lesbians or Other Women Who Have Sex with Women at Risk for HIV?

Case reports of female-to-female transmission of HIV are rare. The well-documented risk of female-to-male transmission shows that vaginal fluids and menstrual blood may contain the virus and that exposure to these fluids through mucous membranes (in the vagina or mouth) could potentially lead to HIV infection.

Is the Risk of HIV Different for Different People?

Some groups of people in the United States are more likely to get HIV than others because of many factors, including the status of their sex partners, their risk behaviors, and where they live.

When you live in a community where many people have HIV infection, the chances of having sex or sharing needles or other injection equipment with someone who has HIV are higher. You can use Centers for Disease Control and Prevention's (CDC) HIV, STD, hepatitis, and tuberculosis (TB) atlas to see the percentage of people with HIV ("prevalence") in different U.S. communities. Within any community, the prevalence of HIV can vary among different populations.

Gay and bisexual men have the largest number of new diagnoses in the United States. Blacks/African Americans and Hispanics/Latinos are disproportionately affected by HIV compared to other racial and ethnic groups. Also, transgender women who have sex with men are among the groups at highest risk for HIV infection, and injection drug users remain at significant risk for getting HIV.

Risky behaviors, like having anal or vaginal sex without using a condom or taking medicines to prevent or treat HIV, and sharing needles or syringes play a big role in HIV transmission. Anal sex is the highest-risk sexual behavior. If you don't have HIV, being a receptive partner (or bottom) for anal sex is the highest-risk sexual activity for getting HIV. If you do have HIV, being the insertive partner (or top) for anal sex is the highest-risk sexual activity for transmitting HIV.

But there are more tools available to prevent HIV than ever before. Choosing less risky sexual behaviors, taking medicines to prevent and treat HIV, and using condoms with lubricants are all highly effective ways to reduce the risk of getting or transmitting HIV.

Chapter 9

Risky Behaviors and HIV

Chapter Contents

Section 9.1

Alcohol, Drugs, and HIV Risk

This section includes text excerpted from documents
published by two public domain sources. Text under the headings
marked 1 are excerpted from "HIV and Substance Use in the
United States," Centers for Disease Control and Prevention (CDC),
March 6, 2018; Text under the heading marked 2 is excerpted
from "Prevention—HIV Basics," Centers for Disease Control
and Prevention (CDC), February 27, 2018.

Substance use disorders, which are problematic patterns of using
alcohol or another substance, such as crack cocaine, methamphetamine
("meth"), amyl nitrite ("poppers"), prescription opioids, and heroin,
are closely associated with human immunodeficiency virus (HIV) and
other sexually transmitted diseases (STDs).

Injection drug use (IDU) can be a direct route of HIV transmission
if people share needles, syringes, or other injection materials that are
contaminated with HIV. However, drinking alcohol and ingesting,
smoking, or inhaling drugs are also associated with increased risk
for HIV. These substances alter judgment, which can lead to risky
sexual behaviors (e.g., having sex without a condom, having multiple
partners) that can make people more likely to get and transmit HIV.

In people living with HIV, substance use can hasten disease progression, affect adherence to antiretroviral therapy or ART therapy
(HIV medicine), and worsen the overall consequences of HIV.

Commonly Used Substances and HIV Risk[1]

Some of the commonly used substances that can lead to HIV risk
includes:

- **Alcohol.** Excessive alcohol consumption, notably binge drinking,
  can be an important risk factor for HIV because it is linked to
  risky sexual behaviors and, among people living with HIV, can
  hurt treatment outcomes.

- **Opioids.** Opioids, a class of drugs that reduce pain, include both
  prescription drugs and heroin. They are associated with HIV
  risk behaviors such as needle sharing when infected and risky
  sex, and have been linked to one of the HIV outbreak.

- **Methamphetamine.** "Meth" is linked to risky sexual behavior
  that places people at greater HIV risk. It can be injected,

which also increases HIV risk if people share needles and other injection equipment.

- **Crack cocaine.** Crack cocaine is a stimulant that can create a cycle in which people quickly exhaust their resources and turn to other ways to get the drug, including trading sex for drugs or money, which increases HIV risk.

- **Inhalants.** Use of amyl nitrite ("poppers") has long been linked to risky sexual behaviors, illegal drug use, and sexually transmitted diseases among gay and bisexual men.

How Can I Prevent Getting HIV from Drug Use?[2]

Stopping injection and other drug use can lower your chances of getting or transmitting HIV a lot. If you keep injecting drugs, use only sterile needles and works. Never share needles or works.

You are at very high risk for getting HIV if you use a needle or works after someone with HIV has used them. Also, when people are high, they're more likely to have risky sex, which increases the chance of getting or transmitting HIV.

The best way to reduce your risk of HIV is to stop using drugs. You may need help to stop or cut down using drugs, but many resources are available. Talk with a counselor, doctor, or other healthcare provider about substance abuse treatment. To find a treatment center near you, check out the locator tools on the websites of Substance Abuse and Mental Health Services Administration (SAMHSA) (www.samhsa.gov) or HIV.gov, or call 800-662-HELP (800-662-4357).

If you keep injecting drugs, here are some things you can do to lower your risk for getting HIV and other infections:

- Use only new, sterile needles and works each time you inject. Many communities have needle exchange programs where you can get new needles and works, and some pharmacies may sell needles without a prescription.

- Never share needles or works.

- Clean used needles with bleach only when you can't get new ones. Bleaching a needle may reduce the risk of HIV but doesn't eliminate it.

- Use sterile water to fix drugs.

- Clean your skin with a new alcohol swab before you inject.

- Be careful not to get someone else's blood on your hands or your needle or works.

- Dispose of needles safely after one use. Use a sharp container or keep used needles away from other people.

- Get tested for HIV at least once a year.

- Ask your doctor about taking daily medicine to prevent HIV (called PrEP).

- Don't have sex if you're high. If you do have sex, use a condom the right way every time. Learn the right way to use a male condom.

Prevention Challenges[1]

A number of behavioral, structural, and environmental factors make it difficult to control the spread of HIV among people who use or misuse substances:

- **Complex health and social needs.** People who are alcohol dependent or use drugs often have other complex health and social needs. Research shows that people who use substances are more likely to be homeless, face unemployment, live in poverty, and experience multiple forms of violence, creating challenges for HIV prevention efforts.

- **Stigma and discrimination associated with substance use.** Often, illicit drug use is viewed as a criminal activity rather than a medical issue that requires counseling and rehabilitation. Fear of arrest, stigma, feelings of guilt, and low self-esteem may prevent people who use illicit drugs from seeking treatment services, which places them at greater risk for HIV.

- **Lack of access to the healthcare system.** Since HIV testing often involves questioning about substance use histories, those who use substances may feel uncomfortable getting tested. As a result, it may be harder to reach people who use substances with HIV prevention services.

- **Poor adherence to HIV treatment.** People living with HIV who use substances are less likely to take ART as prescribed due to side effects from drug interaction. Not taking ART as prescribed can worsen the effects of HIV and increase the likelihood of spreading HIV to sex and drug-sharing partners.

Section 9.2

Injection Drug Use and HIV Risk

This section includes text excerpted from "Injection
Drug Use and HIV Risk," Centers for Disease Control and
Prevention (CDC), March 16, 2018.

Sharing needles, syringes, or other injection equipment (works)
to inject drugs puts people at risk for getting or transmitting human
immunodeficiency virus (HIV) and other infections. About 1 in 10 new
HIV diagnoses in the United States are attributed to injection drug
use or male-to-male sexual contact and injection drug use.

Risk of Human Immunodeficiency Virus (HIV)

The risk for getting or transmitting HIV is very high if an HIV-negative person uses injection equipment that someone living with HIV
has used. This is because the needles or works may have blood in them,
and blood can carry HIV. HIV can survive in a used needle for up to
42 days, depending on temperature and other factors.

Substance misuse can also increase the risk of getting HIV through
sex. When people are high, they are more likely to have risky anal or
vaginal sex, such as having sex without a condom or without medicines
to prevent or treat HIV, having sex with multiple partners, or trading
sex for money or drugs.

Risk of Other Infections and Overdose

Sharing needles or works also puts people at risk for getting viral
hepatitis. People who inject drugs should talk to a doctor about getting
vaccinated for hepatitis A and B and getting a blood test for hepatitis
B and C.

In addition to being at risk for HIV and viral hepatitis, people who
inject drugs can get other serious health problems, like skin infections or
abscesses. People can also overdose and get very sick or even die from having too many drugs in their body or from products that may be mixed with
the drugs without their knowledge (for example, illegally made fentanyl).

Reducing the Risk

The best way to reduce the risk of getting or transmitting HIV
through injection drug use is to stop injecting drugs. Talk with a

counselor, doctor, or other healthcare provider about substance use disorder treatment, including medication-assisted treatment. To find a treatment center near you, check out the locator tools on Substance Abuse and Mental Health Services Administration (SAMHSA) or www. hiv.gov, or call 800-662-4357.

If you continue injecting drugs, never share needles or works. Many communities have syringe services programs (SSPs) where you can get free sterile needles and syringes and safely dispose of used ones. They can also refer you to substance use disorder treatment and help you get tested for HIV and hepatitis. Contact your local health department or North American Syringe Exchange Network (NASEN) to find an SSP. Also, some pharmacies may sell needles without a prescription.

Other things you can do to lower your risk of getting or transmitting HIV, if you continue to inject drugs, include:

- Cleaning used needles with bleach. This may reduce the risk of HIV but doesn't eliminate it.

- Using sterile water to fix drugs

- Cleaning your skin with a new alcohol swab before you inject

- Being careful not to get someone else's blood on your hands or your needle or works

- Disposing of needles safely after one use. Use a sharps container, or keep used needles away from other people.

- Getting tested for HIV at least once a year

- Asking your doctor about taking daily medicine to prevent HIV (called preexposure prophylaxis or PrEP)

- Using a condom the right way every time you have anal or vaginal sex

Will Cleaning Intravenous (IV)-Drug Needles and Syringes with Bleach before Using Them Prevent You from Getting HIV?*

You can be infected with HIV if you use needles and syringes contaminated with blood from a person who is HIV positive. One way to avoid getting HIV from Intravenous (IV) drug use is to stop injecting drugs. Another effective way is to always use new, sterile syringes and needles and also to be sure not to use any shared injecting equipment (cookers, spoons, cotton, etc.). But what if you can't get into a drug treatment program, it hasn't worked for you, or you can't get your hands on sterile equipment?

There is some evidence that cleaning your needles and syringes with laundry bleach can lower your risk of getting HIV. In laboratory studies, HIV in syringes was killed after contact with undiluted bleach for at least 30 seconds. Watered-down bleach did not work, and neither did contact with bleach for less than 30 seconds.

Does this process work outside the lab? It's hard to know because this is very difficult to study. But it's probably a lot better than not doing anything at all to kill the HIV in drug-injecting equipment. Note: It is important to rinse the syringes and needles with water after cleaning them with bleach so that you won't inject the bleach into your body. And how do you know when 30 seconds are up? Use a watch or a clock, or hum the song "Happy Birthday to You," all the way through, three times over.

*Source: "Frequently Asked Questions about HIV," U.S. Department of Veterans Affairs (VA), February 9, 2018.

Section 9.3

Sexual Risk Factors and HIV Transmission

This section includes text excerpted from "HIV Risk and Prevention," Centers for Disease Control and Prevention (CDC), March 16, 2018.

Oral Sex and Human Immunodeficiency Virus (HIV) Risk

Oral sex involves using the mouth to stimulate the penis (fellatio), vagina (cunnilingus), or anus (anilingus).

Risk of HIV

The chance an human immunodeficiency virus (HIV)-negative person will get HIV from oral sex with an HIV-positive partner is extremely low. However, it is hard to know the exact risk because a lot of people who have oral sex also have anal or vaginal sex. The type of oral sex that may be the riskiest is mouth-to-penis oral sex. But the risk is still very low, and much lower than with anal or vaginal sex. Though the risk of HIV transmission through oral sex is low, several factors may increase that risk, including sores in the mouth or vagina or on the penis, bleeding gums, oral contact with menstrual blood, and the presence of other sexually transmitted diseases (STDs).

Risk of Other Infections

Other STDs, such as syphilis, herpes, gonorrhea, and chlamydia, can be transmitted during oral sex. Anilingus can also transmit hepatitis A and B, intestinal parasites like Giardia, and bacteria like *E. coli*.

Reducing the Risk

Individuals can further reduce the already low risk of HIV transmission from oral sex by keeping their male partners from ejaculating in their mouth. This could be done by removing the mouth from the penis before ejaculation, or by using a condom. Using a barrier like a condom or dental dam during oral sex can further reduce the risk of transmitting HIV, other STDs, and hepatitis. A dental dam is a thin, square piece of latex or silicone that is placed over the vagina or anus during oral sex. A latex condom can also be cut length-wise and used like a dental dam.

The risk of HIV transmission through oral sex is even lower if the HIV-negative partner is taking medicine to prevent HIV (preexposure prophylaxis or PrEP) or the HIV-positive partner is taking medicine to treat HIV (antiretroviral therapy or ART) and is virally suppressed.

Anal Sex and HIV Risk

The risk of getting HIV varies widely depending on the type of sexual activity. Anal sex (intercourse), which involves inserting the penis into the anus, carries the highest risk of transmitting HIV if either partner is HIV-positive. You can lower your risk for getting and transmitting HIV by using condoms correctly and consistently, choosing lower risk sexual activities, taking daily medicine to prevent HIV, called PrEP; and taking medicines to treat HIV if living with

HIV, called ART. Using more than one of these options at the same time provides even greater protection.

Risk of HIV

Anal sex is the highest-risk sexual behavior for HIV transmission. Vaginal sex has a lower risk, and activities like oral sex, touching, and kissing carry little to no risk for getting or transmitting HIV. The vast majority of men who get HIV get it through anal sex. However, anal sex is also one of the ways women can get HIV.

Receptive versus Insertive Sex

During anal sex, the partner inserting the penis is called the insertive partner (or top), and the partner receiving the penis is called the receptive partner (or bottom).

Receptive anal sex is much riskier for getting HIV. The bottom partner is 13 times more likely to get infected than the top. However, it's possible for either partner to get HIV through anal sex from certain body fluids—blood, semen (cum), preseminal fluid (precum), or rectal fluids—of a person who has HIV. Using condoms or medicines to protect against transmission can decrease this risk.

Being a receptive partner during anal sex is the highest-risk sexual activity for getting HIV. The bottom's risk of getting HIV is very high because the lining of the rectum is thin and may allow HIV to enter the body during anal sex.

The insertive partner is also at risk for getting HIV during anal sex. HIV may enter the top partner's body through the opening at the tip of the penis (or urethra) or through small cuts, scratches, or open sores on the penis.

Risk of Other Infections

In addition to HIV, a person can get other STDs like chlamydia and gonorrhea from anal sex without condoms. Even if a condom is used, some STDs can still be transmitted through skin-to-skin contact (like syphilis or herpes). One can also get hepatitis A, B, and C; parasites like Giardia and intestinal amoebas; and bacteria like *Shigella*, *Salmonella*, *Campylobacter*, and *E. coli* from anal sex without a condom because they're transmitted through feces. Getting tested and treated for STDs reduces a person's chances of getting or transmitting HIV through anal sex. If one has never had hepatitis A or B, there are vaccines to prevent them. A healthcare provider can make recommendations about vaccines.

Reducing the Risk

Condoms and Lubrication

Latex or polyurethane male condoms are highly effective in preventing HIV and certain other STDs when used correctly from start to finish for each act of anal sex. People who report using condoms consistently reduced their risk of getting HIV through insertive anal sex with an HIV-positive partner, on average, by 63 percent, and receptive anal sex with an HIV-positive partner, on average, by 72 percent. Condoms are much less effective when not used consistently. It is also important that sufficient water- or silicone-based lubricant be used during anal sex to prevent condom breakage and tearing of tissue. Female nitrile condoms can also prevent HIV and some other STDs. Since condoms are not 100 percent effective, consider using other prevention methods to further reduce your risk.

Preexposure Prophylaxis (PrEP)

People who are HIV-negative and at very high risk for HIV can take daily medicine to prevent HIV. PrEP, if taken consistently, can reduce the risk of getting HIV from sex by more than 90 percent. PrEP is much less effective when it is not taken consistently. Since PrEP is not 100 percent effective at preventing HIV, consider using other prevention methods to further reduce your risk. Only condoms can help protect against other STDs.

Postexposure Prophylaxis (PEP)

Postexposure prophylaxis (PEP) means taking antiretroviral medicines—medicines used to treat HIV—after being potentially exposed to HIV during sex to prevent becoming infected. PEP should be used only in emergency situations and must be started within 72 hours after a possible exposure to HIV, but the sooner the better. PEP must be taken once or twice daily for 28 days. When administered correctly, PEP is effective in preventing HIV, but not 100 percent. To obtain PEP, contact your healthcare provider, your local or state health department, or go to an emergency room.

Antiretroviral Therapy (ART)

For those living with HIV, ART can reduce the amount of virus in the blood and body fluids to very low levels, if taken the right way, every day. When taken consistently, ART can reduce the risk of HIV transmission to a negative partner by 96 percent. Since ART is not 100 percent effective at preventing HIV, consider using other prevention methods to further reduce your risk. Only condoms can help protect against some other STDs.

Other Ways to Reduce the Risk

People who engage in anal sex can make other behavioral choices to lower their risk of getting or transmitting HIV. These individuals can:

- choose less risky behaviors like oral sex, which has little to no risk of transmission

- get tested and treated for other STDs

Vaginal Sex and HIV Risk

Vaginal sex (intercourse) involves inserting the penis into the vagina. HIV can be transmitted during this activity if either partner is living with HIV. You can lower your risk for getting and transmitting HIV by using condoms correctly and consistently; taking daily medicine to prevent HIV, called PrEP; and taking medicines to treat HIV if living with HIV, called ART. Using more than one of these options at the same time provides even greater protection.

Risk of HIV

Some sexual activities are riskier than others for getting or transmitting HIV. For an HIV-negative person, the riskiest activity for getting HIV is being the receptive partner ("bottom") in anal sex. Being the insertive partner ("top") in anal sex or having vaginal sex (insertive or receptive) is less risky, though either partner can get HIV through those activities as well. Activities like oral sex, touching, and kissing carry little to no risk for getting or transmitting HIV.

A woman can get HIV during vaginal sex because the lining of the vagina and cervix may allow HIV to enter her body if her male partner's body fluids carry HIV, including blood, semen (cum), and preseminal fluid (precum). Using condoms or medicines to protect against transmission can decrease this risk.

Men can also get HIV from having vaginal sex with a woman who's HIV-positive because vaginal fluid and blood can carry HIV. Men can get HIV through the opening at the tip of the penis (or urethra); the foreskin if they're not circumcised; or small cuts, scratches, or open sores anywhere on the penis. Using condoms or medicines to protect against transmission can decrease this risk.

Risk of Other Infections

In addition to HIV, a person can get other STDs like chlamydia and gonorrhea from vaginal sex if condoms are not used correctly. Even if a condom is used, some STDs can still be transmitted through skin-to-skin contact (like syphilis or herpes). Hepatitis A and B can also be transmitted through vaginal sex. Getting tested and treated for STDs reduces a person's chances of getting or transmitting HIV through vaginal sex. If one has never had hepatitis A or B, there are vaccines to prevent them. A healthcare provider can make recommendations about vaccines.

Reducing the Risk

Condoms and Lubrication

Latex or polyurethane male condoms are highly effective in preventing HIV and certain other STDs when used correctly from start to finish for each act of vaginal sex. People who report using condoms consistently reduced their risk of getting HIV through vaginal sex, on average, by 80 percent. Condoms are much less effective when not used consistently. It is also important that sufficient water- or silicone-based lubricant be used during vaginal sex to prevent condom breakage and tearing of tissue. Female nitrile condoms can also prevent HIV and some other STDs. Since condoms are not 100 percent effective, consider using other prevention methods to further reduce your risk.

PrEP

People who are HIV-negative and at very high risk for HIV can take daily medicine to prevent HIV. PrEP, if taken consistently, can reduce the risk of getting HIV from sex by more than 90 percent. PrEP is much less effective when it is not taken consistently. Since PrEP is not 100 percent effective at preventing HIV, consider using other prevention methods to further reduce your risk. Only condoms can help protect against other STDs.

PEP

PEP means taking antiretroviral medicines—medicines used to treat HIV—after being potentially exposed to HIV during sex to prevent becoming infected. PEP should be used only in emergency situations and must be started within 72 hours after a possible exposure to HIV, but the sooner the better. PEP must be taken once or twice daily for 28 days. When administered correctly, PEP is effective in preventing HIV, but not 100 percent. To obtain PEP, contact your healthcare provider, your local or state health department, or go to an emergency room.

ART

For those living with HIV, ART can reduce the amount of virus in the blood and body fluids to very low levels, if taken the right way, every day. When taken consistently, ART can reduce the risk of HIV transmission to a negative partner by 96 percent. Since ART is not 100 percent effective at preventing HIV, consider using other prevention methods to further reduce your risk. Only condoms can help protect against some other STDs.

Other Ways to Reduce the Risk

People who engage in vaginal sex can make other behavioral choices to lower their risk of getting or transmitting HIV. These individuals can:

- choose less risky behaviors like oral sex, which has little to no risk of transmission

- get tested and treated for other STDs

Section 9.4

Sexually Transmitted Diseases and HIV Risk

This section includes content from "HIV and
Opportunistic Infections, Coinfections, and Conditions,"
AIDS*info*, U.S. Department of Health and Human
Services (HHS), September 27, 2017.

What Is Sexually Transmitted Disease (STD)?

STD stands for sexually transmitted disease. Sometimes STDs are
called sexually transmitted infections (STIs). STDs are infections that
spread from person to person through sexual contact, including anal,
vaginal, or oral sex. STDs are caused by bacteria, parasites, yeasts, and
viruses. Human immunodeficiency virus (HIV) is an STD. Chlamydia,
gonorrhea, human papillomavirus (HPV) infection, and syphilis are
examples of other STDs.

What Is the Connection between Human Immunodeficiency Virus (HIV) and Other STDs?

Behaviors that put people at risk for HIV also increase their risk
for infection with other STDs. These risky behaviors include the
following:

- having anal, vaginal, or oral sex without a condom

- having sex with many partners

- having sex while using drugs or alcohol. Using drugs and alcohol
  affects the brain, which can lead to poor decisions and risky
  behaviors.

Having an STD can make it easier to get HIV. For example, an
STD can cause a sore or break in the skin, which can make it easier
for HIV to enter the body. Having HIV and another STD may increase
the risk of HIV transmission.

How Can I Reduce My Risk of Getting an STD?

Sexual abstinence (never having sex) is the only way to eliminate
any chance of getting an STD. But if you are sexually active, you can
take the following steps to lower your risk for STDs, including HIV.

Avoid risky behaviors.

- Reduce the number of people you have sex with
- Don't drink alcohol or use drugs before and during sex
- Use condoms every time you have vaginal, anal, or oral sex
- Use latex or polyurethane condoms.

I Have HIV. How Can I Prevent Passing HIV to My Partner?

To protect your partner from HIV, avoid risky behaviors and use condoms. In addition, take HIV medicines daily. Treatment with HIV medicines (called antiretroviral therapy or ART) helps people with HIV live longer, healthier lives. ART can't cure HIV infection, but it can reduce the amount of HIV in the body. Having less HIV in your body will reduce your risk of passing HIV to your partner during sex.

Also, talk to your partner about taking preexposure prophylaxis or PrEP. PrEP is an HIV prevention option for people who don't have HIV but who are at high risk of becoming infected with HIV. PrEP involves taking one pill (an HIV medicine called Truvada) daily to prevent HIV infection.

What Are the Symptoms of STDs?

Symptoms of STDs may be different depending on the STD, and men and women with the same STD can have different symptoms. Examples of possible STD symptoms include painful urination (peeing), unusual discharge from the vagina or penis, and fever.

Some STDs may not cause any symptoms. Even if a person has no symptoms from an STD, it is still possible to pass the STD on to other people. Talk to your healthcare provider about getting tested for STDs and ask your sex partner to do the same. Sexually active individuals with HIV should get tested for STDs at least once every year, and more often depending on individual risk factors or symptoms.

To find STD information and testing sites near you, call CDC INFO at 800-232-4636 or visit CDC's GetTested webpage (gettested.cdc.gov).

What Is the Treatment for STDs?

STDs caused by bacteria, yeast, or parasites can be treated with antibiotics. There's no cure for STDs caused by viruses, but treatment can relieve symptoms and help keep the STD under control. For example, although there's no cure for HIV, ART can prevent HIV from advancing to acquired immunodeficiency syndrome (AIDS).

Untreated STDs may lead to serious complications. For example, untreated gonorrhea in women can cause problems with pregnancy and infertility. Untreated HIV will eventually advance to AIDS and cause death.

Chapter 10

HIV Risk in the Healthcare Setting

Chapter Contents

Section 10.1

Occupational Exposure

This section contains text excerpted from "Occupational HIV Transmission and Prevention among healthcare Workers," Centers for Disease Control and Prevention (CDC), November 7, 2016.

Only 58 cases of confirmed occupational transmission of human immunodeficiency virus (HIV) to healthcare workers have occurred in the United States. The proper use of gloves and goggles, along with safety devices to prevent injuries from sharp medical devices, can help minimize the risk of exposure to HIV in the course of caring for patients with HIV. When workers are exposed, the Centers for Disease Control and Prevention (CDC) recommends immediate treatment with a short course of antiretroviral drugs to prevent infection.

The Numbers

As of December 31, 2013, 58 confirmed occupational transmissions of HIV and 150 possible transmissions had been reported in the United States. Of these, only one confirmed case has been reported since 1999. Underreporting of cases to CDC is possible, however, because case reporting is voluntary.

Healthcare workers who are exposed to a needlestick involving HIV-infected blood at work have a 0.23 percent risk of becoming infected. In other words, 2.3 of every 1,000 such injuries, if untreated, will result in infection. Risk of exposure due to splashes with body fluids is thought to be near zero even if the fluids are overtly bloody. Fluid splashes to intact skin or mucous membranes are considered to be extremely low risk of HIV transmission, whether or not blood is involved.

Prevention Strategies

To prevent transmission of HIV to healthcare workers in the workplace, healthcare workers must assume that blood and other body fluids from all patients are potentially infectious. They should, therefore, follow these infection control precautions at all times:

- Routinely use barriers (such as gloves and/or goggles) when anticipating contact with blood or body fluid.

- Immediately wash hands and other skin surfaces after contact with blood or body fluids.

- Carefully handle and dispose of sharp instruments during and after use.

Safety devices have been developed to help prevent needlestick injuries. If used properly, these types of devices may reduce the risk of exposure to HIV. Many percutaneous injuries, such as needlesticks and cuts, are related to the disposal of sharp-ended medical devices.

All used syringes or other sharp instruments should be routinely placed in "sharps" containers for proper disposal to prevent accidental injuries and risk of HIV transmission.

Although the most important strategy for reducing the risk of occupational HIV transmission is to prevent occupational exposures, plans for postexposure management of healthcare personnel should be in place. CDC issued updated guidelines in 2013 for the management of healthcare worker exposures to HIV and recommendations for postexposure prophylaxis (PEP): *Updated U.S. Public Health Service Guidelines for the Management of Occupational Exposures to HIV and Recommendations for Postexposure Prophylaxis.*

Occupational exposure is considered an urgent medical concern and should be managed immediately after possible exposure—the sooner the better; every hour counts. The CDC guidelines outline considerations in determining whether healthcare workers should receive PEP (antiretroviral medication taken after possible exposure to reduce the chance of infection with HIV) and in choosing the type of PEP regimen. For most HIV exposures that warrant PEP, a basic 4-week, two-drug regimen is recommended, starting as soon as possible after exposure (within 72 hours). For HIV exposures that pose an increased risk of transmission (based on the infection status of the source and the type of exposure), a three-drug regimen may be recommended. Special circumstances, such as a delayed exposure report, unknown source person, pregnancy in the exposed person, resistance of the source virus to antiretroviral agents, and toxicity of PEP regimens, are also discussed in the guidelines.

Building Better Prevention Programs for Healthcare Workers

Continued diligence in the following areas is needed to help reduce the risk of occupational HIV transmission to healthcare workers:

- **Administrative efforts.** All healthcare organizations should train healthcare workers in infection control procedures and the importance of reporting occupational exposures immediately after they occur. Organizations should develop and distribute written policies for the management of occupational exposures.

- **Development and promotion of safety devices.** Effective and competitively priced devices engineered to prevent sharps injuries should continue to be developed for healthcare workers who frequently come into contact with potentially HIV-infected blood. Proper and consistent use of such safety devices should be continuously evaluated.

- **Monitoring the effects of PEP.** Data on the safety and acceptability of different regimens of PEP, particularly regimens that include new antiretroviral agents, should be monitored and evaluated continuously. Furthermore, health professionals who administer PEP must communicate possible side effects before treatment starts and follow patients closely to make sure they take their medicine correctly.

Section 10.2

Blood Transfusion

This section contains text excerpted from the following sources: Text begins with excerpts from "Blood Transfusion," National Heart, Lung, and Blood Institute (NHLBI), February 3, 2015; Text under the heading "Blood Transfusion and Human Immunodeficiency Virus (HIV)" is excerpted from "Frequently Asked Questions," U.S. Department of Veterans Affairs (VA), January 11, 2017; Text under the heading "Blood Transfusions Safety" is excerpted from "Keeping Blood Transfusions Safe: FDA's Multi-layered Protections for Donated Blood," U.S. Food and Drug Administration (FDA), March 27, 2018.

A blood transfusion is a safe, common procedure in which blood is given to you through an intravenous (IV) line in one of your blood vessels. Blood transfusions are done to replace blood lost during surgery or due to a serious injury. A transfusion also may be done if your body can't make blood properly because of an illness.

During a blood transfusion, a small needle is used to insert an IV line into one of your blood vessels. Through this line, you receive healthy blood. The procedure usually takes 1 to 4 hours, depending on how much blood you need.

Blood transfusions are very common. Each year, almost 5 million Americans need a blood transfusion. Most blood transfusions go well. Mild complications can occur. Very rarely, serious problems develop.

Blood Transfusion and Human Immunodeficiency Virus (HIV)

Can You Get HIV or Hepatitis C from Blood Received from Another Person?

Blood. All blood donated in the United States undergoes a many-layered process to reduce the risk of passing an infection from the donor to the recipient. That includes interviewing and examining the donor to find out about any risk factors for or symptoms of infectious disease, and then, according to the American Red Cross (ARC), performing laboratory tests on blood samples for viruses and other infectious agents, including tests for:

- Syphilis

- HIV-1 and HIV-2

- Hepatitis B

- Hepatitis C

- West Nile virus

Testing for HIV and hepatitis C is actually done multiple times: once to look for antibodies to these viruses, again to look for nucleic acid (deoxyribonucleic acid (DNA) or ribonucleic acid (RNA)), the virus's genetic material, and once more to look for an HIV antigen. That is because each of these infections is associated with what is known as a "window period"—a short period of time when a recently infected person might test negative for antibodies to these viruses. Using both types of tests improves the chances of finding infection during this early period, although, very rarely, an infectious agent still goes undetected. As of present, the risk of becoming infected with HIV or hepatitis C is about 1 in 2 million for each unit of donated blood. This is extremely low.

Blood Transfusion Safety

Keeping the United States blood supply the world's safest is the ultimate responsibility of the nation's blood establishments that collect and process the units of whole blood donated by volunteers each year. The U.S. Food and Drug Administration (FDA), however, has the vital role of ensuring that patients who receive a blood transfusion are protected by multiple overlapping safeguards. This FDA blood-safety system includes measures in the following areas:

- Donor screening

- Blood testing

- Donor deferral lists

- Quarantine

- Problems and deficiencies

Donor screening. Donor screening plays an important role in ensuring the safety of the U.S. blood supply. The FDA regulations require that a donor be free from any disease transmissible by blood transfusion, in so far as can be determined by health history and examination.

Donors are informed about potential risks and are required to answer questions about factors that may have a bearing on the safety of their blood. For example, donors with a history of intravenous drug abuse are routinely deferred.

In addition to federal regulations, FDA periodically issues guidance documents providing recommendations to decrease the potential for transmission of infectious diseases when information or testing methodologies becomes available. For example, since November 1999, the FDA has recommended that the blood industry defer potential donors who have lived in the United Kingdom and other European countries to reduce the risk of variant Creutzfeldt-Jakob disease (vCJD), the human form of "mad cow disease."

Blood testing. The FDA reviews and approves all test kits used to detect infectious diseases in donated blood. After donation, each unit of donated blood is required to undergo a series of tests for infectious diseases, including:

- Hepatitis B and C viruses

- HIV, types 1 and 2

- Human T-Lymphotropic virus, types I and II

- *Treponema pallidum* (syphilis)

Additionally, FDA recommends testing for the following infectious diseases:

- West Nile virus

- *Trypanosoma cruzi* (Chagas disease)

Donor deferral lists. Blood establishments must keep current a list of deferred donors and use it to make sure that they do not collect blood from anyone on the list.

Quarantine. Donated blood must be quarantined until it is tested and shown to be free of infectious agents.

Problems and deficiencies. Blood centers must investigate manufacturing problems, correct all deficiencies, and notify the FDA when product deviations occur in distributed products.

If anyone of these safeguards is breached, the blood component is considered unsuitable for transfusion and is subject to recall.

Section 10.3

Organ Transplantation

This section contains text excerpted from the following sources: Text begins with excerpts from "Frequently Asked Questions about HIV," U.S. Department of Veterans Affairs (VA), February 9, 2018; Text beginning with the heading "Risk Associated with Specific Exposures" is excerpted from "Understanding the Risk of Transmission of HIV, Hepatitis B, and Hepatitis C from U.S. PHS Increased Risk Donors," Organ Procurement and Transplantation Network (OPTN), Health Resources and Services Administration (HRSA), June 2017.

Four people were infected with HIV and hepatitis C in 2007 after receiving organs from a person who turned out to be infected with both viruses. The cases raised concerns in the public's mind about these medical procedures, but are an unfortunate but extremely rare occurrence.

Organs. Blood from potential tissue or organ donors is also tested for antibodies to HIV and hepatitis C before decisions about whether to transplant tissue or organs into waiting recipients are made. People who know a potential donor are also asked to furnish information about the donor's medical history. Transplanting organs from HIV-positive donors is prohibited. Organs from donors with hepatitis C may be transplanted in certain situations, such as those in which the recipient also has hepatitis C.

The antibody tests are quite good at detecting most cases of HIV and hepatitis C infection in the donors, but there is a small risk that an infection might go undetected during the window period. Unfortunately, although antibody testing can be done very rapidly, performing a follow-up nucleic acid test is sometimes not possible because it takes longer to obtain results, during which time the available donor organ might deteriorate too much, the patient needing the transplant might die of disease complications or both.

From 1985 through 2009, it appears that 8 organ or tissue recipients have infected with HIV from HIV antibody-negative donors. However, given that more than 400,000 organs have been transplanted in the past 20 years, the risk of infection remains low.

Risk Associated with Specific Exposures

A potential donor may be labeled as increased risk for a variety of different exposures, and these exposures carry very different risks of transmitting recent infection with HIV, HBV, or HCV. For example, a potential donor who was in a county jail 10 months ago for a period of 3 days would be at much lower risk of acquiring HCV or HIV in the preceding week as compared to a potential donor whose cause of death was opioid overdose from IVDU. Table 3 below is based on modeling data and describes the estimated risk of window period infection (both as risk per 10,000 donors and as a percentage). The table is designed to estimate the average risk irrespective of when the test was completed (remote infection should result in a positive antibody test). The ELISAs refer to the number of donors in the serological window period based on serology (antibody) testing only; the NAT refers to the number of donors with negative NAT who are in the NAT window period. NAT reduces the risk of serological window period infection by about 10-fold for most exposures.

Even with NAT, there is still some risk of transmission. However, not all donors with the PHS characteristics carry the same risk of window period infection. For example, donors with recent IVDU with negative serological testing still have a risk of undetected HCV of 300.6 per 10,000 donors (3%). Having both negative serology and negative NAT reduces this risk to 32.4 out of 10,000 donors (0.3%). In contrast, donors with a history of incarceration within the previous 12 months and negative NAT and serology testing would have only a 0.8 per 10,000 donors (0.008%) risk of infection with transmissible HCV.

Even with the increased sensitivity offered by NAT, this testing may not, for example, detect an HCV exposure that occurred several days prior to testing. Accordingly, a donor that died with an immediate needle exposure has a risk significantly higher than NAT may reflect, possibly as high as 3% for HCV, although lower for HBV and HIV.

Disclosure of the donor's risk behavior is currently up for debate. Even without disclosing the specific behavior of the donor that results in the increased risk designation, the actual comparative risk associated with that behavior should be communicated by the transplant team when informing a transplant candidate about the various risks associated with accepting an offered organ to optimize recipient's informed consent. Risk can also be explained to patients relating to everyday concepts, as well as by using resources available.

Consequences of Transmission of HIV, Hepatitis B, and Hepatitis C

As treatments for HIV, HBV, and particularly HCV, have improved, the medical consequences of donor derived infection have lessened. Solid organ transplantation of organs from donors who have screened negative for HIV into selected recipients living with HIV infection prior to transplant has become standard.

Overall graft and recipient survival in HIV mono-infected recipients is similar to HIV negative recipients. Current treatments for HCV have demonstrated high cure rates in the posttransplant setting in those infected with HCV pretransplant. HBV, if chronic infection develops, can be successfully suppressed. Nonetheless, the psychological consequence of donor-derived infection, particularly HIV, may have significant impact on recipient quality of life. Finally, if appropriate monitoring is not conducted after transplantation and donor-derived infection is not recognized early, significant clinical consequences may occur and treatment of the infection may be less efficacious.

Risk of Declining the Organ from a Donor with the PHS Characteristics for Increased Risk of HIV, HCV or HBV Infection and Remaining on the Waiting List

In communicating the risk of donor-derived infection from any donor, including those associated with donors bearing the behavioral risk factors identified by the PHS, it is important to consider the risks to the potential recipient of not accepting that organ and continuing to wait for another offer.

This risk-benefit calculation should be individualized, based on organ type, underlying disease, and patient factors, such as blood type and immunologic profile. Local organ wait times also vary. For example, the Scientific Registry for Transplant Recipients (SRTR) reported that waiting list mortality rates varied by DSA from approximately two to eight deaths occurring per year for every 100 candidates on the kidney transplant waitlist in 2015.

The Johns Hopkins Increased Risk Donor Tool uses model-based predictions to calculate risks based on particular recipient characteristics.

In one analysis of candidates on the kidney waiting list, accepting or declining an increased risk donor organ resulted in five year survival differences that varied from 6.4% to +67.3% depending on specific recipient characteristics.

The risks of continuing to wait are likely even greater for liver or heart candidates. Given the recent availability of highly effective HCV treatments, older estimates may overestimate mortality associated with HCV transmission.

Pediatric Organ Transplant Considerations

There may be unique considerations when evaluating an increased risk pediatric donor. The benefits of accepting an increased risk donor organ should be weighed against pediatric-specific organ, and disease mortality and morbidity data, where possible. Though in smaller numbers as compared to adult deceased donors, OPTN data does note an increase in pediatric deceased donors that met increase risk guidelines during the period of 2005–2016.

During the same period, there was an increase in transplants performed on pediatric recipients using organs from increased risk deceased donors, up from 4.5% to 10.6%. There have been no reported transmissions involving HIV, HBV, or HCV from pediatric organ donors. Furthermore, no cases of donor-derived HIV or HCV have been identified in pediatric recipients. Having said this, less is known about treatment options, particularly for HCV infected pediatric transplant recipients, should infection occur.

Chapter 11

HIV/AIDS Risks and Prevention Strategies

An estimated 37,600 human immunodeficiency virus (HIV) infections are diagnosed each year, according to the Centers for Disease Control and Prevention (CDC) data. The federal approach to reducing further additions in HIV infections is based on the best available scientific evidence and modeling studies have informed decisions about the allocation of resources with regard to the strategies employed, geography, and the populations at greatest risk. In short, these data have indicated that the best ways to prevent addition of HIV infections are to ensure timely diagnosis and engagement in care and treatment for those who are living with HIV to increase the percentage of persons with HIV who have achieved viral suppression; target prevention resources to the places with the largest burden of disease and populations at greatest risk; and ensure that the most effective prevention strategies are prioritized and widely implemented.

Activities of the federal government also include research to evaluate updated prevention methods such as vaccines, microbicides, and long-acting formulations of preexposure prophylaxis or PrEP and to improve the efficient and effective delivery of HIV prevention, care, and treatment. In addition, the federal government supports a range of services that are essential for reducing risk behavior and making

---

This chapter includes text excerpted from "Reducing New HIV Infections," HIV.gov, U.S. Department of Health and Human Services (HHS), May 20, 2017.

it possible for people living with HIV to be maintained in HIV medical care and treatment. These include substance abuse treatment and other behavioral health services, housing assistance, transportation, and other services shown to address risks associated with HIV transmission or interfere with the ability of people living with HIV to achieve viral suppression. This evidence-based approach is reflected in the updated National HIV/acquired immunodeficiency syndrome (AIDS) strategy that incorporates the updated scientific evidence. The first goal of the strategy is to reduce further HIV infections. Across the federal government, agencies are engaged in a wide variety of efforts to prevent HIV acquisition and transmission. Results show that further addition in HIV infections have declined overall, in most subgroups, and in all states for which data are available. Exceptions are some subgroups of men who have sex with men.

Human Immunodeficiency Virus (HIV) Does Not Impact All Americans Equally

While anyone can become infected with or, if they are living with HIV and have not achieved viral suppression, transmit HIV, the epidemic in the United States is concentrated in certain key populations and geographic areas:

- Gay, bisexual, and other men who have sex with men of all races and ethnicities (with a particularly high burden of HIV among African American/Black gay and bisexual men)
- African American/Black women and men
- Latino men and women
- People who inject drugs
- Youth aged 13–24 years (with a particularly high burden of HIV among young African American/Black gay and bisexual men)
- People in the southern United States
- Transgender women (with a particularly high burden of HIV among African American/Black transgender women)

HIV Prevention Toolbox

There are now more options than ever before to reduce the risk of acquiring or transmitting HIV and the updated methods are even more effective than those that were available earlier. These include personal actions that people can take to protect themselves like abstinence, having only one partner with the same HIV status, and choosing less risky behaviors, as well as risk reduction tools, services, and interventions that are delivered by healthcare providers, public health departments, community-based organizations and others. As of now available tools that have been shown to significantly reduce the risk of HIV transmission or acquisition include:

- HIV testing (to detect undiagnosed infection)
- HIV medications to prevention transmission
- Treatment as prevention
- Prevention of mother-to-child transmission
- Preexposure prophylaxis (PrEP)
- Postexposure prophylaxis (PEP)
- Interventions to improve access to prevention tools:
  - Syringe services programs
  - Laws allowing sterile syringe purchase
  - Condom distribution programs
  - Drug treatment (including medication-assisted therapy)
  - Sexually transmitted diseases (STDs) diagnosis and treatment
  - Medical male circumcision

Mass media campaigns, behavioral interventions, medication reminders, and other strategies have been shown to effectively encourage people to adopt and maintain risk reduction strategies including condom use, adherence to HIV treatment, and sterile injection practices. Education, training, and capacity building for healthcare providers are also important activities that can improve the ability of healthcare providers and systems and community-based organizations and their staff to provide high-quality HIV prevention, care, and treatment services efficiency and effectively.

For example, final results from research funded by the National Institutes of Health (NIH) that were released in 2016 provided the most compelling evidence to date that early HIV treatment reduces HIV transmission by 93 percent among heterosexual couples. Other studies have reported similar findings in diverse populations that included gay and bisexual men. Most importantly, none of these studies has found a case where HIV was transmitted sexually by someone with a suppressed viral load. These research findings, coupled with the results of earlier studies showing that starting HIV treatment as early as possible is good for the health of people living with HIV and modeling studies that have been done to predict the impact that various interventions can have on HIV transmission, make "treatment as prevention" the top priority of the federal response to HIV in the United States.

Given this priority, a wide range of federally funded programs conducted by the CDC, Health Resources and Services Administration (HRSA), Substance Abuse and Mental Health Services Administration (SAMHSA), U.S. Department of Veterans Affairs (VA), Medicaid, Medicare, the Indian Health Service (IHS), the Bureau of Prisons (BOP), and others provide HIV testing, linkage to HIV care, retention in care, and adherence to care. Federally-funded programs also support the provision of HIV care and treatment through HRSA's Ryan White Care Act Program that provides services to about half of all living people who have been diagnosed with HIV. Other federally-funded efforts provide HIV medical care in health centers, support the training of healthcare providers and other allied health professional, and provide behavioral health, housing, transportation, employment, legal assistance, and other services that make it possible for people living with HIV to achieve the outcomes in HIV care that are necessary to prevent emergency room visits, hospitalizations, illness, disability, and death as well as the onward transmission of HIV.

The NIH-funded research has also proven the important role that HIV medications can play when taken by someone who does not have the virus to prevent infection. Multiple studies have shown that taking PrEP, a daily antiretroviral pill, is more than 90 percent effective in preventing HIV acquisition if it is used as prescribed. It can also reduce infection by 70 percent or more among people who inject drugs. Multiple program across the federal government provide education about PrEP to healthcare providers and community members and provide laboratory testing, medications, and other services that improve access to PrEP. A comprehensive framework to improve access to PrEP (HIV-PrEP Framework) serves as a blueprint for federal activities to scale up PrEP as a strategy to prevent HIV transmission and reduce further additions in number of cases of infections in the United States.

Research has also shown other methods that can effectively reduce HIV risk and in many cases are cost saving, including access to condoms and sterile syringes, substance abuse treatment, screening and treatment for other sexually transmitted infections, as well as choosing less risky sexual behaviors and limiting one's number of sexual partners.

HIV Testing: A Key Prevention Strategy

Widespread HIV testing, timely diagnosis, and linkage to treatment and care remain critical to federal HIV prevention efforts and to federal efforts to improve the health of people living with HIV. HIV testing is the only way to identify the nearly one in seven Americans currently living with HIV in 2014 who did not know they had HIV. Not knowing that they had the virus placed these women and men at risk for serious health problems and premature death, and for unknowingly transmitting the virus to others. Developments in HIV testing technologies have enhanced the ability to diagnose HIV sooner after infection and have broadened the window of opportunity for effective interventions during the acute phase of infection—a time immediately after infection when HIV viral load is high and increases the risk of HIV transmission to others. Early diagnosis and linkage to treatment with antiretroviral therapy (ART) also substantially improves health outcomes for people living with HIV, making it possible for someone in their 20s who is diagnosed and begins HIV treatment soon after infection to live practically as long as a peer who does not have HIV. HIV treatment is also a powerful and highly effective prevention tool that significantly reduces the risk of onward HIV transmission.

National Priority: Reduce Further Addition of HIV Infections

Scientific advances in HIV prevention have fundamentally changed our ability to prevent further additions of cases of infections and the approaches that are needed to make this happen. These led to the National HIV/Acquired Immunodeficiency Syndrome (AIDS) Strategy: Updated to 2020 that is based on this evidence and calls for intensified prevention efforts in communities where HIV is most heavily concentrated; expanded efforts to prevent HIV infection using a combination of effective, evidence-based approaches; and sustained efforts to educate all Americans about HIV risks, prevention, and transmission. Research on the effects of HIV medical care, treatment, and the effects of housing, food instability, and other factors on the ability of people to stay in care and take HIV medications as prescribed were also addressed in the updated Strategy. The updated Strategy also calls for steps to ensure timely linkage to and retention in medical care and social services that can both maximize the benefits of early treatment for people living with HIV and prevent transmission of fresh cases of infections.

Additional efforts focus on continuing to improve the response to HIV among racial and ethnic minority groups that have been hit hardest by HIV. The Minority AIDS Initiative (MAI) serves as an important resource to improve U.S. Department of Health and Human Services (HHS) agencies and offices' ability to improve HIV-related outcomes and reduce HIV-related disparities among racial and ethnic minority communities. Established by Congress in 1999, the legislation allocates MAI resources to the CDC, Health Resources and Services Administration (HRSA), SAMHSA and the HHS Secretary's Minority AIDS Initiative Fund (SMAIF). Resources awarded to the HHS agencies support the delivery of services that are designed to complement, not duplicate, those supported by other funding. Two of areas of special emphasis of the MAI are building capacity of community-based organizations and improving the quality of care. The SMAIF plays a unique role in improving the quality of prevention and care for racial and ethnic minorities. SMAIF supports cross-agency demonstrations and agency-administered projects that serve as laboratories of innovation, testing out updated approaches before innovations are introduced more broadly across prevention, testing, or care systems. The work includes evaluating how efficiency and quality of services can be improved to better serve people who need HIV services. The SMAIF-supported demonstration projects help health departments implement PrEP for gay and bisexual men of color and help health centers expand HIV testing. The successes generated from SMAIF activities create lasting changes across the federal HIV prevention and care portfolio, improving efficiency, further reducing HIV infection, and saving lives and healthcare dollars.

Across the federal government, agencies are developing, planning, and implementing these and other HIV prevention programs targeted to populations at risk; disseminating educational resources and messages on HIV risks and prevention; educating healthcare professionals about evidence-based HIV prevention strategies; conducting research to develop, test, and improve cutting-edge tools and techniques that can prevent HIV in diverse populations around the world; and numerous other activities to achieve the vision of a future free of increase in HIV infections.

Chapter 12

HIV/AIDS Prevention

Chapter Contents

Section 12.1

Safer Sex

This section includes text excerpted from "Stop STIs: Six Steps to Safer Sex," National Women's Health Information Center (NWHIC), Office on Women's Health (OWH), April 12, 2015.

Stop Sexually Transmitted Infections (STIs): Six Steps to Safer Sex

Whether you call them sexually transmitted infections (STIs) or sexually transmitted diseases (STDs), one thing is true: Women are at risk of infection. Not only does a woman's anatomy make her vulnerable to STIs, women are less likely to have symptoms than men. Untreated STIs can lead to serious health issues, including infertility, cancer, and even death. It's not fun to think about, but protecting yourself from STIs like genital herpes, genital warts, chlamydia, syphilis, gonorrhea, and human immunodeficiency virus (HIV) is an important part of staying healthy.

Here are six ways to protect yourself from STIs:

1. **Get the facts.** About 20 million additions of STIs occur in the United States every year, affecting people of all ages and backgrounds. Many STIs are spread through intimate sexual contact, but you don't have to have vaginal or anal sex to be at risk—some common STIs are spread easily by oral sex and genital touching. And because many STIs have only mild symptoms or no symptoms at all, you can't tell by looking at someone whether or not they have an infection.

2. **Talk to your partner.** It's important to talk with your partner about STIs and practicing safe sex before you have sex. Get tips for talking with your partner, and set the ground rules together. Also, don't assume you're at low risk for STIs if you have sex with only one partner at a time. That person may be having sex with others. If you have been forced, pressured, or coerced into having sexual contact without protection, there are people who can help you. Everyone deserves to be in control of their own health, including their sexual health.

3. **Get tested.** It's important to know whether or not you have an infection—to make sure it's treated quickly and to avoid spreading it to others. If you are infected, you can take steps

to protect yourself and your partner(s). Many STIs can be easily diagnosed and treated, and under the Affordable Care Act (ACA), STI prevention, screening, and counseling services are fully covered by most insurance plans, at no cost to you. Talk to your healthcare provider at your annual well-woman visit about which STIs tests you might need. Having an STI can also increase your risk for getting HIV. The same behaviors and situations that put you at risk for STIs also put you at increased risk for getting HIV. Plus, some types of STIs may cause sores or breaks in your skin that make HIV transmission easier. If you test positive for an STI, you should also get tested for HIV.

4. **Practice monogamy.** This means being in a sexual relationship with only one partner who is also faithful to you. Make sure you've both been tested for STIs and know each other's results. Condoms should be used with any partner outside of a long-term, monogamous sexual relationship.

5. **Use condoms.** Use a condom correctly every time you have anal, vaginal, or oral sex to reduce the risk of STI transmission. Get tips for using male and female condoms correctly.

6. **Get vaccinated.** Safe and effective vaccines are available to help prevent the spread of the human papillomavirus (HPV). While it's recommended for kids who are 11 or 12, young women can receive the series of shots through the age of 26. HPV vaccines can help protect you from the types of HPV that cause most cervical cancers. Vaccines for HPV are covered as preventive services under the ACA, which means most insurers must cover them at no cost to you. Learn about HPV, then talk to your doctor about whether the vaccines are right for you.

Thanks to the ACA, taking steps to protect yourself is easier than ever. Most insurers must cover STI screening, counseling, and HPV vaccination services at no cost to you, even if you haven't met your yearly deductible. If you think you may have been exposed to infection, get tested right away. The sooner you get a diagnosis, the sooner you can start treatment and reduce the risk of spreading it to others. Find a testing site near you. Remember, it's your body. By taking steps to protect yourself, you can lower your risk for STIs.

Section 12.2

Circumcision

This section contains text excerpted from the following sources: Text
in this section begins with excerpts from "What Care Do Newborns
Receive in the Hospital?" *Eunice Kennedy Shriver* National Institute
of Child Health and Human Development (NICHD), December 1,
2016; Text beginning with the heading "What We Know about Male
Circumcision" is excerpted from "Male Circumcision," Centers for
Disease Control and Prevention (CDC), December 7, 2015.

Some male infants will be circumcised shortly after birth. Circumcision is a surgical procedure that removes foreskin from the penis.
Foreskin is the fold of skin that covers the tip of the penis of an uncircumcised male.

According to the American Academy of Pediatrics (AAP), scientific
evidence shows some potential medical benefits of male circumcision.
Possible benefits include a lower risk of urinary tract infections (UTI),
penile cancer, and sexually transmitted diseases (STDs). On the other
hand, there is a possibility that the infant will experience pain, and
there is a low risk of bleeding or infection. The AAP states that the
health benefits of newborn male circumcision justify access to the
procedure for those families who choose it.

Parents and families should start thinking about circumcision
before the infant is born. To make an informed choice, parents of all
male infants should be given accurate information about the potential
risks and benefits of the procedure. They should also have an opportunity to discuss the decision with healthcare providers.

If the parents decide to have their son circumcised, the procedure
usually is performed in the first 48 hours after birth, before discharge
from the hospital. Some boys are circumcised in the first few days after
birth at home as part of religious or cultural traditions. Some form
of pain relief, such as a numbing cream, can be used to minimize the
discomfort of circumcision.

Preterm infants (born before 37 completed weeks of pregnancy) and
infants born with health problems should not be circumcised until their
condition is stable. Parents and caregivers should follow advice from
their infant's healthcare provider about how to care for the penis as
it heals from a circumcision. If a male infant is not circumcised, the
parent or caregiver can wash the penis with soap and water without
pulling back (retracting) the foreskin. A newborn's foreskin may not
retract completely. Over time it retracts on its own.

What We Know about Male Circumcision

When men are circumcised, they're less likely than uncircumcised men to get human immunodeficiency virus (HIV) from their HIV-positive female partners. There are biological reasons why, for some men, male circumcision may decrease the risk of getting HIV during vaginal sex with an HIV-positive female partner. Male circumcision also reduces the risk of a man getting herpes and human papillomavirus (HPV) from a woman who has those infections. However, there is no evidence that circumcision decreases the risk of HIV-negative receptive partners getting HIV from a circumcised HIV-positive partner.

The evidence about the benefits of circumcision among gay and bisexual men is inconclusive. More studies are underway.

What Can You Do?

Male circumcision is known to decrease the risk getting HIV only for HIV-negative circumcised men who have sex with HIV-positive women. Also, circumcised men and their partners can still get other sexually transmitted diseases. Take other actions, like using condoms the right way every time you have sex or taking medicine to prevent or treat HIV to further reduce your chances of getting HIV.

If you're a parent, talk to your healthcare provider about the potential risks and benefits of male circumcision to your newborn.

Section 12.3

Syringe Exchange Programs

This section includes text excerpted from "Syringe Services Programs," Centers for Disease Control and Prevention (CDC), February 27, 2018.

, Persons who inject drugs can substantially reduce their risk of getting and transmitting HIV, viral hepatitis, and other blood-borne infections by using a sterile needle and syringe for every injection.

In many jurisdictions, persons who inject drugs can access sterile needles and syringes through syringe services programs (SSPs) and through pharmacies without a prescription. Though less common, access to sterile needles and syringes may also be possible through a prescription written by a doctor and through other healthcare services.

SSPs, which have also been referred to as syringe exchange programs (SEPs), needle exchange programs (NEPs) and needle-syringe programs (NSPs) are community-based programs that provide access to sterile needles and syringes free of cost and facilitate safe disposal of used needles and syringes. As described in the Centers for Disease Control and Prevention (CDC) and U.S. Department of Health and Human Services (HHS) guidance, SSPs are an effective component of a comprehensive, integrated approach to HIV prevention among People who inject drugs (PWID). These programs have also been associated with reduced risk for infection with hepatitis C virus. Most SSPs offer other prevention materials (e.g., alcohol swabs, vials of sterile water, condoms) and services, such as education on safer injection practices and wound care; overdose prevention; referral to substance use disorder treatment programs including medication-assisted treatment (MAT); and counseling and testing for HIV and hepatitis C. Many SSPs also provide linkage to critical services and programs, such as HIV care, treatment, preexposure prophylaxis (PrEP), and postexposure prophylaxis (PEP) services; hepatitis C treatment, hepatitis A, and B vaccinations; screening for other sexually transmitted diseases and tuberculosis; partner services; prevention of mother-to-child HIV transmission; and other medical, social, and mental health services.

What Are Syringe Services Programs (SSPs)?

SSPs, which have also been referred to as SEPs, NEPs, and NSPs are community-based programs that provide, access to sterile needles and syringes free of cost, facilitate safe disposal of used needles and syringes, and offer safer injection education. Many SSPs also provide linkages to critical services and programs, including substance use disorder treatment programs; overdose prevention education; screening, care, and treatment for HIV and viral hepatitis; HIV PrEP and PEP; prevention of mother-to-child transmission; hepatitis A and hepatitis B vaccination; screening for other sexually transmitted diseases (STDs) and tuberculosis (TB); partner services; and other medical, social, and mental health services.

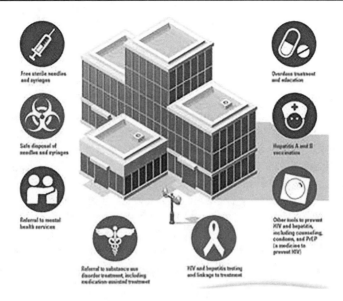

Figure 12.1. *What Is an SSP?* (Source: "HIV and Injection Drug Use: Syringe Services Programs for HIV Prevention," Centers for Disease Control and Prevention (CDC).)

What Are the Benefits of SSPs?

Based on existing evidence, the U.S. Surgeon General has determined that SSPs, when part of a comprehensive prevention strategy, can play a critical role in preventing HIV among PWID; can facilitate entry into drug treatment and medical services, and do not increase the unsafe illegal injection of drugs. These programs have also been associated with reduced risk for infection with hepatitis C virus.

Many SSPs offer other infection prevention materials (e.g., alcohol swabs, vials of sterile water), condoms, and services, such as education on safer injection practices and wound care; overdose prevention; referral to substance use disorder treatment programs including medication-assisted treatment (MAT); and counseling and testing for HIV and viral hepatitis. SSPs also provide linkages to other critical services and programs, including screening, care, and treatment for HIV and viral hepatitis, HIV PrEP and PEP, prevention of mother-to-child transmission, hepatitis A and hepatitis B vaccination, screening for other STDs and TB, partner services, and other medical, social, and mental health services. SSPs also protect the public and first responders by providing safe needle disposal and by reducing the number of people living with HIV and hepatitis C virus infections who could transmit those infections to others.

Do SSPs Increase Drug Use in a Community?

No. Based on existing evidence, the U.S. Surgeon General has determined that SSPs, when part of a comprehensive HIV prevention strategy, do not increase the illegal use of drugs by injection. The opportunity to expand HIV and viral hepatitis prevention services through SSPs will support communities in their efforts to identify and prevent further additions in number of infections. SSPs are an effective public health intervention that can reduce the transmission of HIV and facilitate entry into drug treatment and medical services, without increasing illegal injection of drugs. SSPs often provide other services important to improving the health of PWID, including referrals to substance use disorder and mental health services, physical healthcare, social services, overdose prevention, and recovery support services. Studies also show that SSPs protect the public and first responders by providing safe needle disposal.

Section 12.4

Harm Reduction to Lessen HIV Risks

This section includes text excerpted from "Harm Reduction to Lessen HIV Risks," Centers for Disease Control and Prevention (CDC), February 9, 2016.

Harm reduction strategies aim to lessen harms associated with drug use and related behaviors that increase the risk of human immunodeficiency virus (HIV) infection. Sharing needles and syringes raises the risk of blood-borne HIV transmission. Drug use is associated with risky sexual behaviors including unprotected sex and the exchange of sex for drugs or money, which are linked to an increased risk of HIV infection.

Harm reduction strategies can reduce behaviors resulting in elevated risk of HIV infection among injecting and noninjecting drug users. Research has shown that many people receiving treatment for substance use disorders stop or reduce their drug use and related behaviors, including unsafe sex.

Research also has shown that for people who inject drugs, medication-assisted treatment (MAT) can reduce risky behaviors, helping to prevent HIV infection. For example, findings from the National Institute of Allergy and Infectious Diseases (NIAID)-supported HIV Prevention Trials Network, 058 trial suggested that use of the MAT buprenorphine/naloxone reduces risks related to HIV transmission.

Needle exchange programs contribute to decreased needle sharing and more hygienic injection practices. Numerous studies have indicated that such programs effectively reduce the number of additions in HIV infections. For example, according to findings from an National Institutes of Health (NIH)-funded study published in late 2015, the average monthly rate of further additions in HIV infections among drug users in Washington, D.C., dropped by approximately 70 percent after the city implemented a needle exchange program in 2008.

However, preventing HIV transmission among people who use drugs remains an urgent public health issue. NIH is working to develop interventions that reduce the risk of drug use-associated and sexual transmission of HIV among injecting and noninjecting drug users. NIH also supports development of interventions designed to overcome structural and community-level barriers to accepting and implementing effective HIV prevention strategies.

Chapter 13

Preventing Mother-to-Child Transmission of HIV

Chapter Contents

Section 13.1

HIV Medicines during Pregnancy and Childbirth

This section includes content from "HIV Medicines during Pregnancy and Childbirth," AIDS*info*, U.S. Department of Health and Human Services (HHS), November 28, 2017.

Frequently Asked Questions

Should Women with Human Immunodeficiency Virus (HIV) Take HIV Medicines during Pregnancy?

Yes. All pregnant women with human immunodeficiency virus (HIV) should take HIV medicines during pregnancy to prevent mother-to-child transmission of HIV. HIV medicines work by preventing HIV from multiplying, which reduces the amount of HIV in the body (also called the viral load). A low viral load during pregnancy reduces the chances that any HIV will pass from mother to child during pregnancy and childbirth. Having less HIV in the body also helps keep the mother-to-be healthy.

Are HIV Medicines Safe to Use during Pregnancy?

Most HIV medicines are safe to use during pregnancy. In general, HIV medicines don't increase the risk of birth defects. When recommending HIV medicines for pregnant women with HIV, healthcare providers carefully consider the benefits and risks of specific HIV medicines.

When Should Pregnant Women with HIV Start Taking HIV Medicines?

All pregnant women with HIV should start taking HIV medicines as soon as possible during pregnancy. In general, women who are already taking HIV medicines when they become pregnant should continue taking those HIV medicines throughout their pregnancies.

What HIV Medicines Should a Pregnant Woman with HIV Take?

The choice of an HIV regimen to use during pregnancy depends on several factors, including a woman's current or past use of HIV medicines, other medical conditions she may have, and the results of drug resistance testing. In general, pregnant women with HIV can use the same HIV regimens recommended for nonpregnant adults—unless the risk of any known side effects to a pregnant woman or her baby outweighs the benefit of a regimen. Also, the regimen must be able to control a woman's HIV even with pregnancy-related changes that can affect how the body processes medicine.

In most cases, women who are already on an effective HIV regimen should continue on the same regimen throughout their pregnancies. But sometimes a woman's HIV regimen may change during pregnancy. For example, a change in HIV medicines may be needed to avoid the increased risk of a side effect during pregnancy. Sometimes, changing the dose of an HIV medicine can help offset pregnancy-related changes that make it harder for the body to absorb the medicine. But before making any changes to an HIV regimen, women should always talk to their healthcare providers.

Do Women with HIV Continue to Take HIV Medicines during Childbirth?

Yes. The risk of mother-to-child transmission of HIV is greatest during a vaginal delivery when a baby passes through the birth canal and is exposed to any HIV in the mother's blood and other fluids. During childbirth, HIV medicines that pass from mother to baby across the placenta prevent mother-to-child transmission of HIV, especially near delivery.

Women who are already taking HIV medicines when they go into labor should continue taking their HIV medicines on schedule as much as possible during childbirth.

Women with a high viral load (more than 1,000 copies/mL) or an unknown viral load near the time of delivery should receive an HIV medicine called zidovudine (brand name: Retrovir) by intravenous (IV) injection.

Zidovudine passes easily from a pregnant woman to her unborn baby across the placenta. Once in a baby's system, zidovudine protects the baby from any HIV that passes from mother to child during childbirth. For this reason, the use of zidovudine during childbirth prevents mother-to-child transmission of HIV even in women with high viral loads near the time of delivery.

Can a Cesarean Delivery Reduce the Risk of Mother-to-Child Transmission of HIV?

Yes. A scheduled cesarean delivery (sometimes called a C-section) can reduce the risk of mother-to-child transmission of HIV in

DELIVERY

| Women with HIV take HIV medicines during pregnancy and childbirth. Their babies are given HIV medicine for 4 to 6 weeks after birth. | Women with a high or unknown level of HIV in their blood may have a C-section to reduce the risk of HIV transmission during delivery. | HIV can spread through breast milk. Women with HIV give their babies formula instead of breastfeeding. |

For more information, visit: aidsinfo.nih.gov **AIDS**info

Figure 13.1. *Protecting Your Baby from HIV* (Source: "AIDS Info—HIV and Pregnancy," AIDS*info*, U.S. Department of Health and Human Services (HHS).)

women who have a high viral load (more than 1,000 copies/mL) or an unknown viral load near the time of delivery. A cesarean delivery to reduce the risk of mother-to-child transmission of HIV is scheduled for the 38th week of pregnancy, 2 weeks before a woman's expected due date.

It's unclear whether a scheduled C-section can reduce the risk of mother-to-child transmission of HIV in pregnant women with a viral load of less than 1,000 copies/mL. Of course, regardless of her viral load, a woman with HIV may have a C-section for other medical reasons.

With the help of their healthcare providers, women can decide which HIV medicines to use during childbirth and whether they should schedule a C-section to prevent mother-to-child transmission of HIV.

Do Women with HIV Continue to Take HIV Medicines after Childbirth?

Prenatal care for women with HIV includes counseling on the benefits of continuing HIV medicines after childbirth. Life-long use of HIV medicines prevents HIV from advancing to acquired immunodeficiency syndrome (AIDS) and reduces the risk of transmitting HIV. Together with their healthcare providers, women with HIV make decisions about continuing or changing their HIV medicines after childbirth.

In general, babies born to women with HIV receive zidovudine for 4–6 weeks after birth. (In certain situations, a baby may receive other HIV medicines in addition to zidovudine.) The HIV medicine protects the babies from infection by any HIV that may have passed from mother to child during childbirth.

Section 13.2

Preventing Mother-to-Child Transmission of HIV After Birth

This section includes content from "Preventing Mother-to-Child Transmission of HIV after Birth," AIDS*info*, U.S. Department of Health and Human Services (HHS), November 28, 2017.

Frequently Asked Questions

After Childbirth, Do Babies Born to Women with Human Immunodeficiency Virus (HIV) Receive HIV Medicines to Prevent Mother-to-Child Transmission of HIV?

Babies born to women with human immunodeficiency virus (HIV) receive an HIV medicine called zidovudine within 6–12 hours after birth. In certain situations, a baby may receive other HIV medicines in addition to zidovudine. The HIV medicine protects the babies from infection with any HIV that may have passed from mother to child during childbirth.

The use of HIV medicines and other strategies before and after childbirth have greatly reduced the rate of mother-to-child transmission of HIV. Fewer than 200 babies with HIV are born each year in the United States.

How Long Do Babies Born to Women with HIV Receive Zidovudine to Prevent Mother-to-Child Transmission of HIV?

In general, babies born to women with HIV receive zidovudine for 4- to 6-weeks after birth.

Once the 4- to 6-week course of zidovudine is finished, the babies receive a medicine called sulfamethoxazole/trimethoprim (brand name:

Bactrim). Bactrim helps prevent *Pneumocystis jirovecii* pneumonia (PCP), which is a type of pneumonia that can develop in people with HIV. If HIV testing shows that a baby is not infected with HIV, Bactrim is stopped.

How Soon after Birth Are Babies Born to Women with HIV Tested for HIV?

After birth, care for babies born to women with HIV includes HIV testing, usually at 14–21 days of life, at 1–2 months, and again at 4–6 months. The HIV test used (called a virologic test) looks for HIV in the blood.

Results from at least two HIV virologic tests are needed to know for certain whether a baby is HIV negative or HIV positive.

- To know for certain that a baby is HIV negative (not infected with HIV):

  - Results on two virologic tests must be negative. The first negative result must be from a test done when a baby is 1 month or older, and the second result must be from a test done when a baby is 4 months or older.

- To know for certain that a baby is HIV positive (infected with HIV):

  - Results on two virologic tests must be positive

If testing shows that a baby is HIV positive, the baby is switched from zidovudine to a combination of HIV medicines (called antiretroviral therapy or ART). ART helps people with HIV live longer, healthier lives.

How Can I Prevent Passing HIV to My Baby?*

If you have HIV, the most important thing you can do is to take medicines to treat HIV infection (called ART) the right way, every day.

If you're pregnant, talk to your healthcare provider about getting tested for HIV and other ways to keep you and your child from getting HIV. Women in their third trimester should be tested again if they engage in behaviors that put them at risk for HIV.

If you are HIV-negative but you have an HIV-positive partner and are considering getting pregnant, talk to your doctor about taking PrEP to help keep you from getting HIV. Encourage your partner to take medicines to treat HIV (ART), which greatly reduces the chance that he will transmit HIV to you.

If you have HIV, take medicines to treat HIV (ART) the right way, every day. If you are treated for HIV early in your pregnancy, your risk of transmitting HIV to your baby can be 1 percent or less. After delivery, you can prevent transmitting HIV to your baby by avoiding breastfeeding, since breast milk contains HIV.

*Source: "Prevention—HIV Basics," Centers for Disease Control and Prevention (CDC), February 27, 2018.

What Other Steps Protect Babies from HIV?

Because HIV can spread in breast milk, women with HIV who live in the United States should not breastfeed their babies. In the United States, infant formula is a safe and healthy alternative to breast milk.

There are reports of children becoming infected with HIV by eating food that was previously chewed by a person with HIV. To be safe, babies should not be fed prechewed food.

Chapter 14

HIV Vaccines and Microbicides

Chapter Contents

Section 14.1

Preventive Vaccines

This section includes text excerpted from documents
published by two public domain sources. Text under the headings
marked 1 are excerpted from "HIV and Immunizations," AIDS*info*,
U.S. Department of Health and Human Services (HHS), February 6,
2018; Text under the heading marked 2 is excerpted from
"Prevention—HIV Basics," Centers for Disease Control
and Prevention (CDC), February 27, 2018.

What Are Vaccines?[1]

Vaccines protect people from diseases such as chicken pox, influenza (flu), and polio. Vaccines are given by needle injection (a shot), by mouth, or sprayed into the nose. The process of getting a vaccine is called vaccination or immunization.

When a person gets a vaccine, the body responds by mounting an immune response against the particular disease. (An immune response includes all the actions of the immune system to defend the body against the disease.) In this way, the immune system learns to defend the body if the person is later exposed to the disease. Most vaccines are designed so that a person never gets a particular disease or only gets a mild case of the disease.

Vaccines not only protect individuals from disease, they protect communities as well. When most people in a community get immunized against a disease, there is little chance of a disease outbreak.

Can I Get Vaccinated to Prevent HIV?[2]

No. There is no vaccine available that will prevent HIV infection or treat those who have it.

Is There a Vaccine against Human Immunodeficiency Virus (HIV)?[1]

Testing is underway on experimental vaccines to prevent and treat human immunodeficiency virus (HIV), but no HIV vaccines are approved for use outside of clinical trials. Even though there are no vaccines to prevent or cure HIV, people with HIV can benefit from vaccines against other diseases.

Can HIV Infection Affect the Safety and Effectiveness of Vaccines?[1]

Yes. Damage to the immune system due to HIV can reduce the body's immune response to a vaccine. A weakened immune response makes a vaccine less effective. In people with HIV, vaccines generally work best when a person's cluster of differentiation 4 (CD4)count is above 200 copies/mm^3.

By stimulating the immune system, vaccines may also cause a person's HIV viral load to increase temporarily. Because HIV medicines strengthen the immune system and reduce HIV viral load, people with HIV may want to start antiretroviral therapy (ART) before getting vaccinated whenever possible. In some situations, however, immunizations should be given even if ART has not been started. For example, it's important for people with HIV to get vaccinated against the flu at the time of year when the risk of flu is greatest.

Are All Types of Vaccines Safe for People with HIV?[1]

The design of a vaccine depends on several factors, such as how a microbe infects the body and how the immune system responds. For this reason, there are several types of vaccines, including live, attenuated vaccines, and inactivated vaccines.

Live, Attenuated Vaccines

A live, attenuated vaccine contains a weakened but live form of a disease-causing microbe. Although the attenuated (weakened) microbe cannot cause the disease (or can cause only mild disease), the vaccine can still trigger an immune response. However, to be safe and avoid even the remote chance of getting a disease from a live, attenuated vaccine, people with HIV who have CD4 counts lower than 200 cells/mm^3 or certain symptoms of HIV should not get live, attenuated vaccines.

Inactivated Vaccines

Inactivated vaccines are made from microbes that have been killed with chemicals, heat, or radiation. There is no chance that an inactivated vaccine can cause the disease it was designed to prevent.

Do Vaccines Cause Side Effects?[1]

Side effects from vaccines are generally minor (for example, soreness at the location of an injection or a low-grade fever) and go away within a few days. Severe reactions to vaccines are rare. Before getting a vaccine, talk to your healthcare provider about the benefits and risks of the vaccine and possible side effects.

Which Vaccines Are Recommended for People with HIV?[1]

The following vaccines are recommended for people with HIV:

- Hepatitis B
- Human papillomavirus (HPV) (for those up to age 26)
- Influenza (flu)
- Meningococcal
- Pneumococcal (pneumonia)
- Tetanus, diphtheria, and pertussis (whooping cough). A single vaccine called Tdap protects adolescents and adults against the three diseases. Every 10 years, a repeat vaccine against tetanus and diphtheria (called Td) is recommended.

Additional vaccines may be recommended for a person with HIV based on the person's age, previous vaccinations, risk factors for a particular disease, or certain HIV-related factors.

What about Travel and Immunizations?[1]

Regardless of destination, all travelers should be up to date on routine vaccinations. Those traveling to destinations outside the United States may need immunizations against diseases present in other parts of the world, such as cholera or yellow fever.

If you have HIV, talk to your healthcare provider about any vaccines you may need before you travel.

- If your CD4 count is less than 200 copies/mm^3, your healthcare provider may recommend that you delay travel to give your HIV medicines time to strengthen your immune system.

- If your immune system is strong enough to get a required vaccine, your healthcare provider may recommend blood tests to confirm that the vaccine was effective.

Section 14.2

Microbicides

This section includes text excerpted from "Microbicides," HIV.gov, U.S. Department of Health and Human Services (HHS), May 27, 2017.

What Are Microbicides?

Microbicides are experimental products containing drugs that prevent vaginal and/or rectal transmission of human immunodeficiency virus (HIV) and/or sexually transmitted infections (STIs). Researchers are studying microbicides delivered in the form of vaginal rings, gels, films, inserts, and enemas. A safe, effective, desirable, and affordable microbicide against HIV could help to prevent infections.

Can Microbicides Prevent Human Immunodeficiency Virus (HIV) Infection?

The answer to this question now appears to be "Yes, to a modest degree."

Several large-scale research studies over the past decade have investigated the safety and effectiveness of different microbicides.

In 2016, results from the National Institutes of Health (NIH)-funded ASPIRE study (A Study to Prevent Infection with a Ring for Extended Use), a large clinical trial conducted at 15 clinical research sites in Malawi, South Africa, Uganda, and Zimbabwe, showed that a vaginal ring that continuously releases the experimental antiretroviral drug dapivirine provided a modest level of protection against HIV infection in women. The ring reduced the risk of HIV infection by 27 percent in the study population overall and by 61 percent among women ages 25 years and older, who used the ring most consistently.

A second clinical trial called the Ring Study conducted in parallel with the ASPIRE study also tested the dapivirine ring for safety and efficacy in women. Similar to ASPIRE, The Ring Study investigators found an overall effectiveness of 31 percent, with a slightly greater reduction in risk of HIV infection among women older than 21 years.

To build on the findings from these studies, NIH's National Institute of Allergy and Infectious Diseases (NIAID) is funding an open-label extension study of the vaginal ring to see if this experimental product can offer increased protection against HIV in an open-label setting in which all participants are counseled on how effective the ring may be, and are invited to use or not use the dapivirine ring in order to yield insight into why some women may choose to use or not to use the ring. Finding HIV prevention options that are acceptable to women and that can be integrated into their daily lives is a critical component of developing prevention strategies that work for diverse populations.

Other studies are examining potential rectal microbicide gels to reduce the risk of HIV transmission through anal sex. Some are testing microbicides originally formulated for vaginal use to determine if they are safe, effective, and acceptable when used in the rectum; others focus on the development of products designed specifically for rectal use.

Why Are Microbicides Important?

The only currently licensed and available biomedical HIV prevention product comes in the form of a daily pill taken orally (tenofovir-emtricitabine sold as Truvada®) and is called preexposure prophylaxis, or PrEP. But protection from it requires consistent, daily use. A daily pill can be challenging for some people to take, so other forms of biomedical HIV prevention are being explored. A discreet, long-acting, female-initiated method of prevention such as a microbicide may be a good HIV prevention option for some women.

Microbicides may also be preferable to condoms as an HIV prevention option for some women because women would not have to negotiate their use with a partner, as they often must do with condoms. Because women and girls are at particularly high risk for HIV in many parts of the world, it is especially important to have an effective, desirable, woman-initiated HIV prevention tool. Microbicides could make it possible for a woman to protect herself from HIV. In the future, it may be possible to formulate products that combine anti-HIV microbicide agents with contraception.

Rectal microbicides would also offer another HIV prevention option for men or women who engage in anal sex.

Can I Use a Microbicide to Prevent HIV?

Not yet. The ASPIRE study results are promising, but further study is needed, along with approval by drug regulators before the vaginal ring can be used by the public. Meanwhile, research on other formulations and forms of microbicides continues.

For now, available forms of protection against sexual transmission of HIV continue to be:

- Antiretroviral therapy for people who have HIV, to reduce their risk of transmitting the virus to their sexual partners (i.e., treatment as prevention)

- Daily PrEP

- Voluntary medical male circumcision

- HIV testing—so that you know your own HIV status and your partner's, too

- Using condoms consistently and correctly

- Choosing less risky sexual behaviors

- Reducing the number of people you have sex with

The more of these actions you take, the safer you will be.

Chapter 15

HIV Prophylaxis

Chapter Contents

Section 15.1

Preexposure Prophylaxis (PrEP)

This section includes text excerpted from "PrEP," Centers for
Disease Control and Prevention (CDC), March 23, 2018.

Preexposure prophylaxis (PrEP) can stop human immunodeficiency
virus (HIV) from taking hold and spreading throughout your body. It
is highly effective for preventing HIV if used as prescribed, but it is
much less effective when not taken consistently. Daily PrEP reduces
the risk of getting HIV from sex by more than 90 percent. Among
people who inject drugs, it reduces the risk by more than 70 percent.
Your risk of getting HIV from sex can be even lower if you combine
PrEP with condoms and other prevention methods.

Frequently Asked Questions on Preexposure Prophylaxis (PrEP)

What Is Preexposure Prophylaxis (PrEP)?

PrEP is when people at very high risk for HIV take HIV medicines
daily to lower their chances of getting infected. A combination of two
HIV medicines (tenofovir and emtricitabine), sold under the name Tru-
vada®, approved for daily use as PrEP to help prevent an HIV-negative
person from getting HIV from a sexual or injection-drug-using partner
who's positive. Studies have shown that PrEP is highly effective for
preventing HIV if it is used as prescribed. PrEP is much less effective
when it is not taken consistently.

Why Take PrEP?

For those at very high risk for HIV, PrEP can significantly reduce
your risk of HIV infection if taken daily. Daily PrEP use can lower the
risk of getting HIV from sex by more than 90 percent and from injection drug use by more than 70 percent. You can combine additional
strategies with PrEP to reduce your risk even further.

Is PrEP a Vaccine?

No. PrEP does not work the same way as a vaccine. A vaccine
teaches your body to fight off infection for several years. For PrEP,

you take a pill every day by mouth. The pill that was shown to be safe and to help block HIV infection is called "Truvada." Truvada is a combination of two drugs (tenofovir and emtricitabine). If you take PrEP daily, the presence of the medicine in your bloodstream can often stop HIV from taking hold and spreading in your body. If you do not take PrEP every day, there may not be enough medicine in your bloodstream to block the virus.

Should I Consider Taking PrEP?

PrEP is for people without HIV who are at very high risk for getting it from sex or injection drug use. The federal guidelines recommend that PrEP be considered for people who are HIV-negative and in an ongoing sexual relationship with an HIV-positive partner.

This recommendation also includes anyone who isn't in a mutually monogamous relationship with a partner who recently tested HIV-negative, and is a gay or bisexual man who has had anal sex without using a condom or been diagnosed with an STD in the past 6 months, or heterosexual man or woman who does not regularly use condoms during sex with partners of unknown HIV status who are at substantial risk of HIV infection (for example, people who inject drugs or women who have bisexual male partners). PrEP is also recommended for people who have injected drugs in the past 6 months and have shared needles or works or been in drug treatment in the past 6 months.

If you have a partner who is HIV-positive and are considering getting pregnant, talk to your doctor about PrEP if you're not already taking it. PrEP may be an option to help protect you and your baby from getting HIV infection while you try to get pregnant, during pregnancy, or while breastfeeding.

Because PrEP involves daily medication and regular visits to a healthcare provider, it may not be right for everyone. And PrEP may cause side effects like nausea in some people, but these generally subside over time. These side effects aren't life-threatening.

How Well Does PrEP Work?

Studies have shown that PrEP reduces the risk of getting HIV from sex by more than 90 percent when used consistently. Among people who inject drugs, PrEP reduces the risk of getting HIV by more than 70 percent when used consistently.

Is PrEP Safe?

PrEP can cause side effects like nausea in some people, but these generally subside over time. No serious side effects have been observed, and these side effects aren't life-threatening. If you are taking PrEP, tell your healthcare provider about any side effects that are severe or do not go away.

How Can I Start PrEP?

PrEP can be prescribed only by a healthcare provider, so talk to yours to find out if PrEP is the right HIV prevention strategy for you. You must take PrEP daily for it to work. Also, you must take an HIV test before beginning PrEP to be sure you don't already have HIV and every 3 months while you're taking it, so you'll have to visit your healthcare provider for regular follow-ups.

The cost of PrEP is covered by many health insurance plans, and a commercial medication assistance program provides free PrEP to people with limited income and no insurance to cover PrEP care.

How Do I Speak to My Doctor or Other Healthcare Provider about PrEP?

You can ask some questions to your healthcare provider when discussing whether PrEP (taking daily HIV medicines) is right for you.

How Can I Get Help to Pay for PrEP?

The cost of PrEP is covered by many health insurance plans, and a commercial medication assistance program provides free PrEP to people with limited income and no insurance to cover PrEP care.

If I Take PrEP, Can I Stop Using Condoms When I Have Sex?

No, you should not stop using condoms because you are taking PrEP. PrEP doesn't give you any protection against other STDs, like gonorrhea and chlamydia. Also, while PrEP can significantly reduce your risk of HIV infection if taken daily, you can combine additional strategies like condom use with PrEP to reduce your risk even further.

If used the right way every time you have sex, condoms are highly effective in preventing HIV and some STDs you can get through body fluids, like gonorrhea and chlamydia. However, they provide less protection against STDs spread through skin-to-skin contact, like human papillomavirus or HPV (genital warts), genital herpes, and syphilis.

How Long Do I Need to Take PrEP?

You must take PrEP daily for it to work. But there are several reasons people stop taking PrEP. For example,

- If your risk of getting HIV infection becomes low because of changes in your life, you may want to stop taking PrEP.

- If you find you don't want to take a pill every day or often forget to take your pills, other ways of protecting yourself from HIV infection may work better for you.

- If you have side effects from the medicine that are interfering with your life, or if blood tests show that your body is reacting to PrEP in unsafe ways, your provider may stop prescribing PrEP for you.

You should discuss this question with your healthcare provider.

How Long Do I Have to Take PrEP before It Is Effective?

When taken every day, PrEP is safe and highly effective in preventing HIV infection. PrEP reaches maximum protection from HIV for receptive anal sex at about 7 days of daily use. For receptive vaginal sex and injection drug use, PrEP reaches maximum protection at about 20 days of daily use. No data are yet available about how long it takes to reach maximum protection for insertive anal or insertive vaginal sex.

Does Taking PrEP Long-Term Have Harmful Health Effects?

In people who are HIV-negative and have taken PrEP for up to 5 years, no significant health effects have been seen.

Can You Start PrEP after You Have Been Exposed to HIV?

PrEP is only for people who are at ongoing very high risk of HIV infection. But PEP (postexposure prophylaxis) is an option for someone who thinks they've recently been exposed to HIV during sex or through sharing needles and works to prepare drugs.

PEP means taking antiretroviral medicines after a potential exposure to HIV to prevent becoming infected. PEP must be started within 72 hours of possible exposure to HIV. If you're prescribed PEP, you'll need to take it once or twice daily for 28 days.

How Can I Locate PrEP in My Area?

Visit the PrEP locator to find a PrEP provider near you (www. preplocator.org).

Section 15.2

Long-Acting PrEP

This section includes text excerpted from "Long-Acting PrEP," HIV.gov, U.S. Department of Health and Human Services (HHS), May 15, 2017.

What Is Long-Acting PrEP and Why Is It Needed?

Preexposure prophylaxis, or PrEP, is a way for people who are at high risk for human immunodeficiency virus (HIV) infection to prevent it by taking a pill every day. When taken daily, the medications in the pill provide a high level of protection against HIV. Studies have shown that PrEP reduces the risk of getting HIV from sex by more than 90 percent when used consistently. Among people who inject drugs, PrEP reduces the risk of getting HIV by more than 70 percent when used consistently. However, many studies of PrEP indicate that PrEP is much less effective if it is not taken consistently and that taking a daily pill can be challenging for some people.

Researchers are working to create new forms of PrEP that do not require people to take a pill every day. This may make it easier for more people to get very high levels of protection from PrEP. To generate new biomedical HIV prevention options that may be more desirable than a daily pill, the National Institutes of Health (NIH) funds the design and testing of new, long-acting forms of PrEP. Scientists are studying long-acting PrEP products that are put inside the body (for example, under the skin, in the vagina). These products are being designed for people who are committed to using PrEP on an ongoing basis and may work for a month or as long as a year. This research aims to provide people with a variety of acceptable, discreet, and convenient choices for highly effective HIV prevention.

What Types of Long-Acting PrEP Are under Study?

Three forms of long-acting PrEP are in design and testing in research studies: intravaginal rings, injectable drugs, and implants.

Intravaginal rings for women. Long-acting PrEP intravaginal rings are polymer-based products that are inserted into the vagina, where they release one or more HIV antiretroviral drugs over time. The intravaginal ring at the most advanced stage of research is the dapivirine ring that was tested in two large clinical trials, including the National Institutes of Health (NIH)-funded ASPIRE study (A Study to Prevent Infection with a Ring for Extended Use). The ring is undergoing further evaluation in the HIV Open-Label Extension (HOPE) study, an open-label extension trial. NIH also is funding the human testing of two more long-acting PrEP intravaginal rings and supporting the design of several others.

Injected PrEP. Long-acting PrEP injectables are select long-acting antiretroviral drugs that are injected into the body. The first large-scale clinical trial of a long-acting PrEP injectable began in December 2016. Called HPTN 083, the NIH-sponsored study—a partnership with ViiV Healthcare and the Bill and Melinda Gates Foundation—is examining whether a long-acting form of the investigational antiretroviral drug cabotegravir, injected once every 8 weeks, can safely protect men and transgender women from HIV infection at least as well as daily PrEP. Results are expected in 2021. A related study called HIV Prevention Trials Network (HPTN) 084 will test whether injectable cabotegravir safely prevents HIV infection in young women. NIH also is funding the design and early clinical testing of additional long-acting PrEP injectable drugs.

Implanted PrEP. Long-acting PrEP implants are small devices that are implanted in the body and release an antiretroviral drug over time. NIH is funding the development of several long-acting PrEP implants, which will undergo laboratory testing before being studied in human trials.

Can I Use Long-Acting PrEP to Prevent HIV Now?

At this time, some forms of long-acting PrEP are being tested in clinical trials. The effectiveness of long-acting PrEP has not yet been proven, and it has not been considered for approval by the U.S. Food and Drug Administration (FDA). The NIH-supported clinical trials may be seeking volunteers to participate in studies on long-acting PrEP. You may be eligible to participate in one of these trials if one is taking place near you. Information about NIH clinical trials can be found at www.clinicaltrials.gov/. It will probably be a number of years before long-acting PrEP is available to the general public. In the meantime, the best forms of prevention against sexual transmission of HIV continue to be:

- HIV testing—so that you know your own HIV status and your partner's too

- Antiretroviral therapy for people who have HIV, to protect their health and reduce their risk of transmitting the virus to their sexual partners

- PrEP for people who do not have HIV but are at very high risk of getting it

- Using condoms consistently and correctly

- Choosing less risky sexual behaviors

- Reducing the number of people you have sex with

- PEP, or postexposure prophylaxis, meaning taking antiretroviral medicines very soon after being potentially exposed to HIV to prevent becoming infected

The more of these actions you take, the safer you will be.

Section 15.3

Postexposure Prophylaxis (PEP)

This section includes text excerpted from "PEP," Centers for Disease Control and Prevention (CDC), May 24, 2018.

Frequently Asked Questions on Postexposure Prophylaxis (PEP)?

What Is Postexposure Prophylaxis (PEP)?

PEP stands for postexposure prophylaxis. It means taking antiretroviral medicines (ART) after being potentially exposed to human immunodeficiency virus (HIV) to prevent becoming infected.

PEP must be started within 72 hours after a recent possible exposure to HIV, but the sooner you start PEP, the better. Every hour counts. If you're prescribed PEP, you'll need to take it once or twice daily for 28 days. PEP is effective in preventing HIV when administered correctly, but not 100 percent.

Is PEP Right for Me?

If you're HIV-negative or don't know your HIV status, and in the last 72 hours you:

- think you may have been exposed to HIV during sex (for example, if the condom broke),

- shared needles and works to prepare drugs (for example, cotton, cookers, water), or

- were sexually assaulted, talk to your healthcare provider or an emergency room doctor about PEP right away.

PEP should be used only in emergency situations and must be started within 72 hours after a recent possible exposure to HIV. It is not a substitute for regular use of other proven HIV prevention methods, such as preexposure prophylaxis (PrEP), which means taking HIV medicines daily to lower your chance of getting infected; using condoms the right way every time you have sex; and using only your own new, sterile needles and works every time you inject.

PEP is effective, but not 100 percent, so you should continue to use condoms with sex partners and safe injection practices while taking PEP. These strategies can protect you from being exposed to HIV again and reduce the chances of transmitting HIV to others if you do become infected while you're on PEP.

I'm a Healthcare Worker, and I Think I've Been Exposed to HIV at Work. Should I Take PEP?

PEP should be considered if you've had a recent possible exposure to HIV at work. Report your exposure to your supervisor, and seek medical attention immediately. Occupational transmission of HIV to healthcare workers is extremely rare, and the proper use of safety devices and barriers can help minimize the risk of exposure while caring for patients with HIV.

A healthcare worker who has a possible exposure should see a doctor or visit an emergency room immediately. PEP must be started within 72 hours after a recent possible exposure to HIV. The sooner, the better; every hour counts. The Centers for Disease Control and Prevention (CDC) issued updated guidelines in 2013 for the management of healthcare worker exposures to HIV and recommendations for PEP.

Clinicians caring for healthcare workers who've had a possible exposure can call the PEPline (888-448-4911), which offers around-the-clock advice on managing occupational exposures to HIV, as well as hepatitis B and C. Exposed healthcare workers may also call the PEPline, but they should seek local medical attention first.

Why Should I Take PEP?

PEP must be started within 72 hours after a possible exposure. The sooner you start PEP, the better; every hour counts. Starting PEP as soon as possible after a potential HIV exposure is important. Research has shown that PEP has little or no effect in preventing HIV infection if it is started later than 72 hours after HIV exposure.

If you're prescribed PEP, you'll need to take it once or twice daily for 28 days.

Does PEP Have Any Side Effects?

PEP is safe but may cause side effects like nausea in some people. These side effects can be treated and aren't life-threatening.

Where Can I Get PEP?

Your healthcare provider or an emergency room doctor can prescribe PEP. Talk to them right away if you think you've recently been exposed to HIV.

How Can I Pay for PEP?

If you're prescribed PEP after a sexual assault, you may qualify for partial or total reimbursement for medicines and clinical care costs through the Office for Victims of Crime (OVC), funded by the U.S. Department of Justice (DOJ).

If you're prescribed PEP for another reason and you cannot get insurance coverage (Medicaid, Medicare, private, or employer-based), your healthcare provider can apply for free PEP medicines through the medication assistance programs run by the manufacturers. Online applications can be faxed to the company, or some companies have special phone lines. These can be handled urgently in many cases to avoid a delay in getting medicine.

If you're a healthcare worker who was exposed to HIV on the job, your workplace health insurance or workers' compensation will usually pay for PEP.

Can I Take a Round of PEP Every Time I Have Unprotected Sex?

PEP should be used only in emergency situations.

PEP is not the right choice for people who may be exposed to HIV frequently—for example, if you often have sex without a condom with a partner who is HIV-positive. Because PEP is given after a potential exposure to HIV, more drugs and higher doses are needed to block infection than with PrEP. PrEP is when people at high risk for HIV take HIV medicines (sold under the brand name Truvada) daily to lower their chances of getting HIV. If you are at ongoing risk for HIV, speak to your doctor about PrEP.

Part Three

Receiving an HIV/AIDS Diagnosis

Chapter 16

HIV Testing

Chapter Contents

Section 16.1

HIV Testing Basics

This section contains text excerpted from the following sources: Text
beginning with the heading "About Human Immunodeficiency Virus
(HIV) Infection Testing" is excerpted from "HIV Testing,"
U.S. Food and Drug Administration (FDA), March 12, 2018;
Text under the heading "FAQs on HIV Testing" is excerpted
from "HIV/AIDS—Testing," Centers for Disease Control
and Prevention (CDC), March 16, 2018.

About Human Immunodeficiency Virus (HIV) Infection Testing

The U.S. Food and Drug Administration (FDA) regulates the tests
that detect infection with human immunodeficiency virus (HIV),
the virus that causes acquired immunodeficiency syndrome (AIDS).
AIDS is a serious disease that can be fatal because the body has
lost the ability to fight infections and cancers. There are a number
of options for people to be tested for HIV, using tests approved by
the FDA:

1. Trained health professionals collect a sample and run the test
   in a professional medical setting. You receive your test results
   from a trained health professional.

2. You collect a sample in the home, forward the sample to a
   medical laboratory, and trained health professionals run the
   test in the medical laboratory

3. You collect a sample, run the test, and obtain your own test
   results in your home

HIV Tests for Screening and Diagnosis

HIV tests are very accurate, but no test can detect the virus immediately after infection. How soon a test can detect infection depends
upon different factors, including the type of test being used. There
are three types of HIV diagnostic tests: antibody tests, combination
or fourth-generation tests, and nucleic acid tests (NATs).

- **Antibody tests** detect the presence of antibodies, proteins that
  a person's body makes against HIV, not HIV itself. Most HIV

tests, including most rapid tests and home tests, are antibody tests. It can take 3–12 weeks for a person's body to make enough antibodies for an antibody test to detect HIV infection. In general, antibody tests that use blood can detect HIV slightly sooner after infection than tests done with oral fluid.

- **Combination or fourth-generation tests** look for both HIV antibodies and antigens. Antigens are a part of the virus itself and are present during acute HIV infection. It can take 2–6 weeks for a person's body to make enough antigens and antibodies for a combination test to detect HIV. Combination tests are now recommended for testing done in labs and are becoming more common in the United States. There is also a rapid combination test available.

- **NATs** detect HIV the fastest by looking for HIV in the blood. It can take 7–28 days for NATs to detect HIV. This test is very expensive and is not routinely used for HIV screening unless the person recently had a high-risk exposure or a possible exposure to early symptoms of HIV infection.

An initial HIV test will either be an antibody test or combination test. It may involve obtaining blood or oral fluid for a rapid test or sending blood or oral fluid to a laboratory. If the initial HIV test is a rapid test and it is positive, the individual will be directed to get follow-up testing. If the initial HIV test is a laboratory test and is positive, the laboratory will usually conduct follow-up testing on the same blood specimen as the initial test. Although HIV tests are generally very accurate, follow-up testing allows the healthcare provider to be sure the diagnosis is right.

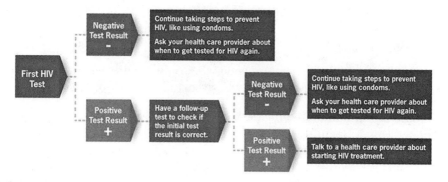

Figure 16.1. *HIV Test Flowchart*

173

FAQs on HIV Testing

The only way to know for sure whether you have HIV is to get tested. The Centers for Disease Control and Prevention (CDC) recommends that everyone between the ages of 13–64 get tested for HIV at least once as part of routine healthcare. Knowing your HIV status gives you powerful information to help you take steps to keep you and your partner healthy.

Should I Get Tested for HIV?

The CDC recommends that everyone between the ages of 13–64 get tested for HIV at least once as part of routine healthcare. About 1 in 7 people in the United States who have HIV don't know they have it.

People at higher risk should get tested more often. If you were HIV-negative the last time you were tested, and that test was more than one year ago, and you answer yes to any of the following questions, you should get an HIV test as soon as possible because these things increase your chances of getting the virus:

- Are you a man who has had sex with another man?
- Have you had sex—anal or vaginal—with an HIV-positive partner?
- Have you had more than one sex partner since your last HIV test?
- Have you injected drugs and shared needles or works (for example, water or cotton) with others?
- Have you exchanged sex for drugs or money?
- Have you been diagnosed with or sought treatment for another sexually transmitted disease (STD)?
- Have you been diagnosed with or treated for hepatitis or tuberculosis (TB)?
- Have you had sex with someone who could answer yes to any of the above questions or someone whose sexual history you don't know?

You should be tested at least once a year if you keep doing any of these things. Sexually active gay and bisexual men may benefit from more frequent testing (for example, every 3–6 months).

If you're pregnant, talk to your healthcare provider about getting tested for HIV and other ways to protect you and your child from getting HIV.

Before having sex for the first time with a new partner, you and your partner should talk about your sexual and drug-use history, disclose your HIV status, and consider getting tested for HIV and learning the results.

How Can Testing Help Me?

The only way to know for sure whether you have HIV is to get tested. Knowing your HIV status gives you powerful information to help you take steps to keep you and your partner healthy.

- If you test positive, you can take medicine to treat HIV to stay healthy for many years and greatly reduce the chance of transmitting HIV to your sex partner

- If you test negative, you have more prevention tools available to prevent HIV than ever before

- If you are pregnant, you should be tested for HIV so that you can begin treatment if you're HIV-positive. If an HIV-positive woman is treated for HIV early in her pregnancy, the risk of transmitting HIV to her baby is very low.

I Don't Believe I Am at High Risk. Why Should I Get Tested?

The CDC recommends that everyone between the ages of 13–64 get tested for HIV at least once as part of routine healthcare, and more often if you do things that might increase your risk for getting HIV.

Even if you are in a monogamous relationship (both you and your partner are having sex only with each other), you should find out for sure whether you or your partner has HIV.

I Am Pregnant. Why Should I Get Tested?

All pregnant women should be tested for HIV so that they can begin treatment if they're HIV-positive. If a woman is treated for HIV early in her pregnancy, the risk of transmitting HIV to her baby can be very low. Testing pregnant women for HIV infection and treating those women who are infected have led to a big decline in the number of children infected with HIV from their mothers.

The treatment is most effective for preventing HIV transmission to babies when started as early as possible during pregnancy. However, there are still great health benefits to beginning preventive treatment even during labor or shortly after the baby is born.

What Kinds of Tests Are Available, and How Do They Work?

There are three types of tests available: nucleic acid tests (NAT), antigen/antibody tests, and antibody tests. HIV tests are typically performed on blood or oral fluid. They may also be performed on urine.

1. A NAT looks for the actual virus in the blood. The test can give either a positive/negative result or an amount of virus present in the blood (known as an HIV viral load test). This test is very expensive and not routinely used for screening individuals unless they recently had a high-risk exposure or a possible exposure and they have early symptoms of HIV infection. Nucleic acid testing is usually considered accurate during the early stages of infection. However, it is best to get an antibody or antigen/antibody test at the same time to help the healthcare provider understand what a negative NAT means. Taking preexposure prophylaxis (PrEP) or postexposure prophylaxis (PEP) may also reduce the accuracy of NAT if you have HIV.

2. An antigen/antibody test looks for both HIV antibodies and antigens. Antibodies are produced by your immune system when you're exposed to bacteria or viruses like HIV. Antigens are foreign substances that cause your immune system to activate. If you're infected with HIV, an antigen called p24 is produced even before antibodies develop. Antigen/antibody tests are recommended for testing done in labs and are now common in the United States. There is also a rapid antigen/antibody test available.

3. Most rapid tests and home tests are antibody tests. HIV antibody tests look for antibodies to HIV in your blood or oral fluid. In general, antibody tests that use blood from a vein can detect HIV sooner after infection than tests done with blood from a finger prick or with oral fluid.

    •   While most laboratories are now using antigen/antibody tests, laboratory-based antibody screening tests are still available. These tests require blood to be drawn from your vein into a tube and then that blood is sent to a laboratory for testing. The results may take several days to be available.

    •   With a rapid antibody screening test, results are ready in 30 minutes or less. These tests are used in clinical and nonclinical settings, usually with blood from a finger prick or with oral fluid.

- The oral fluid antibody self-test provides fast results. You have to swab your own mouth to collect an oral fluid sample and use a kit to test it. Results are available in 20 minutes. The manufacturer provides confidential counseling and referral to follow-up testing sites. These tests are available for purchase in stores and online. They may be used at home, or they may be used for testing in some community and clinic testing programs.

- The home collection kit involves pricking your finger to collect a blood sample, sending the sample by mail to a licensed laboratory, and then calling in for results as early as the next business day. This antibody test is anonymous. The manufacturer provides confidential counseling and referral to treatment.

If you use any type of antibody test and have a positive result, you will need to take a follow-up test to confirm your results. If your first test is a rapid home test and it's positive, you will be sent to a health-care provider to get follow-up testing. If your first test is done in a testing lab and it's positive, the lab will conduct the follow-up testing, usually on the same blood sample as the first test.

Talk to your healthcare provider to see what type of HIV test is right for you.

After you get tested, it's important for you to find out the result of your test so that you can talk to your healthcare provider about treatment options if you're HIV-positive. If you're HIV-negative, continue to take actions to prevent HIV, like using condoms the right way every time you have sex and taking medicines to prevent HIV if you're at high risk.

How Soon after an Exposure to HIV Can an HIV Test Detect If I Am Infected?

No HIV test can detect HIV immediately after infection. If you think you've been exposed to HIV in the last 72 hours, talk to your healthcare provider about postexposure prophylaxis (PEP), right away.

The time between when a person may have been exposed to HIV and when a test can tell for sure whether they have HIV is called the window period. The window period varies from person to person and depends on the type of test used to detect HIV.

- NAT can usually tell you if you are infected with HIV 10–33 days after an exposure.

- An antigen/antibody test performed by a laboratory on blood from a vein can usually detect HIV infection 18–45 days after an exposure. Antigen/ antibody tests done with blood from a finger prick can take longer to detect HIV (18–90 days after an exposure). When the goal is to tell for sure that a person does not have HIV, an antigen/antibody test performed by a laboratory on blood from a vein is preferred.

- Antibody tests can usually take 23–90 days to reliably detect HIV infection. Most rapid tests and home tests are antibody tests. In general, antibody tests that use blood from a vein can detect HIV sooner after infection than tests done with blood from a finger prick or with oral fluid.

Ask your healthcare provider about the window period for the test you're taking. If you're using a home test, you can get that information from the materials included in the test's package. If you get an HIV test after a potential HIV exposure and the result is negative, get tested again after the window period for the test you're taking to be sure. If your healthcare provider uses an antigen/antibody test performed by a laboratory on blood from a vein you should get tested again 45 days after your most recent exposure. For other tests, you should test again at least 90 days after your most recent exposure to tell for sure if you have HIV.

If you learned you were HIV-negative the last time you were tested, you can only be sure you're still negative if you haven't had a potential HIV exposure since your last test. If you're sexually active, continue to take actions to prevent HIV, like using condoms the right way every time you have sex and taking medicines to prevent HIV if you're at high risk.

Where Can I Get Tested?

You can ask your healthcare provider for an HIV test. Many medical clinics, substance abuse programs, community health centers, and hospitals offer them too. You can also find a testing site near you by

- calling 800-CDC-INFO (800-232-4636)

- visiting gettested.cdc.gov

- texting your ZIP code to KNOW IT (566948)

You can also buy a home testing kit at a pharmacy or online.

What Should I Expect When I Go for an HIV Test?

If you take a test in a healthcare setting when it's time to take the test, a healthcare provider will take your sample (blood or oral fluid), and you may be able to wait for the results if it's a rapid HIV test. If the test comes back negative, and you haven't had an exposure for 3 months, you can be confident you're not infected with HIV.

If your HIV test result is positive, you may need to get a follow-up test to be sure you have HIV.

Your healthcare provider or counselor may talk with you about your risk factors, answer questions about your general health, and discuss next steps with you, especially if your result is positive.

What Does a Negative Test Result Mean?

A negative result doesn't necessarily mean that you don't have HIV. That's because of the window period—the time between when a person may have been exposed to HIV and when a test can tell for sure whether they have HIV. The window period varies from person to person and is also different depending on the type of HIV test.

Ask your healthcare provider about the window period for the test you're taking. If you're using a home test, you can get that information from the materials included in the test's package. If you get an HIV test after a potential HIV exposure and the result is negative, get tested again after the window period for the test you're taking to be sure. For example, if your healthcare provider uses an antigen/antibody test performed by a laboratory with blood from a vein you should get tested again 45 days after your most recent exposure. For other tests, you should test again at least 90 days after your most recent exposure to tell for sure if you have HIV.

If you learned you were HIV-negative the last time you were tested, you can only be sure you're still negative if you haven't had a potential HIV exposure since your last test. If you're sexually active, continue to take actions to prevent HIV, like using condoms the right way every time you have sex and taking medicines to prevent HIV if you're at high risk.

If I Have a Negative Result, Does That Mean That My Partner Is HIV-Negative Also?

No. Your HIV test result reveals only your HIV status.

HIV is not necessarily transmitted every time you have sex. Therefore, taking an HIV test is not a way to find out if your partner is infected.

179

It's important to be open with your partners and ask them to tell you their HIV status. But keep in mind that your partners may not know or may be wrong about their status, and some may not tell you if they have HIV even if they are aware of their status. Consider getting tested together so you can both know your HIV status and take steps to keep yourselves healthy.

What Does a Positive Result Mean?

A follow-up test will be conducted. If the follow-up test is also positive, it means you are living with HIV (or HIV-positive).

If you had a rapid screening test, the testing site will arrange a follow-up test to make sure the screening test result was correct. If your blood was tested in a lab, the lab will conduct a follow-up test on the same sample.

It is important that you start medical care and begin HIV treatment as soon as you are diagnosed with HIV. Antiretroviral therapy or ART (taking medicines to treat HIV infection) is recommended for all people with HIV, regardless of how long they've had the virus or how healthy they are. ARTworks by lowering the amount of virus in your body to very low levels called viral suppression. It slows the progression of HIV and helps protect your immune system. If you are on ART and virally suppressed, you can stay healthy for many years, and greatly reduce your chance of transmitting HIV to sex partners.

If you have health insurance, your insurer is required to cover some medicines used to treat HIV. If you don't have health insurance, or you're unable to afford your copay or coinsurance amount, you may be eligible for government programs that can help through Medicaid, Medicare, the Ryan White HIV/AIDS Program, and community health centers. Your healthcare provider or local public health department can tell you where to get HIV treatment.

To lower your risk of transmitting HIV:

- Take medicines to treat HIV (ART) the right way every day. Being on ART and getting and staying virally suppressed is the most effective thing you can do to reduce the chance of transmitting HIV.

- Use condoms the right way every time you have sex.

- If your partner is HIV-negative, encourage them to talk to their healthcare provider to see if taking daily medicine to prevent HIV (called preexposure prophylaxis, or PrEP) is right for them.

- If you think your partner might have been recently exposed to HIV—for example, if the condom breaks during sex and you aren't virally suppressed—they should talk to a healthcare provider as soon as possible within the next 3 days (72 hours) about taking medicines (called postexposure prophylaxis, or PEP) to prevent getting HIV.

- Get tested and treated for STDs and encourage your partner to do the same.

Receiving a diagnosis of HIV can be a life-changing event. People can feel many emotions—sadness, hopelessness, or anger. Allied healthcare providers and social service providers, often available at your healthcare provider's office, will have the tools to help you work through the early stages of your diagnosis and begin to manage your HIV.

Talking to others who have HIV may also be helpful. Find a local HIV support group. Learn about how other people living with HIV have handled their diagnosis.

If I Test Positive for HIV, Does That Mean I Have Acquired Immunodeficiency Syndrome (AIDS)?

No. Being HIV-positive does not mean you have AIDS. AIDS is the most advanced stage of HIV disease. HIV can lead to AIDS if a person does not get treatment or take care of their health.

Will Other People Know My Test Result?

If you take an anonymous test, no one but you will know the result. If you take a confidential test, your test result will be part of your medical record, but it is still protected by state and federal privacy laws.

- **Anonymous testing** means that nothing ties your test results to you. When you take an anonymous HIV test, you get a unique identifier that allows you to get your test results.

- **Confidential testing** means that your name and other identifying information will be attached to your test results. The results will go in your medical record and may be shared with your healthcare providers and your health insurance company. Otherwise, the results are protected by state and federal privacy laws, and they can be released only with your permission.

With confidential testing, if you test positive for HIV, the test result and your name will be reported to the state or local health department to help public health officials get better estimates of the rates of HIV in the state. The state health department will then remove all personal information about you (name, address, etc.) and share the remaining nonidentifying information with the CDC. The CDC does not share this information with anyone else, including insurance companies.

Should I Share My Positive Test Results with Others?

It's important to share your status with your sex partners. Whether you disclose your status to others is your decision.

Partners

It's important to disclose your HIV status to your sex partners even if you're uncomfortable doing it. Communicating with each other about your HIV status means you can take steps to keep both of you healthy. The more practice you have disclosing your HIV status, the easier it will become.

Many resources can help you learn ways to disclose your status to your partners. If you're nervous about disclosing your test result, or you have been threatened or injured by your partner, you can ask your doctor or the local health department to tell them that they might have been exposed to HIV. This is called partner notification services. Health departments do not reveal your name to your partners. They will only tell your partners that they have been exposed to HIV and should get tested.

Many states have laws that require you to tell your sexual partners if you're HIV-positive before you have sex (anal, vaginal, or oral) or tell your drug-using partners before you share drugs or needles to inject drugs. In some states, you can be charged with a crime if you don't tell your partner your HIV status, even if your partner doesn't become infected.

Family and Friends

In most cases, your family and friends will not know your test results or HIV status unless you tell them yourself. While telling your family that you have HIV may seem hard, you should know that disclosure has many benefits—studies have shown that people who disclose their HIV status respond better to treatment than those who don't. And telling friends and family can provide an important source of support in managing your HIV.

If you are under 18, however, some states allow your healthcare provider to tell your parents that you received services for HIV if they think doing so is in your best interest.

Employers

In most cases, your employer will not know your HIV status unless you tell them. But your employer does have a right to ask if you have any health conditions that would affect your ability to do your job or pose a serious risk to others. (An example might be a healthcare professional, like a surgeon, who does procedures where there is a risk of blood or other body fluids being exchanged.)

If you have health insurance through your employer, the insurance company cannot legally tell your employer that you have HIV. But it is possible that your employer could find out if the insurance company provides detailed information to your employer about the benefits it pays or the costs of insurance.

All people with HIV are covered under the Americans with Disabilities Act (ADA). This means that your employer cannot discriminate against you because of your HIV status as long as you can do your job.

Who Will Pay for My HIV Test?

HIV screening is covered by health insurance without a copay, as required by the Affordable Care Act (ACA). If you do not have medical insurance, some testing sites may offer free tests.

Who Will Pay for My Treatment If I Am HIV Positive?

If you have health insurance, your insurer is required to cover some medicines used to treat HIV. If you don't have health insurance, or you're unable to afford your copay or coinsurance amount, you may be eligible for government programs that can help through Medicaid, Medicare, the Ryan White HIV/AIDS Program, and community health centers. Your healthcare provider or local public health department can tell you where to get HIV treatment.

Section 16.2

Frequency of HIV Testing and Time from Infection to Diagnosis Improve

This section includes text excerpted from "Frequency of HIV Testing and Time from Infection to Diagnosis Improve," Centers for Disease Control and Prevention (CDC), November 28, 2018.

A Centers for Disease Control and Prevention (CDC) Vital Signs report finds that HIV is being diagnosed sooner after infection than was previously reported. According to the report, the estimated median time from HIV infection to diagnosis was three years in 2015. The CDC previously estimated that, in 2011, the median time from HIV infection to diagnosis was three years and seven months.

The seven-month improvement is a considerable decrease over a four-year period and reinforces other signs that the nation's approach to HIV prevention is paying off. Overall, 85 percent of the estimated 1.1 million people living with HIV in 2014 knew their HIV status. The CDC estimates about 40 percent of HIV infections originate from people who don't know they have HIV.

"These findings are more encouraging signs that the tide continues to turn on our nation's HIV epidemic," said the CDC Director Brenda Fitzgerald, M.D. "HIV is being diagnosed more quickly, the number of people who have the virus under control is up, and annual infections are down. So while we celebrate our progress, we pledge to work together to end this epidemic forever."

Getting an HIV test is the first step to learning how to reduce future risk for people who do not have HIV and to starting treatment and getting the virus under control for people living with HIV. Taking HIV medications as prescribed allows people with the virus to live a long, healthy life and protect their partners from acquiring HIV.

"If you are at risk for HIV, don't guess—get a test," said Jonathan Mermin, M.D., M.P.H, the director of CDC's National Center for HIV/AIDS, Viral Hepatitis, STD, and TB Prevention (NCHHSTP). "The benefits are clear. Prompt diagnosis is prevention. It is the first step to protecting people living with HIV and their partners."

The CDC recommends testing all people ages 13–64 for HIV at least once in their lifetime, and people at higher risk for HIV at least annually. Healthcare providers may find it beneficial to test some sexually active gay and bisexual men more frequently (e.g., every 3–6 months).

The *Vital Signs* analysis found that the percentage of people at increased risk for HIV who reported getting an HIV test the previous year has increased. Despite that progress, too few are tested. A multi-city study found that people who reported that they did not get an HIV test in the last year included 29 percent of gay and bisexual men, 42 percent of people who inject drugs, and 59 percent of heterosexuals at increased risk for HIV. The same study also found that seven in 10 people at high risk who were not tested for HIV in the past year saw a healthcare provider during that time—signaling a missed opportunity to get high-risk individuals tested as frequently as needed.

The *Vital Signs* analysis suggests that, without increased testing, many people living with undiagnosed HIV may not know they have HIV for many years. A quarter of people diagnosed with HIV in 2015 lived with HIV for seven or more years without knowing it.

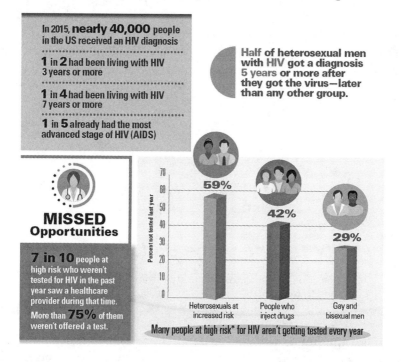

Figure 16.2. *HIV Risk Analysis* (Source: "CDC National Surveillance, 2015; CDC National HIV Behavioural Surveillance, 2014–2016," Centers for Disease Control and Prevention (CDC).)

People with high risk for HIV include: sexually active gay and bisexual men, people who inject drugs, and heterosexuals who have sex with someone who is at high risk for or has HIV.

185

In 2015, estimated timing from HIV infection to diagnosis varied by risk group and by race/ethnicity.

- Estimated timing of HIV infection to diagnosis ranged from a median of five years for heterosexual males to two-and-a-half years for heterosexual females and females who inject drugs. The median was three years for gay and bisexual males.

- Estimated timing of HIV infection to diagnosis ranged from a median of four years for Asian Americans to two years for white Americans and about three years for African Americans and Latinos.

"Ideally, HIV is diagnosed within months of infection, rather than years later," said Eugene McCray, M.D., the director of CDC's Division of HIV/AIDS Prevention (DHAP). "Further increasing regular HIV testing and closing testing, diagnosis, and treatment gaps is essential to stopping HIV in our communities."

The CDC funding supports more than 3 million tests across the country each year that identify on average more than 12,000 people with HIV who were not previously diagnosed—accounting for one-third of all HIV diagnoses a year in the United States.

Section 16.3

HIV Testing in the United States

This section includes text excerpted from "HIV Testing in the United States," Centers for Disease Control and Prevention (CDC), August 2016.

Human immunodeficiency virus infection (HIV) testing is essential for improving the health of people living with HIV and helping to prevent further infections. The Centers for Disease Control and Prevention (CDC) estimates that 13 percent of people infected with HIV in the United States are unaware of their infection—more than 161,200 people. As many as 50,000 HIV infections occur each year, and many of these are transmitted by people who do not know they are HIV-positive.

The CDC recommends all adolescents and adults get tested at least once for HIV as a routine part of medical care, and that gay and bisexual men and others at high risk be tested more frequently. The CDC is working to increase testing in a wide range of settings—outside of the medical system—among people at higher risk for HIV infection.

Benefits of Knowing Your HIV Status

HIV testing has never been quicker or easier than it is today—and it has significant benefits for individuals who are infected with HIV and those who are not.

For those who have HIV, testing is the gateway to treatment and care. Highly effective treatments make it possible to live a long, healthy life with HIV. However, one-third of people learn they are infected with HIV less than a year before being diagnosed with acquired immunodeficiency syndrome (AIDS), meaning they have already been infected for many years and may not fully benefit from treatment.

Testing also helps reduce the transmission of HIV. Early diagnosis allows those infected to take steps to protect their partners from infection, and early treatment can lower viral load, and reduce the risk of transmitting HIV to others by 96 percent. And, for people who do not have HIV, testing is just as critical because this information can help link them with important prevention services so they can remain HIV-free. Thanks to increased testing efforts, of the approximately 1.2 million Americans living with HIV, 87 percent have been diagnosed and are aware of their infection.

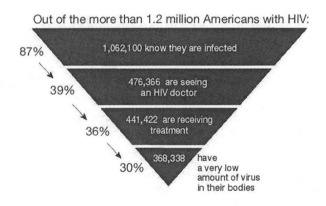

Figure 16.3. *Percentage of HIV-Infected Individuals Engaged in Selected Stages of the Continuum of HIV Care, 2012*

187

- Following are three types of HIV tests. If the first test is positive, a follow-up test is necessary to validate the result.

  1. **Antibody test.** Detects the presence of antibodies against HIV, which typically develop within two to eight weeks after exposure to the virus. An antibody test can be conducted on a sample of blood or oral fluid.

  2. **Combination antigen-antibody test.** Detects both the antibody to HIV and the antigen "p24"—a protein that is part of the virus itself. Because the p24 antigen can be detected within four to seven days before antibodies appear, combination tests can also identify very early infections.

  3. **Ribonucleic acid (RNA) test.** Detects the presence of the virus in the blood. An RNA test can detect very early infection, within 10–15 days of exposure, before antibody tests are able to detect HIV.

HIV Testing Progress and Challenges

While HIV testing rates have steadily increased, more than half of Americans still have not been tested for HIV in their lifetime. Lack of access to healthcare, fear, and misperceptions about HIV risk and the testing process itself are key barriers to increasing HIV testing. In addition, some healthcare settings have not yet made HIV testing a routine part of medical care.

Testing rates remain far too low even among groups at high risk for HIV infection, including men who have sex with men (MSM), African Americans and youth.

- In a study of MSM in 20 U.S. cities, 34 percent of MSM infected with HIV were unaware of their infection. Of those, more than one third (35 percent) had not been tested in the past 12 months, as CDC recommends.

- Although African Americans are more likely to get tested for HIV than Latinos or whites, more than a third have never been tested.

- Nearly half of high school students report having had sex, but the CDC data show that only 22 percent of those have ever been tested for HIV.

Working to Increase HIV Testing and Linkage to Care

HIV testing is a core part of the CDC's commitment to High-Impact Prevention (HIP)—an approach to HIV prevention that aims to achieve a higher level of impact on the epidemic with every federal prevention dollar spent. It is also a key element of the National HIV/AIDS Strategy (NHAS), which seeks to ensure that 90 percent of Americans with HIV are aware of their status and that more people are linked to care within one month of their diagnosis.

The CDC is working to improve testing efforts on many fronts—in both healthcare settings and diverse community venues. For example:

- Providing funding for health departments to implement the CDC's routine testing recommendations and provide free or low-cost testing in other settings

- Piloting HIV testing programs in urban and rural pharmacies

- Guiding individuals to nearby testing sites through HIVtest.cdc. gov

- Updating HIV testing recommendations for laboratories to capitalize on the available testing technology to identify infections earlier

- Launching new phases of the Act Against AIDS (AAA) campaign to increase testing in targeted populations, and supporting the Greater Than AIDS public awareness and information campaign

Section 16.4

HIV Disclosure Policies and Procedures

This section includes text excerpted from "Limits on Confidentiality," HIV.gov, U.S. Department of Health and Human Services (HHS), May 15, 2017.

If your HIV test is positive, the clinic or other testing site will report the results to your state health department. They do this so that public health officials can monitor what's happening with the HIV epidemic in your city and state. (It's important for them to know this, because federal and state funding for HIV services is often targeted to areas where the epidemic is strongest.)

Your state health department will then remove all of your personal information (name, address, etc.) from your test results and send the information to the Centers for Disease Control and Prevention (CDC). CDC is the federal agency responsible for tracking national public health trends. CDC does not share this information with anyone else, including insurance companies.

Many states and some cities have partner-notification laws—meaning that, if you test positive for HIV, you (or your healthcare provider) may be legally obligated to tell your sex or needle-sharing partner(s). In some states, if you are HIV-positive and don't tell your partner(s), you can be charged with a crime. Some health departments require healthcare providers to report the name of your sex and needle-sharing partner(s) if they know that information—even if you refuse to report that information yourself.

Some states also have laws that require clinic staff to notify a "third party" if they know that person has a significant risk for exposure to HIV from a patient the staff member knows is infected with HIV. This is called "duty to warn." The Ryan White HIV/AIDS Program requires that health departments receiving money from the Ryan White program show "good faith" efforts to notify the marriage partners of a patient with HIV.

Disclosure Policies in Correctional Facilities

Any individual who believes that his or her employment rights have been violated may file a charge of discrimination with the Federal Equal Employment Opportunity Commission (EEOC). In addition, an individual, an organization, or an agency may file a charge on behalf of another person in order to protect the aggrieved person's identity.

Section 16.5

An Opt-Out Approach to HIV Screening

This section includes text excerpted from "Pregnant Women,
Infants and Children," Centers for Disease Control and
Prevention (CDC), March 9, 2017.

What Do We Know?

• Many women across the United States do not get tested for HIV
during pregnancy.

• HIV-infected women who do not get tested often transmit HIV
to their infants. 2005 CDC data show that among HIV-infected
infants born in the 33 states which report HIV-exposed infants,
31 percent of the mothers of HIV-infected infants had not been
tested for HIV until after delivery.

• Studies show that more women are tested when the HIV test is
included in the standard group of tests that all pregnant women
receive routinely, and when providers recommend HIV testing
early in pregnancy to all their pregnant patients.

• Since 1995, CDC has recommended all pregnant women be
tested for HIV and, if found to be infected, offered treatment for
themselves to improve their health and to prevent passing the
virus to their infant.

What Testing Approaches Are Available?

There are two different ways to approach pregnant women about
HIV testing:

• Opt-in:

  • Pregnant women are given pre-HIV test counseling.

  • They must agree to receiving an HIV test, usually in writing.

• Opt-out:

  • Pregnant women are told that an HIV test will be included in
  the standard group of prenatal tests (that is to say, tests given
  to all pregnant women), and that they may decline the test.

  • Unless they decline, they will receive an HIV test.

Statistics published in the November 15, 2002, Morbidity Mortality Weekly Report (MMWR) showed that in eight states using the opt-in approach in 1998-1999, testing rates ranged from 25% to 69%. In Tennessee, which uses an opt-out approach, the testing rate was 85%. Other studies support this evidence that, of the voluntary approaches to prenatal HIV testing, more women are tested with the opt-out approach. An evaluation of opt-out testing in Birmingham, Ala. prenatal clinic showed that HIV testing increased from 75% to 88% after opt-out testing was implemented in August 1999. At the Denver Health Medical Center, 98.2% of women who delivered received HIV testing between 1998 and 2001, using opt-out testing.

Which Approach Does CDC Recommend?

In the 2006 *Revised Recommendations for HIV Testing of Adults, Adolescents, and Pregnant Women in Health-Care Settings*, CDC recommended the opt-out approach to testing for all adult and adolescent patients in healthcare settings, including pregnant women.

These recommendations emphasize:

- Universal "opt-out" HIV testing for all pregnant women early in every pregnancy;

- A second test in the third trimester in certain geographic areas or for women who are known to be at high risk of becoming infected (e.g., injection-drug users and their sex partners, women who exchange sex for money or drugs, women who are sex partners of HIV-infected persons, and women who have had a new or more than one sex partner during this pregnancy);

- Rapid HIV testing at labor and delivery for women without a prenatal test result; and

- Exploration of reasons that women decline testing.

Studies show that the opt-out approach can:

- Increase testing rates among pregnant women; thereby, increasing the number of pregnant women who know their HIV status;

- Increase the number of HIV-infected women who are offered treatment; and

- Reduce HIV transmission to their babies.

How Is Opt-Out Implemented in the Healthcare Setting?

Opt-out has three steps for healthcare providers to follow to put this approach into practice (CDC recommends all three steps):

- Tell all pregnant women that an HIV test will be performed as part of the standard group of tests for pregnant women.

- Tell all pregnant women that they may decline this test.

- Give all pregnant women information about how to prevent HIV transmission during pregnancy and provide information about treatment for pregnant women who are HIV-positive.

Section 16.6

Counseling for People Diagnosed with HIV

This section includes text excerpted from "2015 Sexually Transmitted Diseases Treatment Guidelines," Centers for Disease Control and Prevention (CDC), June 4, 2015.

Counseling for Persons with Human Immunodeficiency Virus Infection (HIV) and Referral to Support Services

Providers should expect persons with human immunodeficiency virus infection (HIV) to be distressed when first informed of a positive test result. Such persons face multiple major adaptive challenges, including coping with the reactions of others to a stigmatizing illness, developing and adopting strategies for maintaining physical and emotional health, initiating changes in behavior to prevent HIV transmission to others, and reducing the risk for acquiring additional sexually transmitted diseases (STDs). Many persons will require assistance with making reproductive choices, gaining access to health services, and coping with changes in personal relationships. Therefore, behavioral and psychosocial services are an integral part of healthcare for persons with HIV infection.

Persons testing positive for HIV infection have unique needs. Some require referral for specific behavioral interventions (e.g., a substance abuse program), mental health disorders (e.g., depression), and emotional distress, while others require assistance with securing and maintaining employment and housing. Women should be counseled or appropriately referred regarding reproductive choices and contraceptive options, and persons with multiple psychosocial problems might be candidates for comprehensive risk-reduction counseling and other support services.

The following are specific recommendations for HIV counseling and linkage to services that should be offered to patients before they leave the testing site.

- Persons who test positive for HIV should be counseled, either on-site or through referral, concerning the behavioral, psychosocial, and medical implications of HIV infection.

- Healthcare providers should assess the need for immediate medical care and psychosocial support.

- Providers should link persons with newly diagnosed HIV infection to services provided by healthcare personnel experienced in the management of HIV infection. Additional services that might be needed include substance abuse counseling and treatment, treatment for mental health disorders or emotional distress, reproductive counseling, risk-reduction counseling, and case management. Providers should follow up to ensure that patients have received services for any identified needs.

- Persons with HIV infection should be educated about the importance of ongoing medical care and what to expect from these services.

Several successful, innovative interventions to assist persons with HIV infection to reduce the possibility of transmission to others have been developed for diverse at-risk populations, and these can be locally replicated or adapted. Involvement of nongovernment and community-based organizations might complement such efforts in the clinical setting.

Chapter 17

Types of HIV Diagnostic Tests

Chapter Contents

Section 17.1

HIV Diagnostic Tests: An Overview

This section includes text excerpted from "Types of HIV Tests," Centers for Disease Control and Prevention (CDC), December 7, 2015.

What We Know about the Types of Human Immunodeficiency Virus Infection (HIV) Tests

Human immunodeficiency virus infection (HIV) tests are very accurate at detecting HIV, but no HIV test can detect HIV immediately after infection. How soon a test can detect infection depends upon different factors, including the type of test being used. In general, nucleic acid tests (NAT) can detect HIV the soonest, followed by combination or fourth generation tests, and then antibody tests.

Most HIV tests, including most rapid tests and home tests, are antibody tests. Antibodies are produced by your immune system when you're exposed to viruses like HIV and bacteria. Antibody tests look for these antibodies to HIV in your blood or oral fluid. In general, antibody tests that use blood can detect HIV slightly sooner after infection than tests done with oral fluid. With a rapid antibody screening test, results are ready in 30 minutes or less.

Home tests are antibody tests you can buy at a pharmacy or online. There are only two U.S. Food and Drug Administration (FDA)—approved home test kits:

1. the Home Access HIV-1 Test System

2. the OraQuick In-Home HIV Test

The **Home Access HIV-1 Test System** is a home collection kit, which involves pricking your finger to collect a blood sample, sending the sample to a licensed laboratory, and then calling in for results as early as the next business day. This test is anonymous. If the test is positive, a follow-up test is needed to confirm your results. The manufacturer provides confidential counseling and referral to treatment.

The **OraQuick In-Home HIV Test** provides fast results in the home. You have to swab your mouth for an oral fluid sample and use a kit to test it. Results are available in 20 minutes. If you test positive, you will need a follow-up test to confirm your results. The manufacturer provides confidential counseling and referral to follow-up testing sites. Because the level of antibody in oral fluid is lower than it is in blood, blood tests find infection sooner after exposure than oral fluid tests.

If you use any type of antibody test and have a positive result, you will need to take a follow-up test to confirm your results. If your first test is a rapid home test and it's positive, you will be sent to a health-care provider to get follow-up testing. If your first test is done in a testing lab and it's positive, the lab will conduct the follow-up testing, usually on the same blood sample as the first test. It can take 3–12 weeks (21–84 days) for an HIV-positive person's body to make enough antibodies for an antibody test to detect HIV infection. This time range is called the window period. If you get a negative HIV antibody test result during the window period, you should be retested 3 months after your possible exposure to HIV.

A combination or fourth-generation test looks for both HIV antibodies and antigens. Antigens are foreign substances that cause your immune system to activate. The antigen is part of the virus itself and is present during acute HIV infection. If you're infected with HIV, an antigen called p24 is produced even before antibodies develop. Combination screening tests are now recommended for testing done in labs and are becoming more common in the United States. There is now a rapid combination test available. It can take 2–6 weeks (13–42 days) for a person's body to make enough antigens and antibodies for a combination, or fourth-generation test to detect HIV. This time range is called the window period. If you get a negative combination test result during the window period, you should be retested 3 months after your possible exposure.

Nucleic acid tests (NAT) look for HIV in the blood. The test can give either a positive/negative result or an actual amount of virus present in the blood (known as a viral load test). This test is very expensive and not routinely used for screening individuals unless they recently had a high-risk exposure or a possible exposure to early symptoms of HIV infection. It can take 7–28 days for a NAT to detect HIV. Nucleic acid testing is usually considered accurate during the early stages of infection. However, it is best to get an antibody or combination test at the same time to help the doctor interpret the negative NAT. This is because a small number of people naturally decrease the amount of virus in their blood over time which can lead to an inaccurate negative NAT result. Taking preexposure prophylaxis (PrEP) or postexposure prophylaxis (PEP) may also reduce the accuracy of NAT if you have HIV.

What You Can Do

Talk to your healthcare provider to see what type of HIV test is right for you. They can tell you the window period for the type of test you take. If you're using a home test, you can get that information from the materials included in the test's package.

After you get tested, it's important for you to find out the result of your test so that you can talk to your healthcare provider about treatment options if you're HIV-positive or learn ways to prevent getting HIV if you're HIV-negative.

Section 17.2

Rapid Oral HIV Tests

This section contains text excerpted from the following sources: Text beginning with the heading "What Is a Rapid Oral Human Immunodeficiency Virus (HIV) Test?" is excerpted from "Rapid Oral HIV Test—Patient Fact Sheet," U.S. Department of Veterans Affairs (VA), March 2017; Text under the heading "How Accurate Is the Rapid Oral HIV Test?" is excerpted from "HIV/AIDS— Frequently Asked Questions," U.S. Department of Veterans Affairs (VA), January 11, 2017.

What Is a Rapid Oral Human Immunodeficiency Virus Infection (HIV) Test?

This is a test for human immunodeficiency virus infection (HIV), the virus that causes acquired immunodeficiency syndrome (AIDS). With a rapid oral test, results take about 20 minutes. There are also rapid tests that use a blood sample. Rapid tests are usually used when results need to be delivered within a few minutes, like in an outreach center or homeless clinic; otherwise, a traditional blood test is used. The rapid oral test is quite good at detecting chronic (long-standing) HIV infection but not so good at detecting very recent HIV infection.

How Does the Rapid Oral HIV Test Work?

When HIV enters the body, antibodies are produced. The test looks for HIV antibodies in your oral fluids. The test uses a swab to collect a sample from the inside of your mouth.

What Happens When You Agree to Be Tested?

The test is explained to you by a health provider. A health provider will ask you to swab your gums with a special swab. Results are ready in about 20 minutes. You will learn your HIV result and discuss what it means. Your provider will give you information about how to protect yourself and others from HIV. If your test result is positive, you will do a second, different, test using a blood sample that is sent to the lab. Your test result will be confidential (results will only be discussed with you).

What Does a Negative Rapid Oral HIV Test Result Mean?

This means that HIV antibodies have not been found in your system. This could mean one of two things:

1. You do not have HIV, or

2. You have HIV but it was not detected by the rapid oral test (this is a false-negative result).

It can take up to 3 months for your system to produce enough antibodies to be detected by the rapid oral test. If you have engaged in activities that might put you at risk of HIV infection in the past 3 months, you should repeat the test in a few weeks, or talk with your provider about doing a standard blood test for HIV right away.

What Does a Positive Rapid Oral HIV Test Result Mean?

This means that HIV antibodies may be in your system. Positive results on the rapid test must always be confirmed by doing a second HIV test. This is because sometimes (rarely) the rapid oral test gives a false-positive result. A person is considered to be HIV positive only if two different test results are positive. The second HIV test is a blood test that is sent to the lab; the results may take up to 1–2 weeks to return.

If your positive result is confirmed by a second test, that means:

- You have HIV and should be evaluated right away for treatment

- Your testing site will refer you to a clinic that has expertise in caring for people with HIV. They may also refer you for counseling and other support services.

- HIV treatment (medication) greatly improves health and can prevent transmission (infection) to others

Why Should You Get Tested?

Many HIV-positive people do not know they are infected with HIV because they have never been tested. Knowing your HIV status helps you protect yourself and others. Getting diagnosed early can greatly improve your health. Although there is no cure for HIV, there are many effective medicines that can control it. Most people with HIV who take their medication every day can live long, healthy lives. If you test negative, you may feel less anxious after testing, and you may be more committed to preventing yourself from becoming infected.

An HIV test is part of routine medical care.

How Accurate Is the Rapid Oral HIV Test?

The rapid oral HIV test detects antibodies made by the immune system in response to HIV infection, just like the standard blood antibody test. The rapid oral test, however, detects these antibodies in oral fluid and doesn't require a blood sample.

The rapid oral HIV test has similar accuracy to the standard blood antibody test for persons with chronic, or long-standing, HIV infection. But, like any antibody test for HIV, the rapid oral HIV test is not reliable during the "window period" (lasting several weeks to months) between the time a person is infected and the time the body has made enough antibodies for the test to detect. During this window period, someone who is infected might test negative for antibodies (a false-negative result). The "window period" for the rapid oral test is longer than it is for some HIV blood tests, meaning that for someone with acute or new HIV infection certain blood tests can detect HIV earlier than the oral rapid tests can.

It also is possible to have false-positive results (a person may have a positive rapid oral HIV test result but not be actually infected with

HIV). That's why anyone who has a positive result with a rapid oral HIV test must have a more specific "confirmatory" blood test before a diagnosis of HIV infection can be made.

Section 17.3

HIV Home Test Kits

This section contains text excerpted from the following sources: Text in this chapter begins with excerpts from "HIV/AIDS—Home Tests," Centers for Disease Control and Prevention (CDC), October 16, 2015; Text under the heading "Home Access Human Immunodeficiency Virus Infection (HIV)-1 Test System" is excerpted from "Information Regarding the Home Access HIV-1 Test System," U.S. Food and Drug Administration (FDA), March 7, 2018; Text under the heading "OraQuick In-Home HIV Test" is excerpted from "Information Regarding the OraQuick In-Home HIV Test," U.S. Food and Drug Administration (FDA), February 5, 2018.

As of now, there are only two home HIV tests: the Home Access HIV-1 Test System and the OraQuick In-home HIV test. If you buy your home test online make sure the HIV test is U.S. Food and Drug Administration (FDA)-approved.

The **Home Access HIV-1 Test System** is a home collection kit, which involves pricking your finger to collect a blood sample, sending the sample to a licensed laboratory, and then calling in for results as early as the next business day. This test is anonymous. If the test is positive, a follow-up test is performed right away, and the results include the follow-up test. The manufacturer provides confidential counseling and referral to treatment. The tests conducted on the blood sample collected at home find infection later after infection than most lab-based tests using blood from a vein, but earlier than tests conducted with oral fluid.

The **OraQuick In-Home HIV Test** provides rapid results in the home. The testing procedure involves swabbing your mouth for an oral fluid sample and using a kit to test it. Results are available in 20 minutes. If you test positive, you will need a follow-up test. The manufacturer provides confidential counseling and referral to follow-up testing sites. Because the level of antibody in oral fluid is lower than it is in blood, oral fluid tests find infection later after exposure than do blood tests. Up to 1 in 12 infected people may test false-negative with this test.

Home Access Human Immunodeficiency Virus Infection (HIV)-1 Test System

What Is the Home Access HIV-1 Test System?

The Home Access HIV-1 Test System is a laboratory test sold over-the-counter (OTC) that uses fingerstick blood mailed to the testing laboratory. The test kit consists of multiple components, including materials for specimen self-collection, prepaid materials for mailing the specimen to a laboratory for testing, testing directions, an information booklet, an anonymous registration system, and a call center to receive your test results and follow-up counseling by telephone.

This approved system uses a finger prick process for home blood collection which results in dried blood spots on special paper. The dried blood spots are mailed to a laboratory with a confidential and anonymous unique personal identification number (PIN) and are analyzed by trained clinicians in a laboratory using the same tests that are used for samples taken in a doctor's office or clinic. Test results are obtained through a toll-free number using the PIN, and posttest counseling is provided by telephone when results are obtained.

When Should I Take a Test for HIV?

If you actively engage in behavior that puts you at risk for HIV infection, or your partner engages in such behavior, then you should consider testing on a regular basis. It may take some time for the immune system to produce sufficient antibodies for the test to detect, and this time period can vary from person to person. This time-frame is commonly referred to as the "window period," when a person is infected with HIV but antibodies to the virus cannot be detected, however, the person may be able to infect others. According to the Centers for Disease Control and Prevention (CDC), it can take up to 6 months to develop antibodies to HIV, although most people (97%) will develop detectable antibodies in the first 3 months following the time of their infection.

How Reliable Is the Home Access HIV-1 Test System?

Clinical studies reported to FDA showed that the sensitivity (i.e., the percentage of results that will be positive when HIV is present) was estimated to be greater than 99.9 percent. The specificity (i.e., the percentage of results that will be negative when HIV is not present) was also estimated to be greater than 99.9 percent. Results reported as positive have undergone testing using both a screening test and another test to confirm the positive result.

What about Counseling?

The Home Access HIV-1 Test System has a built-in mechanism for pretest and posttest counseling provided by the manufacturer. This counseling is anonymous and confidential. Counseling, which uses both printed material and telephone interaction, provides the user with an interpretation of the test result. Counseling also provides information on how to keep from getting infected if you are negative, and how to prevent further transmission of disease if you are infected. Counseling provides you with information about treatment options if you are infected, and can even provide referrals to doctors who treat HIV-infected individuals in your area.

If the Test Results Are Positive, What Should I Do?

The counselors can provide you with information about treatment options and referrals to doctors who treat HIV-infected individuals in your area.

Do I Need a Confirmatory Test?

No, a positive result from the Home Access HIV-1 Test System means that antibodies to the HIV-1 virus are present in the blood sample submitted to the testing laboratory. The Home Access HIV-1 Test System includes confirmatory testing for HIV-1, and all confirmation testing is completed before the results are released and available to users of the test system.

How Quickly Will I Get the Results of the Home Access HIV-1 Test System?

You can anonymously call for the results approximately 7 business days (3 business days for the Express System) after shipping your specimen to the laboratory by using the unique PIN on the tear-off label included with your test kit. This label includes both the unique PIN and the toll-free number for the counseling center.

How Are Unapproved Test Systems Different?

The manufacturers of unapproved test systems have not submitted data to FDA to review to determine whether or not their test systems can reliably detect HIV infection. Therefore, FDA cannot give the public any assurance that the results obtained using an unapproved test system are accurate.

OraQuick In-Home HIV Test

What Is the OraQuick In-Home HIV Test and How Does It Work?

The OraQuick In-Home HIV Test is a rapid self-administered over-the-counter (OTC) test. The OraQuick In-Home HIV Test kit consists of a test stick (device) to collect the specimen, a test tube (vial) to insert the test stick (device) and complete the test, testing directions, two information booklets, a disposal bag, and phone numbers for consumer support.

This approved test uses oral fluid to check for antibodies to HIV Type 1 and HIV Type 2, the viruses that cause AIDS. The kit is designed to allow you to take the HIV test anonymously and in private with the collection of an oral fluid sample by swabbing your upper and lower gums with the test device. After collecting the sample you insert the device into the kit's vial which contains a developer solution, wait for 20–40 minutes, and read the test result. A positive result with this test does not mean that an individual is definitely infected with HIV but rather that additional testing should be done in a medical setting to confirm the test result. Additionally, a negative test result does not mean that an individual is definitely not infected with HIV, particularly when exposure may have been within the previous three months. Again an individual should obtain a confirmatory test in a medical setting.

When Should I Take a Test for HIV?

If you actively engage in behavior that puts you at risk for HIV infection, or your partner engages in such behavior, then you should consider testing on a regular basis. It can take some time for the immune system to produce enough antibodies for the test to detect, and this time period can vary from person to person. This timeframe is commonly referred to as the "window period," when a person is infected with HIV but antibodies to the virus can not be detected, however, the person may be able to infect others. According to the Centers for Disease Control and Prevention (CDC), although it can take up to 6 months to develop antibodies for HIV, most people (97%) will develop detectable antibodies in the first 3 months following the time of their infection.

How Reliable Is the OraQuick In-Home HIV Test?

As noted in the package insert, clinical studies have shown that the OraQuick In-Home HIV Test has an expected performance of approximately 92 percent for test sensitivity (i.e., the percentage of results that will be positive when HIV is present). This means that one false negative result would be expected out of every 12 test results in HIV infected individuals. The clinical studies also showed that the OraQuick In-Home HIV Test has an expected performance of 99.98 percent for test specificity (i.e., the percentage of results that will be negative when HIV is not present). This means that one false positive result would be expected out of every 5,000 test results in uninfected individuals.

It is extremely important for those who self-test using the OraQuick In-Home HIV Test to carefully read and follow all labeled directions. Even when used according to the labeled directions, there will be some false negative results and a small number of false-positive results. The OraQuick test package contains step-by-step instructions, and there is also an OraQuick consumer support center (Toll-Free: 866-436-6527) to assist users in the testing process.

If the Test Says I'm HIV Positive, What Should I Do?

A positive test result does not necessarily mean that you are infected with HIV. If you test positive for HIV using the OraQuick In-Home Test, you should see your healthcare provider or call the OraQuick consumer support center, which has support center representatives available 24 hours a day/7 days a week to answer your questions and provide referrals to local healthcare providers for follow-up care. You will be advised to obtain confirmatory testing to confirm a positive result or inform you that the initial result was a false positive result. The test kit also contains an information booklet, "What your results mean to You," which is designed to instruct individuals on what to do once they have obtained their test results.

Do I Need a Confirmatory Test?

A positive test result on the OraQuick In-Home HIV Test indicates that you may be infected with HIV. Additional testing in a medical setting will either confirm a positive test result or inform you that the initial result was a false positive result.

What Is a "False Positive" Result?

A "false positive" result occurs when an individual not infected with the HIV virus receives a test result that indicates that he or she is infected with HIV.

If the Test Says I'm HIV Negative, What Should I Do?

A negative result on this test does not necessarily mean that you are not infected with HIV. The OraQuick test kit contains an information booklet, "What your results mean to You," which is designed to instruct individuals on what to do once they have obtained their test results. The test is relatively reliable if there has been sufficient time for HIV antibodies to develop in the infected person. For the OraQuick In-Home HIV Test, that period of time, called the window period, is about three months. If you have recently been engaging in behavior that puts you at high risk for HIV infection, you should take the test again at a later time. Alternatively, you should see your healthcare provider who can discuss other options for HIV testing.

What Is a "False Negative" Result?

A "false negative" result occurs when an HIV-infected individual receives a test result that incorrectly indicates that he or she is not infected with HIV.

How Quickly Will I Get the Results of the OraQuick Test?

You can read the results of the OraQuick In-Home HIV Test within 20–40 minutes.

How Are Unapproved Test Systems Different?

The manufacturers of unapproved test systems have not submitted data to FDA in order for FDA to review and determine whether their test systems can reliably detect HIV infection. Therefore, FDA cannot give the public any assurance that the results obtained using an unapproved test system are accurate.

Chapter 18

Understanding Your Test Results

What Does a Negative Test Result Mean?

A negative result doesn't necessarily mean that you don't have human immunodeficiency virus (HIV). That's because of the window period—the time between when a person gets HIV and when a test can accurately detect it. The window period varies from person to person and is also different depending on the type of HIV test.

Ask your healthcare provider about the window period for the test you're taking. If you're using a home test, you can get that information from the materials included in the test's package. If you get an HIV test within 3 months after a potential HIV exposure and the result is negative, get tested again in 3 more months to be sure.

If you learned you were HIV-negative the last time you were tested, you can only be sure you're still negative if you haven't had a potential HIV exposure since your last test. If you're sexually active, continue to take actions to prevent HIV, like using condoms the right way every time you have sex and taking medicines to prevent HIV if you're at high risk.

This chapter includes text excerpted from "Understanding HIV Test Results," HIV.gov, U.S. Department of Health and Human Services (HHS), May 15, 2017.

If I Have a Negative Test Result, Does That Mean That My Partner Is HIV-Negative Also?

No. Your HIV test result reveals only your HIV status. HIV is not necessarily transmitted every time you have sex. Therefore, taking an HIV test is not a way to find out if your partner is infected.

It's important to be open with your partner(s) and ask them to tell you their HIV status. But keep in mind that your partner(s) may not know or may be wrong about their status, and some may not tell you if they have HIV even if they know they're infected. Consider getting tested together so you can both know your HIV status and take steps to keep yourselves healthy.

What Does a Positive Test Result Mean?

A follow-up test will be conducted. If the follow-up test is also positive, it means you are HIV-positive.

If you had a rapid screening test, the testing site will arrange a follow-up test to make sure the screening test result was correct. If your blood was tested in a lab, the lab will conduct a follow-up test on the same sample.

It is important that you start medical care and begin HIV treatment as soon as possible after you are diagnosed with HIV. Antiretroviral therapy or ART (taking medicines to treat HIV infection) is recommended for all people with HIV, regardless of how long they've had the virus or how healthy they are. ART slows the progression of HIV and helps protect your immune system. It can keep you healthy for many years and greatly reduces your chance of transmitting HIV to your sex partner(s) if taken the right way, every day.

If you have health insurance, your insurer is required to cover some medicines used to treat HIV. If you don't have health insurance, or you're unable to afford your copay or coinsurance amount, you may be eligible for government programs that can help through Medicaid, Medicare, the Ryan White HIV/AIDS Program, and community health centers. Your healthcare provider or local public health department can tell you where to get HIV treatment.

- To lower your risk of transmitting HIV

- Take medicines to treat HIV (ART) the right way every day

- Use condoms the right way every time you have sex. Learn the right ways to use a male condom and a female condom.

- If your partner is HIV-negative, encourage them to talk to their healthcare provider to see if taking daily medicine to prevent HIV (called preexposure prophylaxis, or PrEP) is right for them

- If you think your partner might have been recently exposed to HIV—for example, if the condom breaks during sex and you are not virally suppressed—they should talk to a healthcare provider right away (no later than 3 days) about taking medicines (called postexposure prophylaxis, or PEP) to prevent getting HIV

Get tested and treated for STDs and encourage your partner to do the same.

Receiving a diagnosis of HIV can be a life-changing event. People can feel many emotions—sadness, hopelessness, and even anger. Allied healthcare providers and social service providers, often available at your healthcare provider's office, will have the tools to help you work through the early stages of your diagnosis and begin to manage your HIV.

Talking to others who have HIV may also be helpful. Find a local HIV support group. Learn about how other people living with HIV have handled their diagnosis.

If I Test Positive for HIV, Does That Mean I Have Acquired Immunodeficiency Syndrome (AIDS)?

No. Being HIV-positive does not mean you have acquired immunodeficiency syndrome (AIDS). AIDS is the most advanced stage of HIV disease. HIV can lead to AIDS if not treated.

Will Other People Know My Test Result?

If you take an anonymous test, no one but you will know the result. If you take a confidential test, your test result will be part of your medical record, but it is still protected by state and federal privacy laws. Most testing is done confidentially.

- Anonymous testing means that nothing ties your test results to you. When you take an anonymous HIV test, you get a unique identifier that allows you to get your test results. These tests are not available at every place that provides HIV testing.

- Confidential testing means that your name and other identifying information will be attached to your test results. The results will go in your medical record and may be shared with your healthcare providers and your health insurance company. Otherwise, the results are protected by state and federal privacy laws, and they can be released only with your permission.

With confidential testing, if you test positive for HIV, the test result and your name will be reported to the state or local health department to help public health officials get better estimates of the rates of HIV in the state. The state health department will then remove all personal information about you (name, address, etc.) and share the remaining nonidentifying information with the Centers for Disease Control and Prevention (CDC). CDC does not share this information with anyone else, including insurance companies.

As a follow up to a positive HIV test, the local health department may contact you to make sure that you received the test results and understood them, and to find out whether you received referrals to HIV medical care and social services and whether you have received HIV medical care and treatment. The health department representative may talk with you about the need to tell your sexual or needle-sharing partner(s) about their possible exposure to HIV. They may also offer partner services to assist you with these conversations. If you want, the health department can try attempt to locate any or all of your partners to let them know they may have been exposed to HIV. They will be able to help them find a place to get tested and give them information about PrEP, PEP, and other ways that they can protect themselves and access other prevention and care services.

Chapter 19

You and Your HIV/AIDS Healthcare Provider: First Steps

Chapter Contents

Section 19.1

Choosing a Healthcare Provider

This section includes text excerpted from "Starting HIV Care—Find
a Provider—Locate a HIV Care Provider," HIV.gov, U.S. Department
of Health and Human Services (HHS), May 15, 2017.

Once you receive a diagnosis of human immunodeficiency virus
(HIV), the most important next step is to get into medical care. Getting into medical care and staying on treatment will help you manage
your HIV effectively and make decisions that can keep you healthy
for many years.

If you received your diagnosis in a healthcare provider's office or
a nonclinical setting (health fair, community organization, or testing
event), you have probably received a lot of information about HIV, its
treatment, and how to stay healthy. Give yourself time to absorb the
information and get into care and on treatment right away.

If you received a diagnosis by taking an HIV test at home, it is
important that you take the next steps to make sure the result is
correct. Both manufacturers provide confidential counseling and will
help you with getting the follow-up test done.

Finding a Human Immunodeficiency Virus (HIV) Care Provider

If you have a primary healthcare provider (someone who manages
your regular medical care and annual tests), that person may have
the medical knowledge to treat your HIV. If not, he or she can refer
you to a healthcare provider who is a specialist in providing HIV care
and treatment.

Here are some other services to help you locate HIV providers and
services near you:

- HIV.gov's HIV Testing Sites and Care Services Locator (locator.
  hiv.gov) can help you find HIV-related services across the United
  States, including HIV medical care, HIV testing, housing assistance,
  and substance abuse and mental health services (from HIV.gov).

- State HIV/AIDS toll-free hotlines (hab.hrsa.gov/get-care/state-
  hivaids-hotlines) are available to help you connect with agencies
  that can help determine what services you are eligible for and
  help you get them (from the Health Resources and Services
  Administration (HRSA)).

- The Ryan White HIV/AIDS Medical Care Provider Locator (findhivcare.hrsa.gov) can help you find medical providers who can help people living with HIV/AIDS access the medical care they need but can't afford (from the HRSA).

- This directory of credentialed HIV care specialists (aahivm. org/ReferralLink/exec/frmAdvSearch.aspx) and members of the American Academy of HIV Medicine (AAHIVM) can help you access HIV practitioners across the country (from the AAHIVM).

It is important that you start medical care and begin HIV treatment as soon as possible after you are diagnosed with HIV. Antiretroviral therapy (ART) is recommended for all people with HIV, regardless of how long they've had the virus or how healthy they are. Starting ART slows the progression of HIV and helps protect your immune system. ART is taken consistently and correctly, it can keep you healthy for many years and greatly reduces your chance of transmitting HIV to sex partners.

Most people living with HIV who do not seek medical care eventually receive an AIDS diagnosis. This happens because, if left untreated, HIV will attack the immune system and allow different types of life-threatening infections and cancers to develop. A cure for HIV does not yet exist, but ART can dramatically prolong the lives of many people living with HIV and lower their chance of infecting others.

Types of Providers

Who Should Be on My Healthcare Team?

Finding a healthcare team that is knowledgeable about HIV care is an important step in managing your care and treatment. If you are able to choose your provider, you should look for someone who has a great deal of experience treating HIV. This matters because the more HIV experience your provider has, the more familiar he or she will be with the full range of treatment options, as well as the unique issues that can come up in HIV care over time.

Who is on your HIV healthcare team will depend on your healthcare needs and the way that the healthcare system, clinic, or office you will get your care from is set up. It should also be based on your preferences and what will work best for you. Don't get hung up on finding the perfect provider the first week after you are diagnosed. The most important thing you can do now for your health is to meet with an HIV provider who can order your first lab tests and start HIV treatment as soon as possible. Don't let the search for the perfect doctor slow you down on this. You can change doctors later if you need to.

Your HIV healthcare provider should lead your healthcare team. That person will help you determine which HIV medicines are best for you, prescribe antiretroviral therapy (ART), monitor your progress, and partner with you in managing your health. He or she can also help put you in touch with other types of providers who can address your needs. Your primary HIV healthcare provider may be a doctor of medicine (MD) or doctor of osteopathic medicine (DO), nurse practitioner (NP), or a physician assistant (PA). On the whole, the patients of providers with more experience in HIV care tend to do better than those who see a provider who only has limited HIV care experience.

In addition to your HIV healthcare provider, your healthcare team may include other healthcare providers, allied healthcare professionals, and social service providers who are experts in taking care of people living with HIV.

The types of professionals who may be involved in your HIV care include:

Healthcare Providers

- **Medical doctors (MD or DO).** Healthcare professionals who are licensed to practice medicine.

- **Nurse practitioners (NP).** Registered nurses, with specialized graduate education, who can diagnose and treat illnesses independently, or as part of a healthcare team.

- **Physician assistants (PA).** Healthcare professionals who are trained to examine patients, diagnose injuries and illnesses, and provide treatment to patients under the supervision of physicians and surgeons.

Allied Healthcare Professionals

- **Nurses.** Healthcare professionals who provide and coordinate patient care as part of a healthcare team.

- **Mental health providers.** Professionals, such as a counselor, psychologist, or psychiatrist, who provide mental healthcare in the form of counseling or other types of therapy.

- **Pharmacists.** Healthcare professionals who provide prescription medicines to patients and offer expertise in the safe use of prescriptions. Pharmacists may also provide advice on how to lead a healthy life; conduct health and wellness screenings; provide immunizations; and oversee medicines given to patients.

- **Nutritionists/dietitians.** Experts in food and nutrition who advise people on what to eat in order to lead a healthy lifestyle or achieve a specific health-related goal.

- **Dentists.** Healthcare professionals who diagnose and treat problems with a person's teeth, gums, and related parts of the mouth. Dentists also provide advice and instruction on taking care of teeth and gums and on diet choices that affect oral health.

Social Service Providers

- **Social workers.** Professionals who help people solve and cope with problems in their everyday lives.

- **Case managers.** Professionals who help people find the support and services they need, develop a services plan, and follow up to make sure that services are provided.

- **Substance use/abuse specialists.** Counselors who provide advice, treatment, and support to people who have problems with substance use.

Patient Navigators

There are a number of different types of navigators who are trained and culturally sensitive workers who provide support and guidance to people by helping them "navigate" through the healthcare system. For example, navigators could be healthcare workers, social workers, those who work for community-based organizations, or peers.

Take Charge of Your Care

How Can I Work Best with My Healthcare Team?

HIV treatment is most successful when you actively take part in your medical care. That means taking your HIV medications every time, at the right time, and in the right way; keeping your medical appointments; and communicating honestly with your healthcare provider. This can be achieved when you:

- **Keep all of your medical appointments.** There are many tools you can use to help you remember and prepare for your appointments. You can:
  - Use a calendar to mark your appointment days
  - Set reminders on your phone
  - Download a free app from the Internet to your computer or smartphone that can help remind you of your medical appointments. Search for "reminder apps" and you will find many choices.
  - Keep your appointment card reminder in a place where you will see it often, such as on a mirror, or on your refrigerator
  - Ask a family member or friend to help you remember your appointment

- **Be prepared for your medical appointments.** Before an appointment, write down questions or concerns you want to discuss with your healthcare provider. Be prepared to write down the answers you receive during your visit.
  - If you can't keep a scheduled appointment, contact your provider to let them know, and make a fresh appointment as soon as possible.

- **Communicate openly and honestly with your healthcare providers.** Your healthcare provider needs to have the most accurate information to manage your care and treatment.

- **Keep track of your medical services.** You may have multiple healthcare providers working on your healthcare team. Keep records of your lab results, medical visits, appointment dates and times, medicines and medicine schedules, and care and treatment plans.

Update your contact information. Make sure your healthcare providers have your correct contact information (telephone number, address, and e-mail address) and let them know if any contact information changes.

Section 19.2

Visiting a Healthcare Provider

This section includes text excerpted from "Staying in HIV
Care—Provider Visits and Lab Tests—Making Care Work
for You," HIV.gov, U.S. Department of Health and
Human Services (HHS), May 15, 2017.

Making Human Immunodeficiency Virus (HIV) Care Work

The first year after being diagnosed, especially the first weeks is challenging at times for most people as they adjust to life with HIV. The process is different for different people. For some people, it is quick. For others, it takes longer. That's ok, as long as you are making progress and are dealing with your HIV by getting HIV care, taking your HIV medication, and getting support and other assistance you may need. It's not ok if you are blocking it out of your mind completely and are not taking any action to protect your health or the health of your sex partners. Not thinking about HIV will not get it under control. Only getting in care, staying in care, and continuing to take your HIV medication every day will do that.

That doesn't mean it will be easy all the time. Staying in care, taking medication every day, and dealing with the other things that come along with HIV can be hard sometimes. HIV is an unwelcome trespasser in your body. It is a part of your life, but it does not need to define your life or who you are.

Taking the steps that are necessary for you to get control over the virus can make it easier for you to put more time and energy toward the other parts of your life. A key to this is figuring out what works for you to make and keep your medical appointments, take your medication every day, and make sure that you are protecting your health and the health of others from risks that can come along with some sexual activities and substance use. It can take time to figure out what works for you. If you don't get it right at first, keep on trying different strategies and approaches. Talking to other people living with HIV, close friends whose judgment you trust, mental health professionals, and your physician can help you find solutions that work for you and give you support along the way. You can also find support and assistance from HIV/acquired immunodeficiency syndrome (AIDS) service organizations that exist in most places.

217

Once you find out what works for you, HIV can become a smaller part of your life. For many people, getting HIV medical care, taking medications, and protecting others can be automatic most of the time. This happens because they've already figured out what to do, they've done it before, and they know they can do it again. Of course, nothing stays the same forever and unexpected things can happen that make it harder to manage life with HIV again. If this happens, step back, think about what has changed and about what you had been doing. Be open to rethinking things and to change what you've been doing. Don't be too hard on yourself, and give up. Get support from others to help think through the issues and learn from their experiences. Think about some of the barriers that you have already overcome, and remind yourself of the strengths, abilities, and support systems that you have built up over time. Some of the other information on this site may be useful to you in figuring this out, especially the information about HIV treatment, mental health, substance use and other topics related to living well with HIV.

Remember, living with HIV is about living. It's not about the fear of what might happen or about feeling bad about the past. It is about living today. It's about being a good friend, family member, partner, or neighbor. It's about doing what you can to do to be healthy and happy and to continue to be a contributing member of society for many years to come.

Seeing Your Healthcare Provider

Managing Your Appointments

HIV is a treatable condition. If you are diagnosed early, get on antiretroviral therapy (ART), and adhere to your medication, you can stay healthy, live a normal lifespan, and reduce the chances of transmitting HIV to others. Part of staying healthy is seeing your HIV care provider regularly so that he or she can track your progress and make sure your HIV treatment is working for you.

Your HIV care provider might be a doctor, nurse practitioner, or physician assistant. Some people living with HIV go to an HIV clinic; others see an HIV specialist at a community health center or other health clinic; and some people see their provider in a private practice. Current guidelines recommend that most people living with HIV see their provider for lab tests every 3–4 months. Some people may see their provider more frequently, especially during the first two years of treatment or if their HIV viral load is not suppressed (i.e., very low or undetectable). The guidelines say that people who take their medication every day and have had a suppressed viral load at every test for more than 2 years only need to have their lab tests done two times a year.

In addition to seeing your HIV care provider, you may need to see other healthcare practitioners, including dentists, nurses, case managers, social workers, psychiatrists/psychologists, pharmacists, and medical specialists. This may mean juggling multiple appointments, but it is all part of staying healthy. You can help make this easier by preparing a plan for yourself.

Before Your Visit

For many people living with HIV, appointments with their HIV care provider become a routine part of their life. These tips may help you better prepare for your visits to your HIV care provider and get more out of them:

- **Start with a list or a notebook.** Write down any questions you have before you go.

- **Make a list of your health and life goals** so that you can talk about them with your HIV provider and how she/he can help you reach them.

- **Make a list of any symptoms or problems** you are experiencing that you want to talk to your provider about.

- **Bring a list of all the HIV and non-HIV medications that you are taking** (or the medications themselves), including over-the-counter (OTC) medications, vitamins, or supplements. Include a list of any HIV medications you may have taken in the past and any problems you had when taking them.

- **Bring along a copy of your medical records** if you are seeing a provider who does not already have them. You have the right to access your medical records and having copies of your records can help you keep track of your lab results, prescriptions, and other health information. It can also help your provider have a better understanding of your health history.

- **Be prepared to talk about any changes in your living situation, relationships, insurance, or employment** that may affect your ability to keep up with your HIV appointments and treatment or to take care of yourself. Your provider may be able to connect you with resources or services that may assist you.

- **Be on time.** Most healthcare providers have full appointment schedules—if you are late, you throw the schedule off for everyone who comes after you. If you are late, there is a chance your provider will not be able to see you the same day.

During Your Visit

The following tips will help you during your visit:

- **Lab tests.** If your provider wants to run some lab tests during your visit, make sure you understand what the lab tests are for and what your provider will do with the results. If you don't understand, ask your provider to explain it in everyday terms. Typically, you will be asked to give a sample (blood, urine) during your visit and your provider's office will call you with your results in a few days. Keep track of your results and call your provider back if you have any questions.

- **Be honest.** Your provider isn't there to judge you, but to make decisions with you based on your particular circumstances. Talk about any HIV medication doses you have missed. Tell your provider about your sexual or alcohol/drug use history. These behaviors can put you at risk of developing drug resistance and getting other sexually transmitted infections (STIs) as well as hepatitis. Your provider will work with you to develop strategies to keep you as healthy as possible.

- **Describe any side effects you may be having from your HIV medications.** Your provider will want to know how the HIV medications are affecting your body in order to work with you to solve any problems and find the right combination of medications for you.

- **Get appointments for your next visit.** Ask your provider about your next visit and what you should bring to that appointment.

- **Ask for a list of your upcoming appointments when you check out.** Work with your case manager, if you have one, to develop a system to help you remember your appointments, such as a calendar, app, or text/e-mail reminders.

Asking Questions and Solving Problems

It's important for you to be an active participant in your own health-care and it's your right to ask questions. You may need to direct your questions to different people, depending on what you need/want to know:

- HIV care providers (doctors, nurse practitioners, physician assistants) can answer specific questions about a wide range of issues that affect your health. They can also help you find resources and solutions to problems you may have that affect your health, including:

  - Your prognosis (how your HIV disease is affecting your body)

  - How to manage any symptoms you may be experiencing

  - Medication issues, including medication changes, newly prescribed medications, and how the HIV medications may interact with other medications you take

  - Sexual health issues, including questions about any sexual symptoms you may be having, and how you can prevent or treat STIs, and how you can prevent transmitting HIV to your partner(s)

  - Family planning considerations, including your goals; birth control options for you and/or your partner, if relevant; your options for having children should you wish to do so; and, if you are an HIV-positive woman who is pregnant or considering getting pregnant, how you can reduce the risk of transmitting HIV to your baby

  - Substance use issues, including how alcohol/drug use can affect your HIV treatment and overall health, and whether you should be referred for substance abuse treatment

  - Mental health issues, including questions about any mental health symptoms you may be having, and whether you should be referred for mental health treatment

  - Referrals for other medical issues you may be experiencing

  - The meaning of lab test results

  - The need for surgical procedures, if relevant

  - Medication adherence strategies (tips for keeping up with your medication and ensuring you take it as scheduled and exactly as prescribed)

  - Any clinical trials or research studies that may be relevant for you

- Information about resources and services that can help you with issues or challenges you may be having that affect your health

- Nurses and case managers often have more time to answer questions about what you discuss with your provider and to help identify solutions to problems that are affecting your health, particularly around:

  - Understanding your HIV treatment plan, including how many pills of each medicine you should take; when to take each medicine; how to take each medicine (for example, with or without food); and how to store each medicine

  - Understanding possible side effects from your HIV medication and what you should do if you experience them

  - Challenges you may have in taking your medications and/ or keeping your medical appointments, and strategies for overcoming these challenges

  - Resources to help you better understand lab reports, tests, and procedures

  - Mental health and/or substance abuse treatment, housing assistance, food assistance, and other resources that exist in your community

  - Insurance and pharmacy benefits, and other aspects of paying for care

  - Understanding other medical conditions you may have

  - How to quit smoking and resources that are available to assist you

  - Information about resources and services that can help you with issues or challenges you may be having that affect your health

Dental Appointments

Dental visits are an extremely important part of your care when living with HIV. Many signs of HIV infection can begin in the mouth and throat, and people with HIV are more likely to develop some serious dental problems. For these reasons, it is important to see a dentist regularly.

Tips for your dental visit:

- **Make sure you have routine dental visits for cleaning and check-ups.** Preventing problems before they occur is always the best approach.

- **Tell your dentist you have HIV.** That's not because your dentist will need to take additional precautions—all healthcare professionals use "universal precautions" to prevent the transmission of bloodborne diseases to patients and vice versa. Rather, it will help the dentist know to look for particular oral health problems that you might be at risk for.

- **Don't wait for problems in your mouth to get out of hand.** When you notice something wrong (such as tooth pain or a mouth sore), call your dentist right away.

- **Be on time for your dental visit.** Try not to miss your appointment, if you can help it—and if you can't, reschedule it as soon as possible.

- **Keep a record of your dental visits, just like you do with your visits to your HIV care provider.** Keep track of when you had dental X-rays (and what was X-rayed), any procedures or treatments you had, and when your next visit is scheduled.

- **Bring copies of your recent test results and lab reports.** Your dentist may need to have information about your cluster of differentiation 4 (CD4) count and platelet count to know how best to treat your dental issue. Also bring a list of any medications you are currently taking, as your dentist needs to know what you are taking to avoid giving you other medications which may have bad interactions.

- **Know your rights.** Any dentist licensed in the United States should be able to provide at least basic dental care to people living with HIV.

Chapter 20

Just Diagnosed: Next Steps after Testing Positive for HIV

What Is the Next Step after Testing Positive for Human Immunodeficiency Virus (HIV)?

Testing positive for human immunodeficiency virus (HIV) often leaves a person overwhelmed with questions and concerns. It's important to remember that HIV is a manageable disease that can be treated with HIV medicines.

The first step after testing positive is to see a healthcare provider, even if you don't feel sick. People with HIV work closely with their healthcare providers to decide when to start HIV medicines and what HIV medicines to take.

The use of HIV medicines to treat HIV infection is called antiretroviral therapy (ART). People on ART take a combination of HIV medicines (called an HIV regimen) every day. ART prevents HIV from multiplying and reduces the amount of HIV in the body. ART can't cure HIV, but it helps people with HIV live longer, healthier lives and reduces the risk of HIV transmission.

People with HIV should start ART as soon as possible. In people with HIV who have certain conditions, such as certain HIV-related illnesses and coinfections, it's especially important to start ART right

---

This chapter includes text excerpted from "HIV Treatment," AIDS*info*, U.S. Department of Health and Human Services (HHS), February 6, 2018.

away. Deciding when to start ART and what HIV medicines to take begins with an HIV baseline evaluation.

What Is an HIV Baseline Evaluation?

An HIV baseline evaluation includes all the information collected during a person's initial visits with a healthcare provider. The HIV baseline evaluation includes a review of the person's health and medical history, a physical exam, and lab tests.

The purpose of an HIV baseline evaluation is to:

- Determine how far a person's HIV infection has progressed. Treatment with HIV medicines can prevent HIV from advancing to acquired immunodeficiency syndrome (AIDS). AIDS is the final stage of HIV infection.

- Evaluate whether the person is ready to start lifelong treatment with HIV medicines

- Collect information to decide what HIV medicines to start

During an HIV baseline evaluation, the healthcare provider explains the benefits and risks of HIV treatment and discusses ways to reduce the risk of passing HIV to others. The healthcare provider also takes time to answer any questions.

What Are Some Questions People Typically Ask during Their First Visits with an HIV Healthcare Provider?

People with newly diagnosed HIV infection can have many questions. If you've just tested HIV positive you may have some of the following questions:

- Because I have HIV, will I eventually get AIDS?

- What can I do to stay healthy and avoid getting other infections?

- How can I prevent passing HIV to others?

- How will HIV treatment affect my lifestyle?

- How should I tell my partner that I have HIV?

- Is there any reason to tell my employer and those I work with that I have HIV?

- Are there support groups for people with HIV?

Many people find it helpful to write down questions before a medical appointment. Some people bring a family member or friend to their HIV appointments to remind them of questions to ask and to write down the answers.

What Lab Tests Are Included in an HIV Baseline Evaluation?

The following lab tests are included in an HIV baseline evaluation.

A cluster of differentiation 4 counts (CD4 count). A CD4 count measures the number of CD4 cells in a sample of blood. CD4 cells are infection-fighting cells of the immune system. HIV destroys CD4 cells, which damages the immune system. A damaged immune system makes it hard for the body to fight off infections. Treatment with HIV medicines prevents HIV from destroying CD4 cells. The higher a person's CD4 count is, the better.

ART is recommended as soon as possible for everyone with HIV, no matter what their CD4 count is. However, a low CD4 count (below 200 cells/mm^3) increases the urgency to start ART.

Viral load. A viral load test measures how much virus is in the blood (HIV viral load). A goal of HIV treatment is to keep a person's viral load so low that the virus can't be detected by a viral load test.

The CD4 count and viral load test are both used to monitor the effectiveness of HIV medicines once ART is started.

Drug-resistance testing. Drug-resistance testing identifies which, if any, HIV medicines will not be effective against a person's strain of HIV. Healthcare providers consider a person's drug resistance test results when recommending an HIV regimen.

Testing for sexually transmitted diseases (STDs). Coinfection with another STD can cause HIV infection to advance faster and increase the risk of HIV transmission to a sexual partner. STD testing makes it possible to detect and treat any STDs promptly.

An HIV baseline evaluation also includes other tests, such as a blood cell count, kidney and liver function tests, tests to check the levels of glucose and certain fats in the blood, and tests for hepatitis.

How Does an HIV Baseline Evaluation Help Determine If a Person Is Ready to Start HIV Treatment?

Before starting treatment, people with HIV must be prepared to take HIV medicines every day for the rest of their lives. A baseline evaluation can help to identify any issues that can make it difficult to take HIV medicines every day and exactly as prescribed (called medication adherence).

Issues, such as lack of health insurance or alcohol or drug use that interferes with the activities of daily life, can make medication adherence difficult. Healthcare providers can recommend resources to help people deal with any issues before they start taking HIV medicines.

Chapter 21

Laboratory Tests

Laboratory Tests for Human Immunodeficiency Virus (HIV)

Laboratory tests can help keep tabs on your health. Some of these tests will be done soon after you learn you are human immunodeficiency virus (HIV) positive. Then depending on your immune status, whether you are on medication or not, and a variety of other factors, your provider will set up a schedule for you.

The lab tests look at:

- how well your immune system is functioning (cluster of differentiation 4 (CD4 count))

- how rapidly HIV is replicating, or multiplying (viral load)

- how well your body is functioning (tests to look at your kidneys, liver, cholesterol, and blood cells)

- whether you have other diseases that are associated with HIV (tests for certain infections)

When done shortly after you find out you have HIV, these tests establish a starting point or "baseline." Future tests will let you know how far from this baseline you have moved. This can help you tell how

This chapter includes text excerpted from "Understanding Laboratory Tests," U.S. Department of Veterans Affairs (VA), February 8, 2018.

fast or slow the disease is moving and indicate whether treatments are working.

Most labs include a "normal" range (high and low values) when they report test results. The most important results are the ones that fall outside these normal ranges. Test results often go up and down over time so don't worry about small changes. Instead look for overall trends.

What follows are descriptions of the most common tests:

CD4 Count (or T-Cell Count)

The CD4 count is like a snapshot of how well your immune system is functioning. CD4 cells (also known as CD4+ T cells) are white blood cells (WBCs) that fight infection. The more you have, the better. These are the cells that the HIV virus kills. As HIV infection progresses, the number of these cells declines. When the CD4 count drops below 200 due to advanced HIV disease, a person is diagnosed with acquired immunodeficiency syndrome (AIDS). A normal range for CD4 cells is about 500–1,500. Usually, the CD4 cell count increases as the HIV virus is controlled with effective HIV treatment. The higher your CD4 count, the better.

The same test that measures your CD4 count often includes a cluster of differentiation (CD) 8 cell count, too. CD8 cells (also known as CD8+ T cells) are another type of white blood cell that seeks out and destroys cells infected with viruses, including HIV-infected cells.

HIV Viral Load (or HIV Ribonucleic Acid (RNA))

HIV viral load tests measure the amount of HIV in the blood. Lower levels are better than higher levels. The main goal of HIV drugs is to reduce the HIV viral load to an "undetectable" level, meaning that the HIV RNA is below the level that the test is able to count.

The lower limit of HIV RNA detection depends on the test used, some go down to 50 copies/ml, while others go as low as 20. High viral loads are linked to faster disease progression. Reducing the viral load to "undetectable" levels slows or stops disease progression. Treatment for HIV suppresses the virus but does not eliminate it. Even if HIV levels are not detectable, the HIV is still in the body and will rebind to detectable if the HIV medicines are stopped. The lower your viral load, the better.

CD4 counts and HIV viral load tests are usually done when you first see a medical provider and about every 3 months afterward. Results can help you and your doctor decide how quickly to start taking anti-HIV drugs, and for people on HIV drugs, to tell whether the drugs are working.

Resistance Test (HIV Genotype)

This test determines whether the particular virus in your body is resistant to anti-HIV medications.

HIV reproduces rapidly and, as the virus makes copies of itself, small changes (or mutations) sometimes result. These changes can lead to different HIV strains, particularly if the person is taking HIV medicines but the HIV virus is not completely controlled or suppressed. If a strain that is resistant to your HIV drugs develops, the virus will be able to grow even though you are on medication. Your viral load will start to rise. The resistant virus soon will become the most common strain in your body. If this occurs, your provider may order a resistance test to check for mutations in the HIV virus.

A person can be infected with a drug-resistant strain of HIV if the infection was from an individual with resistant virus. For this reason, an HIV resistance test is recommended for all HIV infected people as soon as they are diagnosed.

Complete Blood Count (CBC)

This test looks at the different cells in your blood, including red blood cells (RBCs), platelets, and WBCs.

- RBCs carry oxygen to other cells in your body. If the level of your red blood cells is too low, you have anemia. Anemia can lead to fatigue. Tests that look at your red blood cells include hemoglobin and hematocrit. Hematocrit refers to the percentage of your blood that consists of RBCs. A normal hematocrit is about 37–47 percent in females and 40–54 percent in males.

- Platelets help with clotting, so if your platelets fall too low, your blood may not clot well. You may bleed more than usual, for example, when you brush your teeth or shave your skin. As the platelet count falls, the chance of internal bleeding rises.

- WBCs come in many types, and all are involved in your immune system's effort to keep you healthy. High white blood cell counts may indicate that you are fighting an infection. Low counts may put you at risk of getting an infection.

These tests are usually done every 3–6 months, unless your lab values are fluctuating a lot, or you have symptoms of HIV disease. Then the tests may be done more often.

Blood Chemistry Tests

Chemistry tests examine the levels of different elements and waste products in the blood and help determine how well different organs are functioning. Usually, the tests are divided into two panels:

- **Electrolyte tests** (sometimes called "lytes") and kidney function—These tests help measure how well your kidneys are working and measure the balance of fluids, acids, and sugar in your body. They include tests for sodium, potassium, chloride, blood urea nitrogen (BUN), creatinine, and glucose.

- **Liver function tests (LFTs)**—These tests measure whether your liver is being damaged. (Things that can damage the liver include viral hepatitis, certain medications, alcohol, and street drugs.) These tests measure alkaline phosphatase, alanine aminotransferase (ALT) test, aspartate aminotransferase (AST) test, albumin, and bilirubin.

- **Blood chemistry tests** are usually done every 3–6 months. It is important to have these done at baseline and while you are on HIV medications because some of the medications can cause kidney or liver abnormalities.

Lipid Profile

The level of certain fatty substances in the blood can give clues to your risk of heart disease. Triglycerides and cholesterol are important for health, but too much of them in the blood can cause fatty deposits to form in the arteries. This increases the chances of a heart attack. Too much triglyceride can also lead to pancreatitis, a serious inflammation of the pancreas. High cholesterol and high triglycerides can occur in people living with HIV. They can also be a side effect of some HIV medications.

Cholesterol is measured by three different tests:

- Total cholesterol

- HDL (high-density lipoprotein), often referred to as "good" cholesterol because high levels lower your risk of heart disease

- LDL (low-density lipoprotein), often referred to as "bad" cholesterol because high levels raise your risk of heart disease

These tests are usually done at least once a year, and more often if your levels are high or you require medication to control triglyceride and cholesterol levels. Your provider may want the lipid panel to be done while you are fasting, which means nothing to eat or drink (except water) after midnight the night before the test. This gives the most accurate evaluation of the cholesterol and triglycerides in the blood. Be sure to ask your provider if the blood tests are recommended to be done fasting.

Tuberculosis (TB) Test

TB is short for tuberculosis, a disease that people with HIV are at higher risk for getting. Most people who are exposed to TB don't get sick from it and the bacteria can live in the body for a long time without causing disease. But some people develop TB disease, and this is more likely if the immune system is weakened.

There are two types of tests for exposure to TB.

1. The TB skin test (also known as purified protein derivative (PPD), which requires the person to return to the clinic 2–3 days after the skin test is placed for the test to be interpreted

2. The other is a blood test called an interferon-gamma release assay (IGRA) (QuantiFERON and TSpotTB are two examples of IGRA blood tests)

HIV can make both types of tests less reliable for diagnosing TB, particularly if the immune system is weak. Neither of these tests can tell the difference between exposure to TB (where a person is not sick with TB) and active TB (where a person is sick with TB). If a person has been exposed to TB, treatment can reduce the risk of becoming sick with TB in the future.

Sexually Transmitted Diseases (STDs) Screening

If you got infected with HIV from unprotected sex, there is a chance you may have become infected with other sexually transmitted diseases (STDs), too. These include syphilis, gonorrhea, and chlamydia. Hepatitis B and C can be sexually transmitted as well, particularly among men who have sex with men.

Infections of syphilis, gonorrhea, and chlamydia can occur in the throat, penis, vagina, and rectum. The bacteria that cause syphilis and gonorrhea can also spread through the blood to other parts of your body. Having one of these other diseases can make your HIV advance faster. They can also make you 2–5 times more likely to pass HIV along to a sexual partner. Syphilis, for example, can cause open sores on your genitals, which allows easy passage of HIV from you to your partner.

Hepatitis A, B, and C

Your liver is an organ that processes almost everything you put into your body, including medications. The three most common types of viral hepatitis (A, B, and C) can damage your liver.

Some of the same behaviors that put people at risk for HIV (unprotected sex, injection drug use) can put them at risk for hepatitis. If you have both HIV and hepatitis B or C, your treatments for either disease can be affected. If you have HIV, your hepatitis may progress faster. If your liver is damaged from hepatitis, it may be harder for your body to process your HIV medications.

What's more, some HIV treatments can damage your liver, so if you have hepatitis, your doctor may want you to avoid certain HIV medicines.

Vaccinations (shots) are available to prevent hepatitis A and hepatitis B. People should be vaccinated against hepatitis A if they have another chronic liver disease (such as hepatitis B or hepatitis C), if they are a man who has sex with men, if they use injection or noninjection drugs, or have certain other risk factors. All people with HIV should receive hepatitis B vaccination.

Chapter 22

FAQs on Testing and the Window Period

The only way to know if you are infected with human immunodeficiency virus (HIV) is to get tested.

Although some people do have a flu-like illness around the time they get infected, many do not. Also, even if you have a flu-like illness from HIV, it's usually pretty difficult to tell it apart from the flu. So, even people who have the symptoms of HIV infection may think they just have the flu.

Many HIV-infected people, including those with AIDS, don't feel or look sick in any way. They find out that they are HIV infected only when they get tested. Sometimes this testing is done as part of routine health exams, like getting your cholesterol checked. Other times, people get tested only when they suddenly become seriously ill with a life-threatening infection, and their doctors need to know whether the infection is a result of a weakened immune system caused by HIV.

Getting tested for HIV is crucial for protecting your health. It's better to find out you are HIV infected when your immune system is still relatively healthy, so that you can start taking medications to control the virus before it makes you sick. Also, finding out you are HIV infected allows you to take steps to avoid infecting your sex partners

This chapter includes text excerpted from "HIV/AIDS—Frequently Asked Questions," U.S. Department of Veterans Affairs (VA), February 9, 2018.

or (for women) to prevent transmission to a fetus or infancy during pregnancy or childbirth.

The U.S. Centers for Disease Control and Prevention (CDC) recommend that every adult in the United States be tested for HIV at least once. The Veterans Health Administration (VHA) recommends that voluntary HIV testing be provided to all patients who receive medical care, and encourages all veterans to be tested.

Would You Know Whether You're Infected with Human Immunodeficiency Virus (HIV) without Getting Tested?

There is no single correct answer to this question. One recommended strategy is to get tested 2–4 weeks, 3 months, and 6 months after a risky exposure. Using a sensitive antigen/antibody HIV test, of those who are infected, most will test positive at 1 month; almost all will test positive at 3 months; and the rest will test positive at 6 months. If you have any symptoms that may be caused by acute HIV infection, you should be retested immediately, with an HIV viral load test included. Newer and more sensitive HIV tests make it more and more likely that HIV will be detected at earlier time points.

How Soon after Risky Sex Can You Be 100 Percent Sure You Are Clear of HIV?

The rapid oral HIV test detects antibodies made by the immune system in response to HIV infection, just like the standard blood antibody test. The rapid oral test, however, detects these antibodies in oral fluid and doesn't require a blood sample.

The rapid oral HIV test has similar accuracy to the standard blood antibody test for persons with chronic, or long-standing, HIV infection. But, like any antibody test for HIV, the rapid oral HIV test is not reliable during the "window period" (lasting several weeks to months) between the time a person is infected and the time the body has made enough antibodies for the test to detect. During this window period, someone who is infected might test negative for antibodies (a false-negative result). The "window period" for the rapid oral test is longer than it is for some HIV blood tests, meaning that for someone with acute or new HIV infection certain blood tests can detect HIV earlier than the oral rapid tests can.

It also is possible to have false-positive results (a person may have a positive rapid oral HIV test result but not be actually infected with

HIV). That's why anyone who has a positive result with a rapid oral HIV test must have a more specific "confirmatory" blood test before a diagnosis of HIV infection can be made.

How Accurate Is the Rapid Oral HIV Test?

When you use a home HIV test, you collect a blood sample at home, usually by sticking your finger with a lancet and blotting the blood onto a piece of filter paper, which you send to a lab for standard HIV antibody testing.

An "inconclusive" result might mean "insufficient" or "indeterminate." "Insufficient" simply means that there was a problem with the sample you provided that prevented it from being tested at all. "Indeterminate" means that the test was run but didn't provide a clear negative or positive result. People with indeterminate HIV test results can be HIV infected and in the process of seroconverting, a time during which an HIV test would show a result somewhere between negative and positive.

Also, for many reasons (other viral infections, or just nonspecific antibodies in the blood), some people can be HIV uninfected and have an indeterminate test. The best course of action would be to repeat the test, but things can get a bit tricky: If the second result is negative, which one do you trust? Ideally, the old blood sample would be retested at the same time as the new one is tested, to see whether there was a problem with the testing method when the first test was run. That isn't always possible. And retesting through home-collection test kits can get very expensive very quickly.

An alternative would be to get retested at a local voluntary testing and counseling site (run by various organizations and searchable on the Internet) or to get tested through your clinic at the U.S. Department of Veterans Affairs (VA). Explain your previous indeterminate result to the staff; they should have a protocol for addressing this situation, whether it involves combining a repeat antibody test with an ribonucleic acid (RNA) test or performing a series of antibody tests.

Part Four

Treatments and Therapies for HIV/AIDS

Chapter 23

Treatment Overview

Human immunodeficiency virus (HIV) treatment involves taking medicines that slow the progression of the virus in your body. HIV is a type of virus called a retrovirus, and the drugs used to treat it are called antiretrovirals (ARV). These drugs are always given in combination with other ARVs; this combination therapy is called antiretroviral therapy (ART). Many ART drugs have been used since the mid-1990s and are the reason why the annual number of deaths related to acquired immunodeficiency syndrome (AIDS) has dropped over the past two decades.

Although a cure for HIV does not yet exist, ART can keep you healthy for many years, and greatly reduces your chance of transmitting HIV to your partner(s) if taken consistently and correctly. ART reduces the amount of virus (or viral load) in your blood and body fluids. ART is recommended for all people living with HIV, regardless of how long they've had the virus or how healthy they are.

Importance of Treatment

To protect your health, it is important to get on and stay on HIV treatment. HIV treatment is important because it helps your body fight HIV. You may hear the phrase "treatment adherence," which means staying on your treatment plan. Most people living with HIV who don't get treatment eventually develop AIDS.

This chapter includes text excerpted from "HIV Treatment," Centers for Disease Control and Prevention (CDC), February 8, 2016.

If left untreated, HIV attacks your immune system and can allow different types of life-threatening infections and cancers to develop. If your cluster of differentiation 4 (CD4) cell count falls below a certain level, you are at risk of getting an opportunistic infection. These are infections that don't normally affect people with healthy immune systems but that can infect people with immune systems weakened by HIV infection. Your healthcare provider may prescribe medicines to prevent certain infections.

HIV treatment is most likely to be successful when you know what to expect and are committed to taking your medicines exactly as prescribed. Working with your healthcare provider to develop a treatment plan will help you know more about HIV, manage it effectively, and make decisions that help you live a longer, healthier life. HIV treatment will also greatly reduce your chance of transmitting HIV to sex partners and injection-drug-use if taken consistently and correctly.

When Should I Start Treatment?

Treatment guidelines from the U.S. Department of Health and Human Services (HHS) recommend that a person living with HIV begin ART as soon as possible after diagnosis. Starting ART slows the progression of HIV and can keep you healthy for many years. If you delay treatment, the virus will continue to harm your immune system and put you at higher risk for developing opportunistic infections that can be life-threatening.

How Antiretroviral Therapy (ART) Works

ART is the use of HIV medicines to treat HIV infection. There are five different types of HIV medicines. Each medicine helps stop HIV at different points in the virus' life cycle.

When taken consistently and correctly ART helps:

- Reduce your viral load (the level of HIV in your body). When you reduce your viral load, you reduce HIV's ability to infect new CD4 cells.

- Keep your immune system healthy by increasing your CD4 count. CD4 cells help protect you from developing infections. The right dose and type of ART medicines can help to keep your viral load low and your CD4 cell levels high.

- Prevent opportunistic infections and other illnesses.

- Reduce, but not eliminate, the chances that you will transmit HIV to others.

- Reduce, but not eliminate, the chances that you will transmit the virus to your baby if you are pregnant or plan on becoming pregnant.

Follow your treatment plan exactly as your healthcare provider has prescribed. Medicines should be taken at specific times of the day, with or without certain kinds of food. If you have questions about when and how to take your medicines, talk to your healthcare provider or pharmacist.

ART is usually taken as a combination of 3 or more drugs to have the greatest chance of lowering the amount of HIV in your body. Ask your healthcare provider about the availability of multiple drugs combined into 1 pill. Your healthcare provider and pharmacist will help you find a treatment combination that works best for you. If the HIV medicines you are taking are not working as well as they should, your healthcare provider may change your prescription. A change is not unusual because the same treatment does not affect everyone in the same way.

Let your healthcare provider and pharmacist know about any medical conditions you may have and any other medicines you are taking. Medicines you are taking for other health conditions may interact with your HIV treatment. These conversations will help you receive the best treatment possible. Additionally, if you or your partner is pregnant or considering getting pregnant, talk to your healthcare provider to determine the right type of ART that can greatly reduce the risk of transmitting HIV to your baby.

Side Effects of ART

Like most medicines, ART can cause side effects. However, not everyone experiences side effects from ART.

Some common side effects of ART that you may experience can include:

- Nausea and vomiting

- Diarrhea

- Difficulty sleeping

- Dry mouth

- Headache

- Rash

- Dizziness

- Fatigue

- Pain

Side effects can differ for each person and each type of ART medicine. Some side effects can occur once you start a medicine and may only last a few days or weeks. Other side effects can start later and last longer.

Contact your healthcare provider or pharmacist immediately if you begin to experience problems or if your treatment makes you sick. Medicines are available to help reduce or eliminate side effects or you can change medicines to find a treatment plan that works for you. Your healthcare provider may prescribe medicines to help manage the side effects or may decide to change your treatment plan.

What I Should Do If I Miss a Dose

Taking your HIV medicines exactly the way your healthcare provider tells you to will help keep your viral load low and your CD4 cell count high. If you skip your medicines, even now and then, you are giving HIV the chance to multiply rapidly. This could weaken your immune system, and you could become sick.

Talk to your healthcare provider if you miss a dose. In most cases, if you realize you missed a dose, take the medicines as soon as you can, then take the next dose at your usual scheduled time (unless your pharmacist or healthcare provider has told you something different).

If you find you miss a lot of doses, talk to your healthcare provider or pharmacist about ways to help you remember your medicines. You and your healthcare provider may even decide to change your treatment regimen to fit your healthcare needs and life situation, which may change over time.

Taking HIV Medicines Even When Viral Load Is Undetectable

ART reduces viral load, ideally to an undetectable level. If your viral load goes down after starting ART, then the treatment is working, and you should always take your medicine as prescribed by your healthcare provider. Even when your viral load is undetectable, HIV can still exist in semen, vaginal and rectal fluids, breast milk, and other parts of your body, so you should continue to take steps to prevent HIV transmission. Taking your HIV medications on schedule will help keep your viral load very low and help you maintain your health. It will also make it more difficult for you to pass HIV on to others.

Before Starting HIV Treatment

Preparing to stay on your treatment plan before you start taking ART is the first step to treatment success. Planning ahead will help you follow your treatment plan once you start treatment.

Begin by talking to your healthcare provider. Make sure you understand why you're starting HIV treatment and why sticking to your treatment plan is important. Discuss these important details about your treatment plan:

- Each HIV medication that you will take
- The dose (amount) of each HIV medication in your plan
- How many pills in each dose
- When to take each medication
- How to take each medication—with or without food
- Possible side effects from each medication, including serious side effects to watch out for
- How to store your medications
- Other medications you are taking and how they may interact with your HIV medications
- Any personal issues such as depression, alcohol or drug abuse, lack of secure housing, or additional medical issues
- Lack of health insurance to pay for anti-HIV medications

Tell your healthcare provider if you have any personal issues, such as depression or alcohol or drug use, that can make staying on your treatment plan difficult. If needed, your healthcare provider can recommend resources to help you address these issues before you start treatment.

Importance of Sticking to Your Treatment Plan

Sticking to your HIV treatment provides many benefits. Among them, it:

- Allows HIV medications to reduce the amount of HIV in your body. If you skip your medications, even now and then, you are giving HIV the chance to multiply rapidly. Keeping the amount of virus in your blood as low as possible is the best way to protect your health.

- Helps keep your immune system stronger and better able to fight infections.

- Reduces the risk of passing HIV to others. Staying on your treatment plan and keeping the amount of HIV in your body as low as possible means that it is less likely that you can pass the virus to others.

- Helps prevent drug resistance. Drug resistance develops when the virus changes form and no longer responds to certain HIV medications. This is a problem because that drug no longer works on your HIV. Skipping your medicines makes it easier for drug resistance to develop. Also, HIV can become resistant to the medications you are taking or to similar ones that you have not yet taken. This limits the options for successful HIV treatment. Drug-resistant strains of HIV can be transmitted to others, too.

HIV Treatment and Challenges

Staying on an HIV treatment plan can be difficult. That is why it is important to understand some of the challenges you may face and to think through how you might address them before they happen. For example, remembering when to take your medicines can be compli-cated. Some treatment plans involve taking several pills every day—with or without food—or before or after other medications. Making a schedule of when and how to take your medicines can be helpful. Or ask your healthcare provider about the availability of multiple drugs combined into one pill.

Other factors can make sticking to your treatment plan difficult:

- Problems taking medications, such as trouble swallowing pills, can make staying on treatment challenging. Your healthcare provider can offer tips and ideas for addressing these problems.

- Side effects from medications, for example, nausea or diarrhea, can make a person not want to take them.

- Talk to your healthcare provider. There are medicines or other support, like nutritional counseling to make sure you are getting important nutrients, which can help with the most common side effects. But don't give up. Work with your healthcare provider to find a treatment that works for you.

- A busy schedule. Work or travel away from home can make it easy to forget to take pills. Planning ahead can help. Or, it may be possible to keep extra medicines at work or in your car for the times that you forget to take them at home. But make sure you talk to your healthcare provider—some medications are affected by extreme temperatures, and it is not always possible to keep medications at work.

- Being sick or depressed. How you feel mentally and physically can affect your willingness to stick to your treatment plan. Again, your healthcare provider is an important source of information to help.

- Alcohol or drug use. If substance use is interfering with your ability to keep yourself healthy, it may be time to seek help to quit or better manage it.

- Treatment fatigue. Some people find that sticking to their treatment plan becomes harder over time. Every time you see your healthcare provider, make it a point to talk about staying on your treatment plan.

Your healthcare provider will help you identify barriers to staying on your plan and ways to address those barriers. Understanding issues that can make staying on your treatment plan difficult will help you and your healthcare provider select the best treatment for you.

Tell your healthcare provider right away if you're having difficulty sticking to your plan. Together you can identify the reasons why you're skipping medications and make a plan to address those reasons. Joining a support group, or enlisting the support of family and friends, can also help you stick to your treatment plan.

Tips for Ensuring Continuation of Treatment Plan

Some tips that may help you stick with your treatment plan are:

- Take your medicine at the same time each day.

- Match your medicine schedule to your life. Add taking your medicines to things you already do each day, like brushing your teeth or eating a meal.

247

- Try a weekly or monthly pill tray with compartments for each day of the week to help you remember whether or not you took your medicine that day.

- Set an alarm on your clock, watch, or phone for the time you take your medicines.

- Use a calendar to check off the days you have taken your medicines.

- Download a free app from the Internet to your computer or on your smartphone that can help remind you when it's time to take your medicines. Search for "reminder apps," and you will find many choices.

- Ask a family member or friend to help you remember to take your medicine.

Chapter 24

FAQs on Treatment

Frequently Asked Questions about Treatment for Human Immunodeficiency Virus (HIV)

I Was Just Diagnosed with HIV and My Clinician Wants Me to Start Treatment Right Away. Does That Sound Like the Right Thing to Do?

You may know that is currently recommended human immunodeficiency virus (HIV) treatment (called antiretroviral therapy, or ART) for everyone with HIV. That's because research studies show that effective ART improves the health of people with HIV no matter the stage of their infection, and it enormously reduces the chance of HIV passing to an HIV-negative sex partner. So, all HIV providers almost always offer ART during one of the first clinic visits.

Some clinics and some local health departments go further and recommend that people with a new diagnosis of HIV start treatment immediately, either that same day or within the next few days. This approach sometimes is called "Treatment on Diagnosis" or "Rapid ART." There are several reasons for starting treatment at the time of HIV diagnosis, but the basic reason is that if early treatment is beneficial, starting treatment at the earliest possible time maybe even better, and patients may get the benefits of ART sooner. This

---

This chapter includes text excerpted from "Frequently Asked Questions about HIV," U.S. Department of Veterans Affairs (VA), February 9, 2018.

may be especially true for people who are diagnosed very soon after they are infected (during the acute HIV infection period). Also, it's known that delays or barriers to getting clinic appointments are common, and if may take a while to get a prescription for ART, which can result in worse health outcomes. So, strategies that get newly diagnosed people straight into care and onto treatment may bypass these barriers.

For individuals with new diagnoses of HIV who are starting ART immediately, clinicians must choose the treatment regimens carefully, and offer extra support and guidance. Please discuss this more with your healthcare provider and decide whether you are ready to start treatment. Remember that this is your decision and you should be comfortable with it.

I Have Hepatitis C and Hope to Start Treatment Soon. Can I Take Hepatitis C Medications along with My HIV Medications?

It's great that you are about to start hepatitis C treatment—good luck with it.

Yes, you can and should continue HIV medications while you take medications for hepatitis C, if at all possible. But, some HIV medications interact with some of the hepatitis C medicines (the so-called direct-acting antivirals, or DAAs). This could cause unwanted increases or decreases of drug levels in your body (depending on the specific interaction) and thus increase the risk of side effects (if a drug level rises) or of treatment failure (if a drug level drops).

So, it is very important for your clinicians to be sure that the two sets of medications are compatible. In some cases, it may be necessary to change the HIV regimen in order to allow treatment with certain DAAs. Please discuss this with your HIV and hepatitis clinicians before you start hepatitis C treatment.

Why Change Your HIV Regimen When You've Been on It for Years and It's Working?

If your HIV medications (antiretrovirals, or ARVs) have kept your HIV viral load suppressed as much as possible (ideally to "undetectable" levels), and your cluster of differentiation 4 (CD4) count is stable (or higher), and your health is stable, then your meds are working well. You may think that "if it ain't broke, don't fix it," but there may be some advantages to changing.

There are many possible reasons why a provider might suggest a change in ARVs to someone whose meds are keeping the HIV viral load under control. Here are a few:

- HIV therapies develop over time, and in recent years a lot of potent and "kinder, gentler" ARVs have become available. In addition, there are a number of combination drugs that decrease the number of individual pills that patients must take, including several that contain an entire regimen in a single pill. So, your provider may want you to switch to meds that have less risk of side effects or switch to a simpler regimen with fewer pills.

- Your provider may have noticed a side effect that you are not aware of or may be concerned about a potential side effect.

- Your provider may want you to start a new medicine that interacts with one of your HIV medicines, so he or she may want to change your ARVs to avoid a problematic interaction.

So, although your current ARVs may be working well to control your HIV virus, there may be good reasons to consider a change of therapy. Talk to your provider about your concerns, ask questions about why he or she wants you to change and about the new ARVs being proposed, and make a decision together about your therapy.

If You Change to New HIV Medicines (ARVs), Can You Go Back to the Old Ones in the Future?

The quick answer is that it depends on why the change was made and whether your virus is resistant (or becomes resistant) to those ARVs.

If your HIV viral load is suppressed (ideally "undetectable") on your old ARVs and you change to new ones, or a new ARV is substituted for one in your old regimen, there is little or no risk of your virus developing new resistance to the drugs, so long as the new ARVs are as "strong" (as potent against the strains of HIV in your body) as the old ones. So, if you develop side effects on the new meds, you theoretically could return to the old ones. (Note that this answer assumes that your provider is knowledgeable about ARVs and selects your medications carefully.)

When Should You Start Antiretroviral Therapy?

The short answer (for almost everyone) is—now!

Treating HIV with antiretroviral medications can have huge benefits for you as an individual, and for anyone who is at risk of being infected with HIV (like a sex partner). HIV therapy helps to:

- Reduce the amount of HIV in your body

- Strengthen your immune system

- Prevent illness

- Help you live longer

- Prevent transmission (passing the virus) to your sex or drug-using partner(s) or during pregnancy and childbirth

In past years, most guidelines recommended waiting until the cluster of differentiation 4 (CD4) (or "T cell") count dropped to a certain level before starting HIV medications. This was because our understanding of the damaging effects of HIV was not as full, and because the available HIV medications were harder to take than they are now (for example, greater numbers of pills, more side effects) and not as likely to be effective.

Many studies have shown that starting HIV treatment earlier lowers the risk of a variety of illnesses related to the effects of HIV. In other words, HIV medications can help people stay healthier if they start the meds when their CD4 counts are higher. Also, there's strong proof that effective HIV therapy dramatically reduces the chance of HIV passing from an HIV-positive person to an HIV-negative sex partner. And—more good news—many of the newer HIV medications are better, easier to take, and consist of fewer pills.

While there may be some individuals in whom it is best to delay treatment temporarily, the guidelines recommend starting therapy for ALL persons with HIV infection, so long as they are willing and able to take the medications.

Are There Once-a-Day Pills for HIV?

Yes. There are six combination pills that include an entire regimen in a single pill. The six once-a-day pills, with their components, are:

1. **Atripla**

   - 600 mg of efavirenz (Sustiva)

   - 300 mg of tenofovir (Viread)

   - 200 mg of emtricitabine (Emtriva)

2. **Complera**
   - 25 mg of rilpivirine (Edurant)
   - 300 mg of tenofovir DF(Viread)
   - 200 mg of emtricitabine (Emtriva)

3. **Odefsey**
   - 25 mg of rilpivirine (Edurant)
   - 300 mg of tenofovir alafenamide
   - 200 mg of emtricitabine (Emtriva)

4. **Stribild**
   - 150 mg of elvitegravir (Vitekta)
   - 150 mg of cobicistat (Tybost)
   - 300 mg of tenofovir DF(Viread)
   - 200 mg of emtricitabine (Emtriva)

5. **Genvoya**
   - 150 mg of elvitegravir (Vitekta)
   - 150 mg of cobicistat (Tybost)
   - 300 mg of tenofovir alafenamide
   - 200 mg of emtricitabine (Emtriva)

6. **Triumeq**
   - 50 mg of dolutegravir (Tivicay)
   - 600 mg of abacavir (Ziagen)
   - 300 mg of lamivudine (Epivir)

People who might benefit from these single-pill combinations include:

- Those starting antiretroviral therapy for the first time
- Those who would like to simplify their regimen from the same or similar individual component medications (for example, Tivicay + Epzicom)
- Those who would like to switch from a more complicated regimen and have not developed resistance to any of the drugs that these single-pill regimens contain

Other one-pill, once-daily regimens may become available in the future.

What Is Drug Resistance in HIV and How Can You Avoid It?

When HIV isn't fully controlled by anti-HIV drugs, the virus makes copies of itself at a very rapid rate. Mistakes (called mutations) can occur, creating new forms of the virus that may not be as sensitive to a particular drug as the original virus. This is called drug resistance because the virus can multiply and cause disease even when a patient is taking the drug.

At present, the standard treatment for HIV usually involves taking at least 3 powerful anti-HIV drugs every day. It is designed to reduce the amount of HIV in the body to a level that cannot be detected by standard lab tests (called "undetectable viral load"). The lower your viral load, the lower your risk of developing resistance because there's less virus to produce mutations. In the early years of HIV, when patients took only 1 or 2 drugs at a time, almost everyone developed some drug resistance. Why? Because these treatments were not powerful enough to stop the virus from making drug-resistant copies of itself.

If your healthcare provider suspects that you have a drug-resistant virus, he or she can do testing (called resistance testing, "HIV genotyping," or "HIV phenotyping") to help identify the drugs to which your virus is resistant. The results of the testing, along with a detailed history of what medications you've taken in the past, help to determine which drugs to use in the future. There are more anti-HIV drugs available now than there used to be, so you have more options for successful treatment.

To reduce your chances of developing drug-resistant HIV:

- Work with your healthcare provider to find an ART drug combination that is effective and that you can tolerate.

- Take every dose of your medications every day, missing as few as possible.

- Keep your appointments with your HIV clinician and have your viral load checked regularly (every 3–4 months for many patients). That will help detect resistance before it affects too many drugs in your regimen.

- Keep a record of which combinations of HIV medications you've taken.

What Should You Do If You Miss a Dose of Your HIV Medicines?

Missing doses of HIV medicines can reduce their usefulness and increase the possibility of developing drug resistance, which makes certain HIV drugs lose their effectiveness.

If you realize you have missed a dose, go ahead and take the medication as soon as you can, then take the next dose at your usual scheduled time. (There may be some exceptions to this general rule—for example, if taking a medicine such as efavirenz (Sustiva) in the daytime could cause unmanageable side effects.)

If you find you are missing doses of your HIV medications, talk to your provider and pharmacist about ways to help you remember to take the medications at the same time every day, or to figure out the most appropriate regimen for you. One simple reminder technique that many people use is to take their HIV medications at the same time as they do another daily task, such as brushing their teeth before bedtime.

Can You Take a Break from Your HIV Medicines?

People may be interested in taking a break from HIV medicines for many reasons, such as becoming tired of taking pills every day, having trouble with side effects, or wishing to avoid being reminded of their HIV infection when taking pills. However, interrupting HIV treatment can be harmful in several ways.

First, HIV drug resistance can develop when patients stop taking certain antiretroviral (ARV) medications, particularly those in the nonnucleoside reverse-transcriptase inhibitors (NNRTIs) class—like efavirenz (Sustiva), nevirapine (Viramune), and rilpivirine (Edurant)—or the combination pills Atripla, Odefsey, and Complera. Once the HIV develops resistance to a medication, that medicine can no longer be used to effectively treat the virus. So, breaks in treatment can jeopardize the availability of some or all of the interrupted medicines for future treatment.

In addition, stopping treatment allows the HIV to actively reproduce and circulate in the blood. That is associated with increased inflammation and with an increased risk of heart attacks and kidney and liver problems. It is known that, once the virus is not being suppressed by HIV medicines, the CD4 cell count (T-cell count) will drop to the same level it was at before treatment was started, which can mean serious immune impairment for people who started taking HIV medicine with a low CD4 cell count.

Finally, increased HIV levels in the blood resulting from treatment discontinuation can lead to a "retroviral syndrome," with fevers, headaches, and swollen glands, similar to the symptoms some people experience when they are newly infected with HIV.

So, even though it may be tempting to take a break from HIV treatment, there may be important health consequences of doing so. If you feel strongly that you need a break or if you have to interrupt your treatment for a period of time (for example, owing to surgery that temporarily prevents you from taking pills by mouth), talk to your provider about the safest way to discontinue the HIV treatment. (To reduce the risk of developing drug resistance, it may be necessary to switch to other medications or to stop taking some drugs before others.)

Will HIV Medicines Cause Changes to Your Fat and Stomach?

The loss of fat in the face, arms, and legs (lipoatrophy) and gain of fat in the belly (lipohypertrophy) and other places in the body (such as at the top of the back, causing a "buffalo hump") are dreaded complications of HIV treatment. Some of these body changes are caused by the HIV medicines, but they rarely occur with the medicines that are most often used nowadays.

Lipoatrophy is most common with medicines such as d4T (stavudine, Zerit) and AZT (ZDV, zidovudine), which are infrequently used in the United States at present. The accumulation of fat in the abdomen may be an effect of HIV, but it is also seen with protease inhibitors such as indinavir (Crixivan), which also is rarely used these days. Therefore, people in the United States who start taking HIV medicines for the first time should not be concerned that they will have unwanted body changes owing to the medicines. On the contrary, many people report that they feel and look healthier once they start taking HIV medications.

People who have already experienced body changes caused by older HIV medications should talk to their providers about the possibility of changing to medicines that may have less impact on fat loss or gain but still control HIV effectively. Fat loss resulting from those older HIV medicines usually does not continue when the offending medicine is discontinued, but some of the changes may be irreversible. There are treatments for facial lipoatrophy, including injections of dermal fillers that can lessen the appearance of these changes. Abdominal fat gain can be reduced in part by diet and exercise, as well as by avoidance of the older medications that may contribute to that change, and specific medical treatments may be appropriate.

Is It True That Someone Has Been Cured of HIV?

It is true that one person appears to have been cured of HIV infection. Known as the "Berlin Patient," he is a man with chronic HIV infection who developed acute leukemia in 2007 while living in Berlin. He underwent intensive chemotherapy and two stem-cell transplants (or "bone marrow transplants"). A stem cell transplant from another person essentially replaces the recipient's immune system with the donor's immune system. Because his donor has a genetic mutation that makes his CD4 cells very resistant to becoming infected with HIV, the Berlin patient was able to discontinue his HIV medications after the first bone marrow transplant and has had no detectable HIV virus since.

It is important to realize that this was an incredibly intensive treatment course that was given for a serious blood cancer, leukemia. It is neither recommended nor feasible to give nonleukemia patients these treatments because the risks involved with chemotherapy and transplantation are very high. Nor is stem-cell transplantation a solution for the worldwide HIV epidemic, with over 33 million people infected.

However, this case has reinvigorated the research and advocacy communities to find strategies for an HIV cure and to understand what aspects of the many treatments the Berlin patient received were key to controlling/curing the infection.

While present antiretroviral HIV medicines are very effective in inhibiting the HIV virus from actively reproducing, present HIV treatment is not able to eliminate the virus. Many different approaches are being investigated as possible avenues towards a cure, including vaccines to control the virus, medicines to change the immune system's response to HIV, medicines to "purge" the dormant HIV from the body, and genetic therapy, where a patient's white cells are altered to prevent the virus from attaching to cells. It is not known if these strategies will work or if they are successful when a cure would be available, but it is heartening that at least one person has been cured and that scientific efforts to find a cure have been intensified.

Chapter 25

Decision Making: To Start Therapy or Not

Human immunodeficiency virus (HIV) drugs are essential in keeping people healthy over the years. For people who are sick from HIV, they can be lifesavers. Effective treatment stops or slows the progression of HIV and has important benefits, even for persons whose immune systems appear to be functioning relatively well. Thus, HIV drugs are recommended for all people with HIV infection, whether they are sick or well. And, in general, starting treatment early after someone is diagnosed with HIV is better than delaying, so long as you are ready to start.

For people whose immune systems are weaker, starting treatment is urgent. For people whose immune systems are still strong, it is important to start HIV medications before their immune systems suffer more. Studies show that starting treatment early is the most effective way to prevent long-term consequences of HIV. And, treatment that suppresses the HIV virus can prevent transmission (spread) of HIV infection to sex partners (or injection drug use partners); for pregnant women, it can prevent infection of the baby in the womb or at birth.

There a couple of things to know about as you decide when to start treatment. First, the current drug regimens usually are very simple and compact (between 1 and 3 pills per day), and they usually work very well, so long as you take them every day. Second, it's really

This chapter includes text excerpted from "HIV/AIDS—Starting Therapy," U.S. Department of Veterans Affairs (VA), February 9, 2018.

important to take the medicines correctly every day or the virus may become resistant to the drugs. That means the virus may change in a way that makes the drugs no longer work. The most common cause of drug resistance is not taking medications correctly every day. So, people need to be ready to commit to taking the medications every day ("adherence"). And third, HIV medicines, like any other drugs, may cause side effects in some people. But people who take the newer HIV drugs usually do not have any problems with them. If you do have side effects, let your healthcare providers know so that they can work with you to solve this problem.

So, as said earlier, treatment of HIV is recommended for all people with the infection. Experts generally advise starting treatment soon after you are diagnosed with HIV, and your clinician may even offer you treatment on the same day you receive your diagnosis. Here are some things your healthcare provider may consider in advising you how quickly to start:

- Symptoms of HIV disease (also called your clinical status, or how well you feel)

- Your cluster of differentiation 4 (CD4) count and HIV viral load

- Whether you have certain other medical conditions that may be helped by HIV treatment

- Whether you can and will stick to your treatment plan (adherence)

- Whether you have sex partner(s) who are HIV-negative and may be at risk of becoming infected through you

- Whether you are pregnant or wish to become pregnant soon.

Symptoms (Clinical Status)

"Clinical status" refers to how well you are doing in general, including how well you feel. Your doctor will look at whether you have symptoms of HIV disease. These symptoms are signs that HIV is weakening your immune system and include things such as weight loss, chronic fevers, and opportunistic infections (OIs). OIs—are infections that can happen in someone with a damaged immune system.

Cluster of Differentiation 4 (CD4) Count and Viral Load

Even though you may not feel it, when you have HIV, the virus and your immune system are at war with each other. The virus is trying to multiply as fast as it can, and your body is trying to stop it. Two tests, the CD4 count, and the HIV viral load help you and your healthcare provider know how strong your immune system is and know whether it is keeping HIV under control.

CD4 cells play a major role in helping your immune system work properly. HIV causes disease by killing off CD4 cells. It does this by infecting the cells and turning them into virus factories. The CD4 count tells us how many CD4 cells you have. The higher the number, the better.

The HIV viral load test indicates how much of the HIV virus is present in your blood, and how fast it is multiplying. The higher the viral load, the faster HIV is infecting and killing your CD4 cells. The lower the viral load, the better.

Your healthcare provider will look at these two things carefully. People whose CD4 count is low, and people whose viral load is high, are more likely to get sick sooner than people with a high CD4 count and low viral load.

CD4 count and viral load tests usually are done before treatment is started and then regularly while someone is on treatment. For people who decide to delay starting treatment, these tests are done every 3 months; they can help you and your healthcare provider decide how urgent it is to start anti-HIV drugs. As said earlier, HIV medicines are recommended for everyone, no matter how high or low their CD4 count is. And HIV treatment is especially urgent if your CD4 count is lower, or if you have symptoms. The lower the CD4, the more important it is to start treatment quickly.

Whether You Have Certain Other Medical Conditions That May Be Helped by HIV Treatment

Starting HIV drugs may be particularly important for people with certain other medical conditions. For example, your doctor will recommend HIV therapy if you are pregnant or plan to become pregnant, if you have kidney disease that is caused by HIV, or if you have hepatitis B or hepatitis C.

Whether You Can and Will Stick to Your Treatment Plan (Adherence)

Before you start medications for HIV, it is very important to make a strong commitment to sticking to a drug therapy plan (or regimen). With an HIV drug regimen, you will need to take medicines every day!

In order for the drugs to work and keep working, you must carefully follow the directions for taking them. If you're not sure you can do this, you might need help in finding ways to stick to the plan.

If you are wondering whether you should start taking treatment for HIV, you should sit down and talk with your provider as soon as possible. Depending on your specific needs, your provider can come up with a personal treatment plan for you.

Risk of Transmitting HIV: To Sex Partners or during Pregnancy

HIV therapy has been shown to greatly reduce the risk of transmitting HIV to uninfected sex partners. In fact, if you take your medicines every day and your HIV treatment is working well, there is almost no risk of transmitting HIV to a sex partner. Thus, if you have a sex partner who is HIV negative, you may consider starting HIV treatment both to protect and improve your own health and to prevent transmission to partners. Similarly, if you are pregnant or intend to become pregnant, it is important to start HIV medications right away both to protect your own health and to reduce the risk of passing HIV to the baby during pregnancy or at the time of birth.

Chapter 26

Antiretroviral Treatment

Chapter Contents

Section 26.1

Starting Anti-HIV Medications

This section includes text excerpted from "When to Start Antiretroviral Therapy," AIDS*info*, U.S. Department of Health and Human Services (HHS), January 24, 2018.

Antiretroviral therapy (ART) is the use of human immunodeficiency virus infection (HIV) medicines to treat HIV infection. ART is recommended for everyone who has HIV. ART helps people with HIV live longer, healthier lives. People with HIV should start ART as soon as possible. In people with HIV who have the following conditions, it's especially important to start ART right away:

- Pregnancy
- Acquired immunodeficiency syndrome (AIDS)
- Certain HIV-related illnesses
- Coinfections
- Recent HIV infection (the period up to 6 months after infection with HIV)

Before starting ART, people with HIV discuss the benefits and risks of ART with their healthcare providers. They also discuss the importance of medication adherence—taking HIV medicines every day and exactly as prescribed.

Right Time to Start Taking Human Immunodeficiency Virus (HIV) Medicine

Treatment with HIV medicines (ART) is recommended for everyone with HIV. ART helps people with HIV live longer, healthier lives and reduces the risk of HIV transmission.

The U.S. Department of Health and Human Services (HHS) guidelines on the use of HIV medicines in adults and adolescents recommend that people with HIV start ART as soon as possible. In people with HIV who have certain conditions, it's especially important to start ART right away.

Conditions That Increase the Urgency to Start Antiretroviral Therapy (ART)

The following conditions increase the urgency to start ART:

Pregnancy

All pregnant women with HIV should take HIV medicines to prevent mother-to-child transmission of HIV. The HIV medicines will also protect the health of the pregnant woman.

All pregnant women with HIV should start taking HIV medicines as soon as possible during pregnancy. In general, women who are already taking HIV medicines when they become pregnant should continue taking HIV medicines throughout their pregnancies. When HIV infection is diagnosed during pregnancy, ART should be started right away.

Acquired Immunodeficiency Syndrome (AIDS)

AIDS is the most advanced stage of HIV infection. People with AIDS should start ART immediately.

A diagnosis of AIDS is based on the following criteria:

- A cluster of differentiation 4 (CD4) count less than 200 cells/mm^3. A low CD4 count is a sign that HIV has severely damaged the immune system. Or

- Illness with an AIDS-defining condition. AIDS-defining conditions are infections and cancers that are life-threatening in people with HIV. Certain forms of lymphoma and tuberculosis are examples of AIDS-defining conditions.

HIV-Related Illnesses and Coinfections

Some illnesses that develop in people with HIV increase the urgency to start ART. These illnesses include HIV-related kidney disease and certain opportunistic infections (OIs). OIs are infections that develop more often or are more severe in people with weakened immune systems, such as people with HIV.

Coinfection is when a person has two or more infections at the same time. Coinfection with HIV and certain other infections, such as hepatitis B or hepatitis C virus infection, increases the urgency to start ART.

Recent HIV Infection

Recent HIV infection is the period up to 6 months after infection with HIV. During recent HIV infection, the level of HIV in the body (called viral load) is very high. A high viral load damages the immune system and increases the risk of HIV transmission.

ART is an important part of staying healthy with HIV. Studies suggest that these benefits begin even when ART is started in recent HIV infection. In addition, starting ART during recent HIV infection reduces the risk of HIV transmission.

Importance of Medication Adherence

Before starting ART, people with HIV discuss the benefits and risks of ART with their healthcare providers. They also discuss the importance of medication adherence—taking HIV medicines every day and exactly as prescribed. Adherence to an HIV regimen prevents HIV from multiplying and destroying the immune system. Taking HIV medicines every day also reduces the risk of HIV transmission.

Before starting ART, it's important to address issues that can make adherence difficult. For example, a busy schedule or lack of health insurance to cover the cost of HIV medicines can make it hard to take HIV medicines consistently. Healthcare providers can recommend resources to help people deal with any issues that may interfere with adherence.

Section 26.2

HIV Treatment Regimens

This section includes text excerpted from the following:
Text under the heading "What to Start: Choosing an Human
Immunodeficiency Virus (HIV) Regimen" is excerpted from "What
to Start: Choosing an HIV Regimen," AIDS*info*, U.S. Department
of Health and Human Services (HHS), March 22, 2018; Text under
the heading "HIV Medicines Approved by the U.S. Food and Drug
Administration (FDA)" is excerpted from "FDA-Approved HIV
Medicines," AIDS*info*, U.S. Department of Health and Human
Services (HHS), April 10, 2018.

What to Start: Choosing an Human Immunodeficiency Virus (HIV) Regimen

What Is an HIV Regimen?

An human immunodeficiency virus infection regimen is a combination of HIV medicines used to treat HIV infection. HIV treatment (also called antiretroviral therapy or ART) begins with choosing an HIV regimen. People on ART take the HIV medicines in their HIV regimens every day. ART helps people with HIV live longer, healthier lives and reduces the risk of HIV transmission.

There are more than 35 HIV medicines approved by the U.S. Food and Drug Administration (FDA) to treat HIV infection. Some HIV medicines are available in combination (in other words, two or more different HIV medicines combined in one pill).

The U.S. Department of Health and Human Services (HHS) provides guidelines on the use of HIV medicines. In general, the guidelines recommend starting ART with a regimen that includes three HIV medicines from at least two different drug classes.

What Are the HIV Drug Classes?

HIV medicines are grouped into seven drug classes according to how they fight HIV. The seven drug classes are:

- Nonnucleoside reverse transcriptase inhibitors (NNRTIs)

- Nucleoside reverse transcriptase inhibitors (NRTIs)

- Protease inhibitors (PIs)

- Fusion inhibitors

- CCR5 antagonists

- Integrase strand transfer inhibitors (INSTIs)

- Postattachment inhibitors

In general, a person's first HIV regimen includes two NRTIs plus an INSTI, an NNRTI, or a PI boosted with cobicistat (brand name: Tybost) or ritonavir (brand name: Norvir). Cobicistat or ritonavir increase (boost) the effectiveness of the PI.

What Factors Are Considered When Choosing an HIV Regimen?

The choice of HIV medicines to include in an HIV regimen depends on a person's individual needs. When choosing an HIV regimen, people with HIV and their healthcare providers consider the following factors:

- Other diseases or conditions that the person with HIV may have, such as heart disease or pregnancy

- Possible side effects of HIV medicines

- Potential interactions between HIV medicines or between HIV medicines and other medicines the person with HIV is taking

- Results of drug-resistance testing (and other tests). Drug-resistance testing identifies which, if any, HIV medicines won't be effective against a person's HIV.

- Convenience of the regimen. For example, a regimen that includes two or more HIV medicines combined in one pill is convenient to follow.

- Any issues that can make it difficult to follow an HIV regimen. For example, a busy schedule can make it hard to take HIV medicines consistently every day.

- Cost of HIV medicines

The HHS guidelines on the use of HIV medicines in adults and adolescents recommend several regimens for people starting ART. The best regimen for a person depends on their individual needs.

How Long Does It Take for Antiretroviral Therapy (ART) to Work?

Viral load is the amount of HIV in a person's blood. A main goal of ART is to reduce a person's viral load to an undetectable level. An undetectable viral load means that the level of HIV in the blood is too low to be detected by a viral load test.

Once effective ART is started, it usually takes 3–6 months for a person's viral load to reach an undetectable level. Having an undetectable viral load doesn't mean a person's HIV is cured. But although there is still some HIV in the person's body, an undetectable viral load shows that ART is working effectively.

HIV Medicines Approved by the U.S. Food and Drug Administration (FDA)

Treatment with HIV medicines is called ART. ART is recommended for everyone with HIV. People on ART take a combination of HIV medicines (called an HIV regimen) every day. A person's initial HIV regimen generally includes three HIV medicines from at least two different drug classes.

ART can't cure HIV, but HIV medicines help people with HIV live longer, healthier lives. HIV medicines also reduce the risk of HIV transmission.

The following table lists HIV medicines recommended for the treatment of HIV infection in the United States based on the HHS-HIV/AIDS medical practice guidelines. All of these drugs are approved by the FDA. The HIV medicines are listed according to drug class and identified by generic and brand names.

Table 26.1. FDA-Approved HIV Medicines

Drug Class	Generic Name (Other Names and Acronyms)	Brand Name
Nucleoside Reverse Transcriptase Inhibitors (NRTIs)		
NRTIs block reverse transcriptase, an enzyme HIV needs to make copies of itself.	abacavir (abacavir sulfate, ABC)	Ziagen
	emtricitabine (FTC)	Emtriva
	lamivudine (3TC)	Epivir
	tenofovir disoproxil fumarate (tenofovir DF, TDF)	Viread
	zidovudine (azidothymidine, AZT, ZDV)	Retrovir
Nonnucleoside Reverse Transcriptase Inhibitors (NNRTIs)		
NNRTIs bind to and later alter reverse transcriptase, an enzyme HIV needs to make copies of itself.	efavirenz (EFV)	Sustiva
	etravirine (ETR)	Intelence
	nevirapine (extended-release nevirapine, NVP)	Viramune Viramune XR (extended release)
	rilpivirine (rilpivirine hydrochloride, RPV)	Edurant

Table 26.1. Continued

Drug Class	Generic Name (Other Names and Acronyms)	Brand Name
Protease Inhibitors (PIs)		
PIs block HIV protease, an enzyme HIV needs to make copies of itself.	atazanavir (atazanavir sulfate, ATV)	Reyataz
	darunavir (darunavir ethanolate, DRV)	Prezista
	fosamprenavir (fosamprenavir calcium, FOS-APV, FPV)	Lexiva
	ritonavir (RTV)*Although ritonavir is a PI, it is generally used as a pharmacokinetic enhancer as recommended in the Guidelines for the Use of Antiretroviral Agents in Adults and Adolescents Living with HIV and the Guidelines for the Use of Antiretroviral Agents in Pediatric HIV Infection.	Norvir
	saquinavir (saquinavir mesylate, SQV)	Invirase
	tipranavir (TPV)	Aptivus
Fusion Inhibitors		
Fusion inhibitors block HIV from entering the CD4 cells of the immune system.	enfuvirtide (T-20)	Fuzeon

Table 26.1. Continued

Drug Class	Generic Name (Other Names and Acronyms)	Brand Name
CCR5 Antagonists		
CCR5 antagonists block CCR5 coreceptors on the surface of certain immune cells that HIV needs to enter the cells.	maraviroc (MVC)	Selzentry
Integrase Inhibitors		
Integrase inhibitors block HIV integrase, an enzyme HIV needs to make copies of itself.	dolutegravir (DTG, dolutegravir sodium)	Tivicay
	raltegravir (raltegravir potassium, RAL)	Isentress Isentress HD
Postattachment Inhibitors		
Postattachment inhibitors block CD4 receptors on the surface of certain immune cells that HIV needs to enter the cells.	ibalizumab (Hu5A8, IBA, Ibalizumab-uiyk, TMB-355, TNX-355)	Trogarzo
Pharmacokinetic Enhancers		
Pharmacokinetic enhancers are used in HIV treatment to increase the effectiveness of an HIV medicine included in an HIV regimen.	cobicistat (COBI)	Tybost

Table 26.1. Continued

Drug Class	Generic Name (Other Names and Acronyms)	Brand Name
Combination HIV Medicines		
Combination HIV medicines contain two or more HIV medicines from one or more drug classes.	abacavir and lamivudine (abacavir sulfate/lamivudine, ABC/3TC)	Epzicom
	abacavir, dolutegravir, and lamivudine (abacavir sulfate/dolutegravir sodium/lamivudine, ABC/DTG/3TC)	Triumeq
	abacavir, lamivudine, and zidovudine (abacavir sulfate/lamivudine/zidovudine, ABC/3TC/ZDV)	Trizivir
	atazanavir and cobicistat (atazanavir sulfate/cobicistat, ATV/COBI)	Evotaz
	bictegravir, emtricitabine, and tenofovir alafenamide (bictegravir sodium/emtricitabine/tenofovir alafenamide fumarate, BIC/FTC/TAF)	Biktarvy
	darunavir and cobicistat (darunavir ethanolate/cobicistat, DRV/COBI)	Prezcobix
	dolutegravir and rilpivirine (dolutegravir sodium/rilpivirine hydrochloride, DTG/RPV)	Juluca
	efavirenz, emtricitabine, and tenofovir disoproxil fumarate (efavirenz/emtricitabine/tenofovir DF, EFV/FTC/TDF)	Atripla

Table 26.1. Continued

Drug Class	Generic Name (Other Names and Acronyms)	Brand Name
	efavirenz, lamivudine, and tenofovir disoproxil fumarate (EFV/3TC/TDF)	Symfi
	efavirenz, lamivudine, and tenofovir disoproxil fumarate (EFV/3TC/TDF)	Symfi Lo
	elvitegravir, cobicistat, emtricitabine, and tenofovir alafenamide fumarate (elvitegravir/cobicistat/emtricitabine/tenofovir alafenamide, EVG/COBI/FTC/TAF)	Genvoya
	elvitegravir, cobicistat, emtricitabine, and tenofovir disoproxil fumarate (QUAD, EVG/COBI/FTC/TDF)	Stribild
	emtricitabine, rilpivirine, and tenofovir alafenamide (emtricitabine/rilpivirine/tenofovir AF, emtricitabine/ rilpivirine/tenofovir alafenamide fumarate, emtricitabine/rilpivirine hydrochloride/tenofovir AF, emtricitabine/rilpivirine hydrochloride/tenofovir alafenamide, emtricitabine/rilpivirine hydrochloride/ tenofovir alafenamide fumarate, FTC/RPV/TAF)	Odefsey
	emtricitabine, rilpivirine, and tenofovir disoproxil fumarate (emtricitabine/rilpivirine hydrochloride/tenofovir disoproxil fumarate, emtricitabine/rilpivirine/ tenofovir, FTC/RPV/TDF)	Complera

Table 26.1. Continued

Drug Class	Generic Name (Other Names and Acronyms)	Brand Name
	emtricitabine and tenofovir alafenamide (emtricitabine/tenofovir AF, emtricitabine/tenofovir alafenamide fumarate, FTC/TAF)	Descovy
	emtricitabine and tenofovir disoproxil fumarate (emtricitabine/tenofovir DF, FTC/TDF)	Truvada
	lamivudine and tenofovir disoproxil fumarate (3TC/TDF)	Cimduo
	lamivudine and zidovudine (3TC/ZDV)	Combivir
	lopinavir and ritonavir (ritonavir-boosted lopinavir, LPV/r, LPV/RTV)	Kaletra

Section 26.3

Deciding Which Drugs to Take

This section includes text excerpted from "Treatment
Decisions for HIV: Entire Section," U.S. Department of
Veterans Affairs (VA), February 9, 2018.

Treatment Decisions

Human immunodeficiency virus (HIV) is a virus that can multiply
quickly in your body and damage your immune system. Even though no
cure exists for HIV infection or the later stage of HIV disease known as
acquired immunodeficiency syndrome (AIDS), there are many different
drugs that can essentially shut down the HIV virus, greatly slow down
the damage it does, and allow the immune system to recover. Today's
treatments allow most people to live long and healthy lives and helps
prevent transmission of HIV to sex partners.

Without treatment, HIV can make your immune system very weak.
Your immune system is what allows your body to fight off infections
and cancers. When it is weakened, you will have a hard time staying
well.

It is important to talk with your healthcare provider, who can help
you make appropriate decisions about HIV treatment.

This section can help you decide:

- Whether and when to start therapy

- What drugs to take

- Whether to continue therapy

Starting Therapy

HIV drugs are very important in keeping people healthy over the
years. For people who are sick from HIV, they can be lifesavers. Effective treatment stops or slows the progression of HIV and has important
benefits, even for persons whose immune systems appear to be functioning relatively well. Thus, in general, HIV drugs are recommended
for all people with HIV infection, whether they are sick or well.

For people whose immune systems are weaker, starting treatment
is urgent. For people whose immune systems are still strong, it is
important to start HIV medications before their immune systems
suffer more. Studies show that starting treatment early may be the

most effective way to prevent long-term consequences of HIV. And, treatment dramatically reduces the risk of passing HIV infection to sex partners (or injection drug use partners); for pregnant women, it greatly reduces the chance of infecting the baby in the womb or at birth.

However, there are reasons some people may be hesitant to start HIV treatment right away. For one thing, the medications must be taken correctly every day or the virus may become resistant to drugs. That means the virus may change in a way that makes the drug no longer work. The most common cause of drug resistance is not taking medications correctly every day. So, people need to be ready to commit to taking the medications every day (referred as "adherence"). Also, HIV medicines, like any other drugs, may cause side effects in some people. But most people who take the newer HIV drugs do not have any problems with them. In addition, the available drug regimens usually are simple and compact (between 1 and 3 pills per day).

So, as mentioned earlier, treatment of HIV is recommended for all people with the infection. Experts generally advise starting treatment soon after you are diagnosed with HIV, but these are some things your healthcare provider may consider in advising you how quickly to start:

- Symptoms of HIV disease (also called your clinical status, or how well you feel)

- Your cluster of differentiation 4 (CD4) count and viral load

- Whether you have certain other medical conditions that may be helped by HIV treatment

- Whether you can and will stick to your treatment plan (adherence)

- Whether you have sex partner(s) who are HIV-negative and may be at risk of becoming infected through you

Symptoms (Clinical Status)

"Clinical status" refers to how well you are doing in general, including how well you feel. Your doctor will look at whether you have symptoms of HIV disease. These symptoms are signs that HIV is weakening your immune system, and include things such as weight loss, chronic fevers, and opportunistic infections. (Opportunistic infections—also called OIs—are infections that happen in someone with a damaged immune system.)

Cluster of Differentiation 4 (CD4) Count and Viral Load

Even though you may not feel it, when you have HIV, the virus and your immune system are at war with each other. The virus is trying to multiply as fast as it can, and your body is trying to stop it. Two tests, the CD4 count and the HIV viral load, help you and your healthcare provider know how strong your immune system is, and know whether it is keeping HIV under control.

CD4 cells play a major role in helping your immune system work properly. HIV causes disease by killing off CD4 cells. It does this by infecting the cells and turning them into virus factories, a process that kills the cell. A test called the CD4 count can tell you how many CD4 cells you have. The higher the number, the better. The test, however, doesn't tell you if those CD4 cells are working properly.

The viral load test indicates how much of the HIV virus is present in your blood, and how fast it is multiplying. The higher the viral load, the faster HIV is infecting and killing your CD4 cells. The lower the viral load, the better.

Your healthcare provider will look at these two things carefully. People whose CD4 count is low, and people whose viral load is high, are more likely to get sick sooner than people with a high CD4 count and low viral load.

CD4 count and viral load tests usually are done every 3 months in people who are not on treatment. Results can help you and your healthcare provider decide how urgent it is to start anti-HIV drugs. The U.S. Department of Health and Human Services (HHS) recommends HIV drugs for everyone, no matter how high or low their CD4 count is. However, they say that HIV treatment is especially important if your CD4 count is lower, or if you have symptoms. The lower the CD4, the more important it is to start treatment quickly.

Other Medical Conditions That May Be Helped by HIV Treatment

Starting HIV drugs may be particularly important for people with certain other medical conditions. For example, your doctor will recommend HIV therapy if you are pregnant or plan to become pregnant, if you have kidney disease that is caused by HIV, or if you have hepatitis B or hepatitis C.

Whether You Can and Will Stick to Your Treatment Plan (Adherence)

Before you start medications for HIV, it is very important to make a strong commitment to sticking to a drug therapy plan (or regimen). With an HIV drug regimen, you will need to take pills every day!

In order for the drugs to work and keep working, you must carefully follow the directions for taking them. If you're not sure you can do this, you might need help in finding ways to stick to the plan.

If you are wondering whether you should start taking drugs for HIV, you should sit down and talk with your provider as soon as possible. Depending on your specific needs, your provider can come up with a personal treatment plan for you.

Risk of Transmitting HIV to Sex Partners

HIV therapy has been shown to greatly reduce the risk of transmitting HIV to uninfected sex partners. In fact, if you take your medicines every day and your HIV treatment is working well, there is almost no risk of transmitting HIV to a sex partner. Thus, if you have a sex partner who is HIV negative, you may consider starting HIV treatment both to protect and improve your own health and to prevent transmission to partners. Similarly, if you are pregnant or intend to become pregnant, it is important to start HIV medications right away both to protect your own health and to reduce the risk of passing HIV to the baby during pregnancy or at the time of birth.

Deciding What Drugs to Take

Your provider will talk with you and together you will come up with a personal treatment plan. You will find it easier to understand your plan if you learn about the different drugs available and what they do.

What Kinds of Drugs Are Available?

Anti-HIV drugs are also called antiretroviral drugs or antiretrovirals (ARVs). A whole treatment regimen is called antiretroviral therapy, or ART. The ARVs work because they attack the HIV virus directly—they cripple the ability of the virus to make copies of itself. Usually, an ART regimen consists of 3 different medicines from at least 2 classes (types) of drugs. This is because it takes a powerful combination of medicines to suppress the HIV virus.

There are 5 main classes of anti-HIV drugs:

- Nucleoside reverse transcriptase inhibitors (NRTIs or "nukes")

- Nonnucleoside reverse transcriptase inhibitors (NNRTIs or "nonnukes")

- Integrase inhibitors

- Protease inhibitors (PIs)

- Entry inhibitors

Each group attacks HIV in its own way and helps your body fight the infection. Most of these drugs come as tablets or capsules. Several of these drugs may be combined into one tablet to make it easier to take your medications. These are known as fixed-dose combinations.

The following is a short description of how each group of drugs works and the names of the individual drugs.

Note: *The names of drugs are long and sometimes hard to pronounce. Don't worry! You can always come back and read this again, and you can talk to your doctor about questions you have.*

Nucleoside Reverse Transcriptase Inhibitors (NRTIs or Nukes)

The first group of antiretroviral drugs is the nucleoside reverse transcriptase inhibitors (NRTIs).

NRTIs were the first type of drug available to treat HIV. They remain effective, powerful, and important medications for treating HIV when combined with other drugs. They are better known as nucleoside analogs or "nukes."

When the HIV virus enters a healthy cell, it attempts to make copies of itself. It does this by using an enzyme called reverse transcriptase. The NRTIs work because they block that enzyme. Without reverse transcriptase, HIV can't make new virus copies of itself.

The following drugs are NRTIs that are in current use; their generic names are listed along with their common names, if they have one, and their brand names. There are several older NRTIs that generally are not used;

- Abacavir (brand name: Ziagen®)

- Emtricitabine (FTC; brand name: Emtriva®)

- Lamivudine (3TC; brand name: Epivir®)

- Tenofovir alafenamide (TAF)

- Tenofovir DF (TDF; brand name: Viread®)

NRTI drugs may be combined into one tablet to make it easier to take your medications. These drugs are known as fixed-dose combinations; here are several examples*:

- Descovy® (tenofovir alafenamide + Emtriva)

- Epzicom® (Epivir + Ziagen)

- Truvada® (Viread + Emtriva)

*Note: *Generic combinations of some currently used NRTIs are available, as well as several combinations of older NRTIs that are not currently recommended.*

Nonnucleoside Reverse Transcriptase Inhibitors (NNRTIs or Nonnukes)

The second type of antiretroviral drugs is the nonnucleoside reverse "nonnukes."

These drugs also prevent HIV from using reverse transcriptase to make copies of itself, but in a different way.

These NNRTIs are available and in use:

- Efavirenz (brand name: Sustiva®)

- Etravirine (brand name: Intelence®)

- Rilpivirine (brand name: Edurant®)

Some NNRTIs are combined with NRTIs in fixed-dose combination tablets.

Protease Inhibitors (PIs)

The third group of drugs is the protease inhibitors (PIs).

Once HIV has infected a cell and made copies of itself, it uses an enzyme called protease to process itself correctly so it can be released from the cell to infect other cells. These medicines work by blocking protease.

There are nine PIs, but only a couple of them are used as of now:

- Atazanavir (brand name: Reyataz®)

- Darunavir (brand name: Prezista®)

- Lopinavir (combined with ritonavir in one table; brand name: Kaletra®)

Many PIs are recommended or approved for use only with another drug that "boosts" their effect. One of these is low-dose Norvir®, the other is a non-HIV drug called Tybost® (cobicistat).

There are three fixed-dose combination tablets that include a "booster" plus a PI:

- Evotaz® (Reyataz® + Tybost®)

- Prezcobix® (Prezista® + Tybost®)

- Kaletra® (lopinavir + Norvir®)

Integrase Inhibitors

This class of anti-HIV drugs works by blocking an enzyme (HIV integrase) that the virus needs in order to splice copies of itself into human deoxyribonucleic acid (DNA).

- Bictegravir

- Dolutegravir (brand name: Tivicay®)

- Elvitegravir (brand name: Vitekta®)*

- Raltegravir (brand name: Isentress®)

Some integrase inhibitors are combined with NRTIs in fixed-dose combination tablets.

***Note:** *Elvitegravir must be "boosted" with a pharmacokinetic enhancer, either cobicistat or ritonavir.*

Chemokine Coreceptor Antagonists (CCR5)

To infect a cell, HIV must bind to two types of molecules on the cell's surface. One of these is called a chemokine coreceptor. Drugs known as chemokine coreceptor antagonists block the virus from binding to the coreceptor.

One CCR5 antagonist is available:

- Selzentry® (maraviroc)

Entry Inhibitors

The three entry inhibitors that are available, work in different ways:

1. Enfuvirtide (T20; brand name: Fuzeon®) prevents HIV from entering the CD4 T cell

2. Ibalizumab (brand name: Trogarzo®) blocks HIV from binding to the CD4 receptor

3. Maraviroc (brand name: Selzentry®) blocks HIV from binding to a coreceptor

Multi-Class Drug Combinations

There are a number of combination tablets that include drugs from two different groups in a complete HIV drug regimen. A patient prescribed one of these combinations takes only one tablet, once a day. Despite the convenience, these combination tablets are not for everyone. Usually, they are just for people who are starting HIV treatment, and each has specific possible side effects or dosing requirements that should be considered. You and your doctor can decide whether these drug combinations are right for you.

- Atripla® (Sustiva + Emtriva + Viread)

- Complera® (Edurant + Emtriva + Viread)

- Genvoya® (Vitekta + Tybost + Emtriva + tenofovir alafenamide)

- Odefsey® (Edurant + Emtriva + tenofovir alafenamide)

- Stribild® (Vitekta + Tybost + Emtriva + Viread)

- Triumeq® (Tivicay + Epzicom + Ziagen)

Which Drugs Should You Take?

Now that you have learned a little about the types of drugs that are available and how they work, you may be wondering how your healthcare provider will know which medicines you should take.

Anti-HIV drugs are used in combination with one another in order to get the best results. The goal is to get the viral load as low as possible (to levels that are undetectable by standard laboratory tests) for as long as possible.

Anti-HIV medicines do different things to the virus—they attack it in different ways—so using the different drugs in combination works better than using just one by itself. Combinations usually include three antiretroviral drugs. Except in very special circumstances, anti-HIV drugs should never be used one or two at a time. Using only one or two drugs at a time can fail to control the viral load and let the virus adapt (or become resistant) to the drug. Once the virus adapts to a drug, the drug won't work as well against the virus, and maybe it won't work at all.

There is no one combination of HIV medications that works best for everyone. Each combination has its pluses and minuses.

When drugs are used together, the therapy is called combination therapy or antiretroviral therapy (ART).

Combination Therapy

So, how will your health provider know which combination to choose? You and your provider can consider the options, keeping certain things in mind, such as possible side effects, the number of pills you'll need to take, and how the drugs interact with each other and with other medications you may take.

Sticking to Your Medicines (Adherence)

"Adherence" refers to how well you stay on your treatment plan—whether you take your medications exactly as your healthcare provider tells you.

If you follow your provider's instructions about how to take your medicine, the anti-HIV drugs will work well to lower the amount of virus in your blood. Taking your drugs correctly increases your likelihood of success.

But, if you miss doses, or don't follow a regular schedule, your treatment may not work, and the HIV virus may become resistant to the medicines.

Before you start a treatment plan, you should:

- Get your healthcare provider to write everything down for you: names of the drugs, what they look like, how to take them (for example, with food or not, with other medications or not), and how often to take them. This way, you'll have something to look at in case you forget what you're supposed to do.

- With your provider's help, develop a plan that works for you.

Questions to Ask about Each Drug

One of the most important things you can do to make sure you take your medicine correctly is to talk with your doctor about your lifestyles, such as your sleeping and eating schedule. If your doctor prescribes a drug, be sure and ask the following questions (and make sure you understand the answers):

- What dose of the drug should be taken? How many pills does this mean?

- How often should the drug be taken?

- Does it matter if it is taken with food, or on an empty stomach?

- Does the drug have to be kept in a refrigerator?

- What are the side effects of the drug?

- What should be done to deal with the side effects?

- How severe do side effects have to be before a doctor is called?

During every visit to your doctor, you should talk about whether you are having trouble staying on your treatment plan. Studies show that patients who take their medicine in the right way get the best results: their viral loads stay down, their CD4 counts stay up, and they feel healthier.

Tips for Staying on Your Treatment Plan

Before you start a treatment plan, you should:

- Get your healthcare provider to write everything down for you: names of the drugs, what they look like, how to take them (for example, with food or not, with other medications or not), and how often to take them. This way, you'll have something to look at in case you forget what you're supposed to do.

- With your provider's help, develop a plan that works for you.

Other Challenges You Might Have While on HIV Therapy

Now that you've thought about adherence and some of the other factors you should consider before starting HIV drug therapy, let's look at some of the other things you will need to know once you are taking the medicine. These involve drug interactions and drug side effects.

What are Drug Interactions?

Your anti-HIV medications can be affected by other medicines, including other prescription drugs you are taking and drugs you buy over the counter at a pharmacy. Even herbal therapies, nutritional supplements, and some things found in common foods can affect your HIV medicines.

When one drug affects how another drug behaves, this is called a drug-drug interaction. For example, some drugs become less effective or cause side effects when they are taken with certain other drugs.

When something in food affects how a drug behaves, it is called a drug-food interaction. For example, grapefruit juice, taken at the same time as certain drugs, can boost the amount of these drugs in your bloodstream to an undesirable level. Everyone taking anti-HIV drugs needs to be very careful about these interactions. Luckily, many of these interactions are well known to your provider, and can be managed.

Your healthcare provider can give you a list of drugs and foods to avoid, depending on what kind of medicine you are taking. Ask for this information for each drug that you are taking.

Also, be sure that you tell your doctor about every single medication, drug, supplement, and herb you are taking—whether you got them by prescription or not.

What Are Side Effects?

Medicines can cause changes (or effects) in the body. Some effects, like making you feel better, are the ones that you want and expect to happen. Other effects are ones that you don't want or don't expect. The effects that you don't want or expect are called side effects.

Almost all medicines may have side effects in some people. Some people take aspirin for a headache, but it gives them an upset stomach. The upset stomach is a side effect of the aspirin. Not all side effects are unpleasant, though. Even the side effects that make you feel sick aren't always bad. Some side effects mean that your medicine has started to work.

Your provider will try to prescribe anti-HIV medicines that fight the HIV virus in your body without causing unpleasant side effects.

How Do You Deal with Side Effects?

Some side effects can be hard to deal with. One way to cope with them is to know what to watch out for and have a plan to deal with problems that come up.

That's why you need to talk to your provider about the risk of side effects from different drugs, before you start therapy.

At the beginning of any treatment, you go through a period of adjustment—a time when your body has to get used to the new drugs you're taking. Sometimes you'll have headaches, an upset stomach, fatigue, or aches and pains. These side effects may go away after a few weeks or so.

If you notice any unusual or severe reactions after starting or changing a drug, report the side effects to your provider immediately.

How Do You Know If the Drugs Are Working?

After you've started taking medicine for your HIV, your healthcare provider will look at how much HIV virus is in your bloodstream (your viral load) to see how well the drug therapy is working. If the medicines are working, your viral load goes down. You will have less of the virus in your bloodstream. A very important goal of treatment is to reduce the viral load to below the level that can be counted by laboratory tests, and to keep it there. This sometimes is called an "undetectable" level of HIV.

Other ways you and your provider can see if the drugs are working are:

- Your CD4 count. This number should stay the same or go up if your drugs are working.

- Your health checkups. Your treatment should help keep you healthy and help you fight off infections and diseases.

Should You Ever Take a 'Holiday' from the Drugs?

In general, taking a "drug holiday" from your anti-HIV medicine for reasons other than a severe reaction to medications may be harmful to your health. Having said that, your doctor may suggest that you temporarily stop your antiretroviral drugs for certain specific reasons. Be sure to talk with your healthcare provider about this issue if you have questions about it. How you stop taking your anti-HIV drugs safely can be a complicated process.

Remember, just skipping doses without your doctor's instructions is dangerous, and you should never change your treatment plan without talking with your doctor.

Should You Ever Switch the Drugs You're Taking?

You should never change the drug plan you're on without talking with your healthcare provider. This is a very important decision and one that must be made with your healthcare provider.

There are a few reasons that your provider may suggest you change your medicines. There may be a fixed-dose combination pill that could simplify your therapy. Or your treatment may not be working well enough and you may need different medicines. Or you may have side effects that are bothering you. Or due to lab tests that show signs of ill effects from the HIV drugs (this is called drug toxicity).

Before changing medicines, you and your provider should talk about:

- All the anti-HIV drugs you have taken before and the ones you haven't taken

- Any drug resistance your HIV virus may have

- The strength of the new drugs that your provider recommends

- Possible side effects of the new medicines

- How well you will be able to follow the new drug treatment plan

Always be sure to talk with your provider about any changes in your drug treatment.

If the Viral Load Is Undetectable, Can You Stop Treatment?

Having a viral load below levels that laboratory tests can measure (this is called a suppressed viral load, or sometimes an "undetectable" viral load) tells us that the anti-HIV medications are working. An undetectable viral load doesn't mean the HIV virus has been eradicated from your body, though. Even though the virus is not detected in the blood, it is still present in other parts of your body, such as the lymph nodes, brain, and reproductive organs. If you stop treatment, the virus will start reproducing again and your viral load will increase, putting your health at risk.

What If Your Treatment Isn't Working?

Sometimes the HIV medications don't work. This may occur because the drugs don't completely stop the virus from reproducing. As the virus makes copies of itself, changes (or mutations) sometimes occur. These changes may result in a new strain of the virus that is resistant to the action of the drugs. If your providers think this has happened, they will do a blood test (called a resistance test, genotype, or phenotype) that can help show which drugs the virus has become resistant to. This can help identify other drugs that might still work against your virus.

If a person has a strain of HIV that is resistant to most or all available drugs, that person may want to consider joining a clinical trial that is testing new drugs that have not yet been approved by the U.S. Food and Drug Administration (FDA).

Chapter 27

HIV/AIDS Treatment Adherence

Chapter Contents

Section 27.1

Importance of Medication Adherence

This section contains text excerpted from the following sources:
Text beginning with the heading "What Is Medication Adherence?"
is excerpted from "HIV Treatment—HIV Medication Adherence,"
AIDS*info*, U.S. Department of Health and Human Services (HHS),
January 17, 2018; Text beginning with the heading "What
Should I Do If I Miss a Dose?" is excerpted from "Taking
Your HIV Medications Every Day," HIV.gov, U.S. Department
of Health and Human Services (HHS), May 15, 2017.

What Is Medication Adherence?

Adherence means "to stick firmly." So for people with human immu-nodeficiency virus (HIV), medication adherence means sticking firmly to an HIV regimen—taking HIV medicines every day and exactly as prescribed.

Why Is Adherence to an HIV Regimen Important?

Adherence to an HIV regimen gives HIV medicines the chance to do their job: to prevent HIV from multiplying and destroying the immune system. HIV medicines help people with HIV live longer, healthier lives. HIV medicines also reduce the risk of HIV transmission.

Poor adherence to an HIV regimen allows HIV to destroy the immune system. A damaged immune system makes it hard for the body to fight off infections and certain cancers. Poor adherence also increases the risk of drug resistance and HIV treatment failure.

What Is Drug Resistance?

Drug resistance can develop as HIV multiplies in the body. When HIV multiplies, the virus sometimes mutates (changes form) and makes variations of itself. Variations of HIV that develop while a person is taking HIV medicines can lead to new, drug-resistant strains of HIV. With drug resistance, HIV medicines that used to suppress the person's HIV are not effective against the new drug-resistant HIV. In other words, the person's HIV continues to multiply.

Once drug-resistant HIV develops, it remains in the body. Drug resistance limits the number of HIV medicines available to include in a current or future HIV regimen.

What Is the Connection between Medication Adherence and Drug Resistance?

Taking HIV medicines every day prevents HIV from multiplying, which reduces the risk that HIV will mutate and produce drug-resistant HIV. Skipping HIV medicines allows HIV to multiply, which increases the risk of drug-resistant HIV developing.

Research shows that a person's first HIV regimen offers the best chance for long-term treatment success. So adherence is important from the start—when a person first begins taking HIV medicines.

Why Is Medication Adherence Sometimes Difficult?

Adherence to an HIV regimen can be difficult for several reasons. For example, side effects from some HIV medicines, such as nausea or diarrhea, can make it hard to follow an HIV regimen. When an HIV regimen includes several HIV medicines, it's easy to forget how many pills to take and when to take them.

The following factors can also make medication adherence difficult:

- Side effects from interactions between HIV medicines and other medicines a person may take

- Trouble swallowing pills or other difficulty taking medicines

- A busy schedule, shift work or travel away from home that makes it hard to take medicines on time

- Having an unstable living or housing situation

- Illness or depression

- Alcohol or drug use that interferes with the activities of daily life

- Fear of disclosing one's HIV-positive status to others

- Lack of health insurance to cover the cost of HIV medicines

Before starting HIV medicines, it helps to have strategies in place to maintain adherence. Strategies may include using a 7-day pill box or using an app, such as the AIDS*info* Drug Database app, to set daily pill reminders. Also, healthcare providers can provide helpful referrals and resources for anticipated adherence challenges. People can work with their healthcare providers to select an HIV regimen that works best for their needs and lifestyle.

What Should I Do If I Miss a Dose?

Taking your HIV medicines exactly the way your healthcare provider tells you to will help keep your viral load low and your CD4 cell count high. If you skip your medicines, even now and then, you are giving HIV the chance to multiply rapidly. This could weaken your immune system, and you could become sick.

Talk to your healthcare provider if you miss a dose. In most cases, if you realize you missed a dose, take the medicines as soon as you can, then take the next dose at your usual scheduled time (unless your pharmacist or healthcare provider has told you something different).

If you find you miss a lot of doses, talk to your healthcare provider or pharmacist about ways to help you remember your medicines. You and your healthcare provider may even decide to change your treatment regimen to fit your healthcare needs and life situation, which may change over time.

Do I Have to Take My Medicines If My Viral Load Is Undetectable?

Yes, antiretroviral therapy (ART) reduces viral load, ideally to an undetectable level. If your viral load goes down after starting ART, then the treatment is working, and you should always take your medicine as prescribed by your healthcare provider. Even when your viral load is undetectable, HIV can still exist in semen, vaginal and rectal fluids, breast milk, and other parts of your body, so you should continue to take steps to prevent HIV transmission. Taking your HIV medications on schedule will help keep your viral load very low and help you maintain your health. It will also make it more difficult for you to pass HIV on to others.

Section 27.2

Following an HIV Regimen: Steps to Take before and after Starting HIV Medicines

This section includes text excerpted from "HIV Treatment—
Following an HIV Regimen: Steps to Take before and after
Starting HIV Medicines," AIDS*info*, U.S. Department of
Health and Human Services (HHS), January 17, 2018.

Before Starting an HIV Regimen, Talk to Your Healthcare Provider about Medication Adherence

Talking with your healthcare provider will help you understand why you're starting human immunodeficiency (HIV) treatment and why medication adherence is important. Medication adherence means sticking firmly to an HIV regimen—taking HIV medicines every day and exactly as prescribed.

Your healthcare provider will explain that taking HIV medicines every day can protect your health and prevent HIV infection from advancing to acquired immunodeficiency syndrome (AIDS). The HIV medicines will also reduce your risk of passing HIV to another person during sex. Your healthcare provider will emphasize that adherence to an HIV regimen reduces the risk of drug resistance and treatment failure.

Information that you share with your healthcare provider will make it easier to select an HIV regimen that suits your needs. The information will also help you and your healthcare provider plan ahead for any issues that may make adherence difficult.

What Should I Tell My Healthcare Provider before Starting an HIV Regimen?

Tell your healthcare provider about other prescription and nonprescription medicines, vitamins, nutritional supplements, and herbal products you are taking or plan to take. Other medicines you take may interact with the HIV medicines in your HIV regimen. A drug interaction can reduce or increase the effect of a medicine or cause side effects.

Tell your healthcare provider about any issues that can make adherence difficult. Issues such as lack of health insurance or alcohol or drug use can make it hard to follow an HIV regimen. If needed, your healthcare provider can recommend resources to help you address any issues before you start treatment.

Describe your schedule at home and at work to your healthcare provider. Working together, you can arrange your HIV medication schedule to match your day-to-day routine.

Ask your healthcare provider for written instructions on how to follow your HIV regimen. The instructions should include the following details:

- Each HIV medicine included in your regimen

- How much of each medicine to take

- When to take each medicine

- How to take each medicine (for example, with or without food)

- Possible side effects from each medicine, including serious side effects

- How to store each medicine

Use small candies to practice following the instructions. This practice will help you identify and address problems with adherence before you start your HIV regimen.

After You Start an HIV Regimen, Use a Variety of Strategies to Maintain Adherence

To maintain adherence over the long-term, try some of the following strategies:

- Use a 7-day pill box. Once a week, fill the pill box with your HIV medicines for the entire week.

- Take your HIV medicines at the same time every day.

- Set the alarm on your cell phone to remind you to take your medicines. (An alarm clock or timer works too.) Or download the AIDS*info* Drug Database App to bookmark your HIV medicines, make notes, and set daily pill reminders.

- Ask your family members, friends, or coworkers to remind you to take your medicines.

- Keep your medicines nearby. Keep a backup supply of medicines at work or in your purse or briefcase.

- Plan ahead for changes in your daily routine, including weekends and holidays. If you're going away, pack enough medicine to last the entire trip.

- Use an app or an online or paper medicine diary to stay on track. Enter the name of each medicine; include the dose, number of pills to take, and when to take them. Record each medicine as you take it. Reviewing your diary will help you identify the times that you're most likely to forget to take your medicines.

- Keep all of your medical appointments. Use a calendar to keep track of your appointments. If you run low on medicines before your next appointment, call your healthcare provider to renew your prescriptions.

- Get additional tips on adherence by joining a support group for people living with HIV.

What Should I Do If I Forget to Take My HIV Medicines?

Unless your healthcare provider tells you otherwise, take the medicine you missed as soon as you realize you skipped it. But if it's almost time for the next dose of the medicine, don't take the missed dose and instead just continue on your regular medication schedule. Don't take a double dose of a medicine to make up for a missed dose.

Discuss Medication Adherence at Each Appointment with Your Healthcare Provider

Tell your healthcare provider if you're having difficulty following your regimen. Don't forget to mention any side effects you're having. Side effects from HIV medicines are a major reason why medication adherence can be difficult.

Let your healthcare provider know if your regimen is too complicated to follow. Your healthcare provider may simplify your regimen by including fewer HIV medicines or by reducing the number of times a day you need to take your HIV medicines.

Discuss any issues that are causing you to skip medicines. Your healthcare provider can recommend resources to help you deal with these issues.

Chapter 28

HIV/AIDS Treatment Interruptions

Discontinuation or Interruption of Antiretroviral Therapy (AVT)

Discontinuation of antiretroviral therapy (ART) may result in viral rebound, immune decompensation, and clinical progression. Thus, planned interruptions of ART are not generally recommended. However, unplanned interruption of ART may occur under certain circumstances as discussed below.

Short-Term Therapy Interruptions

Reasons for short-term interruption (days to weeks) of ART vary and may include drug toxicity; intercurrent illnesses that preclude oral intake, such as gastroenteritis or pancreatitis; surgical procedures; or interrupted access to drugs. Stopping ART for a short time (i.e., less than 1–2 days) because of a medical/surgical procedure can usually be done by holding all drugs in the regimen. Recommendations for some other scenarios are listed below:

This chapter includes text excerpted from "Guidelines for the Use of Antiretroviral Agents in Adults and Adolescents Living with HIV," AIDS*info*, U.S. Department of Health and Human Services (HHS), April 8, 2015.

Unanticipated short-term therapy interruption.

When a patient experiences a severe or life-threatening toxicity or unexpected inability to take oral medications:

- All components of the drug regimen should be stopped simultaneously, regardless of drug half-life.

Planned short-term therapy interruption (Up to 2 Weeks).

When all regimen components have similar half-lives and do not require food for proper absorption:

- All drugs may be given with a sip of water, if allowed; otherwise, all drugs should be stopped simultaneously. All discontinued regimen components should be restarted simultaneously.

When all regimen components have similar half-lives and require food for adequate absorption, and the patient cannot take anything by mouth for a short time:

- Temporary discontinuation of all drug components is indicated. The regimen should be restarted as soon as the patient can resume oral intake.

When the antiretroviral regimen contains drugs with different half-lives:

- Stopping all drugs simultaneously may result in functional monotherapy with the drug with the longest half-life (typically a nonnucleoside reverse transcriptase inhibitor (NNRTI)), which may increase the risk of selection of NNRTI-resistant mutations. Some experts recommend stopping the NNRTI first and the other antiretroviral drugs 2–4 weeks later. Alternatively, the NNRTI may be replaced with a ritonavir- or cobicistat-boosted protease inhibitor (PI/r or PI/c) for 4 weeks. The optimal time sequence for staggered discontinuation of regimen components, or replacement of the NNRTI with a PI/r or PI/c, has not been determined.

Planned Long-Term Therapy Interruptions

Planned long-term therapy interruptions are not recommended outside of controlled clinical trials (AI). Several research studies are evaluating approaches to a functional (virological control in the absence of therapy) or sterilizing (virus eradication) cure of human immunodeficiency virus (HIV) infection. As of now, the only way to reliably test the effectiveness of these strategies may be to interrupt ART and closely monitor viral rebound over time in the setting of a clinical trial.

If therapy must be discontinued, patients should be aware of and understand the risks of viral rebound, acute retroviral syndrome, increased risk of HIV transmission, decline of cluster of differentiation 4 (CD4) count, HIV disease progression, development of minor HIV-associated manifestations such as oral thrush or serious non-AIDS (acquired immunodeficiency syndrome) complications (e.g., renal, cardiac, hepatic, or neurologic complications), development of drug resistance, and the need for chemoprophylaxis against opportunistic infections as a result of CD4 decline.

Patients should be counseled about the need for close clinical and laboratory monitoring during therapy interruptions.

Chapter 29

HIV/AIDS Treatment
Side Effects

Chapter Contents

Section 29.1

Understanding HIV Treatment Side Effects

This section contains text excerpted from the following
sources: Text beginning with the heading "Can Human
Immunodeficiency Syndrome (HIV) Medicines Cause Side Effects?" is
excerpted from "HIV Medicines and Side Effects," AIDS*info*,
U.S. Department of Health and Human Services (HHS), October 9,
2017; Text under the heading "Managing Side Effects" is excerpted
from "Managing Side Effects," U.S. Department of Veterans
Affairs (VA), February 9, 2018.

Can Human Immunodeficiency Syndrome (HIV) Medicines Cause Side Effects?

HIV medicines help people with HIV live longer, healthier lives.
Sometimes HIV medicines can also cause side effects. Most side
effects from HIV medicines are manageable, but a few can be serious. Overall, the benefits of HIV medicines far outweigh the risk of
side effects. In addition, many newer HIV medicines have fewer side
effects than older HIV medicines. As HIV treatment options continue
to improve, people are less likely to experience side effects from their
HIV medicines.

Before starting HIV medicines, people with HIV discuss possible
side effects from HIV medicines with their healthcare providers. They
work together to select an HIV regimen based on the person's individual needs.

Do HIV Medicines Cause the Same Side Effects?

Different HIV medicines can cause different side effects. In addition, people taking the same HIV medicine can have very different
side effects.

Side effects from HIV medicines can last only a few days or
weeks or continue for a much longer time. Some side effects may
not appear until many months or even years after starting an HIV
medicine.

If you are taking HIV medicines, tell your healthcare provider about
any side effects that you are having. Some side effects, like headaches
or occasional dizziness, may not be serious. Other side effects, such
as swelling of the throat and tongue or damage to the liver, can be
life-threatening.

What Are Some Short-Term Side Effects from HIV Medicines?

When starting an HIV medicine for the first time, you may experience side effects that last a couple of weeks. These short-term side effects can include:

- Feeling tired
- Nausea (upset stomach)
- Vomiting
- Diarrhea
- Headache

- Fever
- Muscle pain
- Occasional dizziness
- Insomnia

Sometimes, side effects that may not seem serious, such as fever, rash, nausea, or fatigue, can be a sign of a life-threatening condition. Any swelling of the face, eyes, lips, throat, or tongue is considered a life-threatening side effect that requires immediate medical attention.

People with HIV can have side effects that are not caused by HIV medicines. HIV infection itself, another medical condition, or other medicines a person is taking can also cause side effects. Always tell your healthcare provider about any side effects that you are having. Your healthcare provider can determine the cause of the side effect and recommend ways to treat or manage the side effect.

If you are taking HIV medicines and have any side effects, do NOT cut down on, skip, or stop taking your HIV medicines unless your healthcare provider tells you to. Stopping HIV medicines allows HIV to multiply and damage the immune system. A damaged immune system makes it harder for the body to fight off infections and certain HIV-related cancers. Stopping HIV medicines also increases the risk of drug resistance.

What Are Some Long-Term Side Effects from HIV Medicines?

Some side effects from HIV medicines appear months or even years after starting a medicine and can continue for a long time. Examples of long-term side effects include:

- Kidney problems, including kidney failure
- Liver damage (hepatotoxicity)
- Heart disease

- Diabetes or insulin resistance

- An increase in fat levels in the blood (hyperlipidemia)

- Changes in how the body uses and stores fat (lipodystrophy)

- Weakening of the bones (osteoporosis)

- Nervous system and psychiatric effects, including insomnia, dizziness, depression, and suicidal thoughts

What Are Ways to Manage Side Effects from HIV Medicines?

When taking HIV medicines, it helps to plan ahead. Before starting HIV medicines, talk to your healthcare provider about possible side effects. Tell your healthcare provider about your lifestyle and point out any possible side effects that would be especially hard for you to manage. The information will help your healthcare provider recommend medicines best suited to your needs.

Depending on the HIV medicines you take, your healthcare provider will:

- Tell you which specific side effects to look out for.

- Offer you suggestions on how to deal with those side effects. For example, to manage nausea and vomiting, eat smaller meals more often and avoid spicy foods.

- Tell you about the signs of life-threatening side effects that require immediate medical attention. One example is swelling of the mouth and tongue.

Tell your healthcare provider if you have any side effect that bothers you or that does not go away. Your healthcare provider may recommend that you change HIV medicines. Fortunately, there are many HIV medicines.

Managing Side Effects

Almost all medicines can have side effects, including medicines for HIV. Always let your doctor know if your side effects are severe, especially if you are finding it difficult to stay on your treatment plan.

The following is information on some common side effects and tips on how to deal with them.

- Diarrhea

- Dry mouth

- Fatigue

- Headaches

- Nausea and vomiting

- Pain and nerve problems

- Dry skin

- Rash

- Weight loss

Diarrhea-Treatment

Diarrhea is common in people with HIV, and it can be caused by a variety of things including some anti-HIV medicines. Diarrhea can range from being a small hassle to being a serious medical problem. Talk to your U.S Department of Veteran Affairs (VA) healthcare provider if diarrhea goes on for a long time, if it is bloody, if it is accompanied by fever, or if it worries you.

When you have diarrhea, always be sure to replace the fluids you have lost by drinking fluids, such as broth, herbal tea, or water.

You can also ask your doctor about taking medicines to help with your diarrhea.

Quick Tips: Diarrhea

What to try:

- Try the BRAT diet (bananas, rice, applesauce, and toast).

- Eat foods high in soluble fiber. This kind of fiber can slow diarrhea by soaking up liquid. Soluble fiber is found in oatmeal, grits, and soft bread (but not in whole grain).

- Try psyllium husk fiber bars (another source of soluble fiber). You can find these at health food stores and many groceries. Eating two of these bars and drinking a big glass of water before bedtime may help your diarrhea.

- Your provider may recommend treatments such as calcium, loperamide (Imodium), methylcellulose (Citrucel), or psyllium (Metamucil).

- Drink plenty of clear liquids.

What to avoid:

- Stay away from foods high in insoluble fiber, such as whole grains, brown rice, bran, or the skins of vegetables and fruits. These kinds of foods can make diarrhea worse.

- Avoid milk products.

- Don't eat too many greasy, high-fiber, or very sweet foods.

- Don't take in too much caffeine.

- Avoid raw or undercooked fish, chicken, and meat.

Dry Mouth-Treatment

Certain HIV medicines can cause dry mouth, making it difficult to chew, swallow, and talk.

Treating dry mouth can be simple—start by drinking plenty of liquids during or between meals. If your dry mouth is severe or doesn't go away, talk to your doctor about prescribing a treatment for you.

Quick Tips: Dry Mouth

- Rinse your mouth throughout the day with warm, salted water.

- Carry sugarless candies, lozenges, or crushed ice with you to cool the mouth and give it moisture.

- Try slippery elm or licorice tea (available in health food stores). They can moisten the mouth, and they taste great!

- Ask your VA doctor about mouth rinse and other products to treat your dry mouth.

Treatment for Fatigue

Many people feel tired, especially when they are stressed or their lives are busier than usual. Symptoms of being tired can include: having a hard time getting out of bed, walking up stairs, or even concentrating on something for very long.

If the tiredness (or fatigue) doesn't go away, even after you have given your body and mind time to rest, this tiredness can become a problem. It can get worse if you don't deal with it.

Talk with your VA healthcare provider if your fatigue is not going away or is becoming too hard to deal with. The more information you can give your doctor about how you are feeling, the more likely the two of you will be able to come up with the right treatment for your fatigue.

Quick Tips: Fatigue

- Get plenty of rest.

- Go to sleep and wake up at the same time every day. Changing your sleeping habits too much can actually make you feel tired.

- Drink 8–12 glasses of water per day; if you want a caffeinated beverage, drink it in the morning.

- Try to get some exercise every day.

- Take a short nap during the day.

- Decrease your work schedule if possible.

- Keep prepackaged or easy-to-make food in the kitchen for times when you're too tired to cook.

- Follow a healthy, balanced diet. Your VA healthcare provider may be able to help you create a meal plan.

- Talk to your doctor about the possibility that you have anemia or other medical problems. Anemia means that you have a low red blood cell count, and it can make you feel tired.

Headaches-Treatment

The most common cause of headaches is tension or stress, something we all have from time to time. Medications, including anti-HIV drugs, can cause them, too.

Headaches usually can be taken care of with drugs you can buy without a prescription, such as ibuprofen or acetaminophen. You can also help to prevent future headaches by reducing stress.

Quick Tips: Headaches

For on-the-spot headache relief, try some of these suggestions:

- Lie down and rest in a quiet, dark room.

- Take a hot, relaxing bath.

- Give yourself a "scalp massage"—massage the base of your skull with your thumbs and massage both temples gently.

- Check with your doctor about taking an over-the-counter (OTC) pain reliever, such as acetaminophen (Tylenol) or ibuprofen (Motrin, Advil).

To prevent headaches from happening again, try the following:

- Avoid things that can cause headaches, like chocolate, red wine, onions, hard cheese, and caffeine.
- Reduce your stress level.
- Drink 8–12 glasses of water per day.

Nausea and Vomiting-Treatment

Nausea can be caused by many things, including certain medications used to treat HIV (though severe nausea from HIV medications is rare). This usually goes away within a few weeks after starting a new medication.

Call your doctor if nausea or vomiting keeps you from taking your medication.

Quick Tips: Headaches

For on-the-spot headache relief, try some of these suggestions:

- Lie down and rest in a quiet, dark room.
- Take a hot, relaxing bath.
- Give yourself a "scalp massage"—massage the base of your skull with your thumbs and massage both temples gently.
- Check with your doctor about taking an over-the-counter pain reliever, such as acetaminophen (Tylenol) or ibuprofen (Motrin, Advil).

To prevent headaches from happening again, try the following:
Avoid things that can cause headaches, like chocolate, red wine, onions, hard cheese, and caffeine.

- Reduce your stress level.
- Drink 8—12 glasses of water per day.

Pain and Nerve Problems-Treatment

HIV itself and some older medications for HIV can cause damage to your nerves. This condition is called peripheral neuropathy. When these nerves are damaged, your feet, toes, and hands can feel like they're burning or stinging. It can also make them numb or stiff.

You should talk to your VA doctor if you have pain like this.

Quick Tips: Pain and Nerve Problems

- Massage your feet. This can help make the pain go away for a while.

- Soak your feet in ice water to help with the pain.

- Wear loose-fitting shoes and slippers.

- When you're in bed, don't cover your feet with blankets or sheets. The bedding can press down on your feet and toes and make the pain worse.

- Ask your doctor about taking an over-the-counter pain reliever to reduce the pain.

Dry Skin-Treatment

Dry skin is a common condition and may cause itching.

Quick Tips: Dry Skin

- Drink 8–12 glasses of water per day.

- Avoid long, hot showers or baths.

- Avoid soaps and skin products that contain alcohols or harsh chemicals.

- Use moisturizing lotion after showers (such as Aquaphor, Absorbase, or Lac-Hydrin).

- Use mild, unscented laundry detergents and avoid fabric softeners.

- Use petroleum jelly on dry, itchy areas; your provider may recommend other agents to help.

- Use sunscreen.

Rash-Treatment

Some medications can cause rashes or other skin problems. Most rashes come and go, but sometimes they signal that you are having a bad reaction to the medication, or that you have an infection or another medical issue.

It's important that you check your skin for changes, especially after you start a new medication. Be sure to report any changes to your VA healthcare provider.

Quick Tips: Rash

- Avoid very hot showers or baths. Water that is too hot can irritate the skin.

- Avoid being in the sun. Sun exposure can make your rash worse.

- Try using unscented, nonsoapy cleansers for bathing or showering.

- Try rubbing or pressing on the itchy areas rather than scratching.

- A rash that blisters, or involves your mouth, the palms of your hands, or the soles of your feet, or one that is accompanied by shortness of breath, can be dangerous: contact your care provider right away, or go to an emergency room for evaluation.

Weight Loss-Treatment

Weight loss goes along with some of these other side effects. It can happen because of vomiting, nausea, fatigue, and other reasons.

Talk with your VA healthcare provider if you're losing weight without trying, meaning that you're not on a reducing diet.

Quick Tips: Weight Loss

- Be sure to keep track of your weight, by weighing yourself on scales and writing down how much you weigh. Tell your doctor if there are any changes.

- Create your own high-protein drink by blending together yogurt, fruit (for sweetness), and powdered milk, whey protein, or soy protein.

- Add dried milk powder, whey protein, soy protein, or egg white powder to foods (for example, scrambled eggs, casseroles, and milkshakes).

- Between meals, try store-bought nutritional beverages or bars (such as Carnation Instant Breakfast, Benefit, Ensure,

Scandishake, Boost High Protein, NuBasics). Look for ones that are high in proteins, not sugars or fats.

- Spread peanut butter on toast, crackers, fruit, or vegetables.
- Add cottage cheese to fruit and tomatoes.
- Add canned tuna to casseroles and salads.
- Add shredded cheese to sauces, soups, omelets, baked potatoes, and steamed vegetables.
- Eat yogurt on your cereal or fruit.
- Eat hard-boiled (hard-cooked) eggs. Use them in egg-salad sandwiches or slice and dice them for tossed salads.
- Add diced or chopped meats to soups, salads, and sauces.

Section 29.2

Diabetes

This section includes text excerpted from "HIV and Diabetes," AIDS*info*, U.S. Department of Health and Human Services (HHS), October 6, 2017.

Frequently Asked Questions

What Is Diabetes?

Diabetes is a disease in which levels of blood glucose (also called blood sugar) are too high. Glucose comes from the breakdown of the foods we eat and is our main source of energy.

Diabetes can cause serious health problems, including heart and blood vessel disease, nerve damage, blindness, stroke, and kidney disease. Fortunately, diabetes can be controlled with diet, exercise, and medicines.

How Does Diabetes Develop?

Glucose is carried in the blood to cells throughout the body. A hormone called insulin helps move the glucose into the cells. Once in the cells, glucose is used to make energy. When the body has trouble moving glucose into the cells, glucose builds up in the blood and can lead to diabetes.

There are two main types of diabetes: type 1 diabetes and type 2 diabetes.

In type 1 diabetes, the body's immune system attacks and destroys the cells that produce insulin. Lack of insulin causes glucose to build up in the blood.

In type 2 diabetes, the body can't produce enough insulin or use it effectively to move glucose into the cells. Type 2 diabetes is more common than type 1 diabetes.

What Are the Risk Factors for Type 2 Diabetes?

Risk factors for type 2 diabetes include age over 45, a family history of diabetes, being overweight, and lack of physical activity. People whose family background is African American, Alaska Native, American Indian, Asian American, Hispanic/Latino, or Pacific Islander American are at greater risk of type 2 diabetes.

In people with human immunodeficiency syndrome (HIV), the risk of type 2 diabetes is greater in people who also have hepatitis C.

The use of some HIV medicines in the nucleoside reverse transcriptase inhibitor (NRTI) and protease inhibitor (PI) drug classes may increase the risk of type 2 diabetes in people with HIV. These HIV medicines seem to make it harder for the body to respond to and use insulin (insulin resistance). Insulin resistance leads to high blood glucose levels, which can result in type 2 diabetes.

What Are the Symptoms of Diabetes?

The symptoms of diabetes can include:

- Unusual thirst

- Frequent urination

- Extreme hunger

- Unusual weight loss or weight gain

- Extreme fatigue and irritability

- Frequent infections

- Blurred vision

- Tingling or numbness in the hands and feet

- Slow healing of cuts or bruises

How Is Diabetes Diagnosed?

A common test used to diagnose diabetes is the fasting plasma glucose (FPG) test. The FPG test measures the amount of glucose in the blood after a person has not eaten for 8 hours.

People with HIV should have their blood glucose levels checked before starting treatment with HIV medicines. People with higher-than-normal glucose levels may need to avoid taking some HIV medicines.

Blood glucose testing is also important after starting HIV medicines. If testing shows high glucose levels, a change in HIV medicines may be necessary.

Can Diabetes Be Treated?

Type 2 diabetes can often be controlled with a healthy diet and regular exercise. A healthy diet and daily exercise can help a person maintain a healthy weight. If you are overweight, you may be able to prevent or delay type 2 diabetes by losing weight.

A healthy diet includes lots of vegetables, some fruit, beans, whole grains, and lean meats and is low in processed foods high in sugar and salt. Regular exercise means being active for 30 minutes on most days of the week.

Sometimes people may also need to take medicines to control type 2 diabetes. (Treatment for type 1 diabetes always includes taking insulin.)

If you have HIV, ask your healthcare provider about your risk of diabetes. You can also talk to your healthcare provider about the link between HIV medicines and diabetes. People with HIV who have diabetes may need to avoid taking some HIV medicines and use other HIV medicines instead.

Section 29.3

Hepatotoxicity and Lactic Acidosis

This section contains text excerpted from the following
sources: Text beginning with the heading "Human
Immunodeficiency Virus and Hepatotoxicity" is excerpted from
"HIV and Hepatotoxicity," AIDS*info*, U.S. Department of Health
and Human Services (HHS), October 3, 2017; Text under the heading
"Human Immunodeficiency Virus and Lactic Acidosis" is excerpted
from "HIV and Lactic Acidosis" AIDS*info*, U.S. Department of
Health and Human Services (HHS), October 9, 2017.

Human Immunodeficiency Virus and Hepatotoxicity

What Is Hepatotoxicity?

Hepatotoxicity is the medical term for damage to the liver caused
by a medicine, chemical, or herbal or dietary supplement. Hepatotoxicity can be a side effect of some human immunodeficiency virus
(HIV) medicines.

People taking HIV medicines should know about this potential
side effect of some HIV medicines. In some cases, hepatotoxicity can
be life-threatening.

Are there other factors that can increase the risk of hepatotoxicity?

The following factors may increase the risk of hepatotoxicity due
to HIV medicines:

- Also having hepatitis B and/or hepatitis C infection

- Taking other medicines that can cause liver damage

- Alcohol use

- Past history of liver damage

What Are the Symptoms of Hepatotoxicity?

Symptoms of hepatotoxicity include the following:

- Stomach pain

- Nausea (upset stomach)

- Unusual tiredness

- Dark-colored urine

- Light or clay-colored stools

- Jaundice (yellow skin and eyes)

- Loss of appetite

- Fever

If you are taking HIV medicines and have any of these symptoms, contact your healthcare provider immediately. However, do NOT cut down on, skip, or stop taking your HIV medicines unless your healthcare provider tells you to.

How Is Hepatotoxicity Detected?

Liver function tests (LFTs) are a group of blood tests used to check for damage to the liver. Before treatment with HIV medicines begins, LFTs are done to check for already-existing liver damage. The risk of hepatotoxicity is greater in people who have liver damage before they start taking HIV medicines. If LFT results show preexisting liver damage, HIV medicines that may cause hepatotoxicity should be avoided. There are many other HIV medicines available to use instead.

Once treatment with HIV medicines begins, healthcare providers use LFTs to monitor for signs of hepatotoxicity.

How Is Hepatotoxicity Managed?

Management of hepatotoxicity due to HIV medicines varies depending on the extent of damage to the liver. Sometimes it's necessary to stop taking the HIV medicine that is causing the hepatotoxicity. However, the decision to stop taking an HIV medicine should only be done in consultation with a healthcare provider. If you are taking HIV medicines, do NOT cut down on, skip, or stop taking your HIV medicines unless your healthcare provider tells you to.

If you are taking or plan to take HIV medicines, talk to your healthcare provider about the risk of hepatotoxicity.

Human Immunodeficiency Virus and Lactic Acidosis

What Is Lactic Acidosis?

Lactic acidosis is a condition caused by the buildup of lactic acid in the blood. The condition is a rare but serious side effect of some HIV medicines.

HIV medicines in the nucleoside reverse transcriptase inhibitor (NRTI) drug class can cause the body to produce too much lactic acid.

NRTIs can also damage the liver so that it can't break down a molecule called lactate, leading to a buildup of lactic acid in the blood.

If you are taking NRTIs, it's important to know about lactic acidosis. Although lactic acidosis is a rare side effect of NRTIs, the condition can be life-threatening.

Are There Other Risk Factors for Lactic Acidosis?

In addition to use of some HIV medicines, risk factors for lactic acidosis include the following:

- Being female
- Pregnancy
- Obesity
- Poor liver function
- Lower CD4 count

What Are the Symptoms of Lactic Acidosis?

Lactic acidosis often develops gradually. Early signs of lactic acidosis can include fatigue, nausea and vomiting, stomach pain, and weight loss. These symptoms may not seem serious, but they can be the first signs of life-threatening lactic acidosis. If you are taking HIV medicines, always tell your healthcare provider about any symptoms that you are having—even symptoms that may not seem serious.

Lactic acidosis can advance rapidly. Signs of dangerously high levels of lactate in the blood include:

- Above-normal heart rate
- Rapid breathing
- Jaundice (yellowing of the skin and the whites of the eyes)
- Muscle weakness

If you are taking HIV medicines and have any of these symptoms, get medical help immediately.

What Tests Are Used to Detect Lactic Acidosis?

Tests used to diagnose lactic acidosis include:

- A test to measure the level of lactate in the blood

- Other blood tests to check the functioning of the liver

- An ultrasound or CT scan of the liver

What Is the Treatment for Lactic Acidosis?

An HIV medicine that is causing lactic acidosis should be discontinued. However, stopping an HIV medicine because of lactic acidosis doesn't mean stopping HIV treatment. There are many HIV medicines that can be included in an HIV regimen.

But if you are taking HIV medicines, do NOT cut down on, skip, or stop taking your medicines unless your healthcare provider tells you to.

In the rare cases when lactic acidosis becomes life-threatening, immediate treatment in a hospital is necessary.

Section 29.4

Hyperlipidemia

This section includes text excerpted from "HIV and Hyperlipidemia," AIDS*info*, U.S. Department of Health and Human Services (HHS), October 9, 2017.

Frequently Asked Questions

What Is Hyperlipidemia?

Hyperlipidemia is the medical term for high levels of fat in the blood. Fats in the blood (also called lipids) include cholesterol and triglycerides. The body makes cholesterol and triglycerides. The fats also come from some of the foods we eat.

The body needs cholesterol and triglycerides to function properly, but having too much can cause problems. High levels of cholesterol and triglycerides increase the risk of heart disease, gallbladder disease, and pancreatitis (inflammation of the pancreas).

What Are the Symptoms of Hyperlipidemia?

Usually, hyperlipidemia has no symptoms. A blood test is used to measure levels of fat in the blood and to detect hyperlipidemia.

Testing for hyperlipidemia is recommended both before and after a person starts taking HIV medicines. If blood fat levels are normal, testing is recommended once a year. If blood fat levels are too high, more frequent testing is recommended.

What Are Risk Factors for Hyperlipidemia in People with HIV?

HIV infection and treatment with some HIV medicines can increase the risk of hyperlipidemia by raising blood fat levels.

The following are additional risk factors for hyperlipidemia:

- Family history of hyperlipidemia
- Other medical conditions, including high blood pressure, diabetes, and an underactive thyroid gland
- A high-fat, high-carbohydrate diet
- Being overweight or obese
- Smoking
- Alcohol use
- Lack of physical activity

Many of these risk factors for hyperlipidemia can be controlled by lifestyle choices. For example, maintaining a healthy weight is one way to reduce the risk of hyperlipidemia.

What Are Other Steps a Person Can Take to Prevent Hyperlipidemia?

Here are additional steps to take to reduce the risk of hyperlipidemia. People who already have hyperlipidemia can also follow these steps to lower their blood fat levels.

- Eat foods low in saturated fat, trans fat, and cholesterol. Eat less full-fat dairy products, fatty meats, and desserts high in fat and sugar. Limit foods that are high in cholesterol, such as egg yolks, fatty meats, and organ meat (like liver and kidney). Instead, choose low-fat or fat-free milk, cheese, and yogurt; eat more foods that are high in fiber, like oatmeal, oat bran, beans, and lentils; and eat more vegetables and fresh fruits.

- Get active. Get at least 30 minutes of aerobic physical activity on most days of the week. Aerobic activities include walking quickly, biking slowly, and gardening.

- If you smoke, quit. Nicotine gum, patches, and lozenges can make it easier to quit. Help is also available over the phone and online.

- Drink in moderation. Men should have no more than two alcoholic drinks a day; women no more than one drink. One drink is a glass of wine, a bottle of beer, or a shot of hard liquor.

What Is the Treatment for Hyperlipidemia?

Lifestyle changes may not be enough to reduce blood fat levels.

In people with HIV, treatment for hyperlipidemia may include changing an HIV regimen to avoid taking HIV medicines that can increase blood fat levels.

There are also medicines that can help control blood fat levels. The most common medicines used to reduce cholesterol levels are called statins. Fibrates are a type of medicine used to lower triglycerides.

HIV medicines can interact with medicines that lower blood fat levels. If you have HIV and need medicine to control hyperlipidemia, your healthcare provider can recommend medicines that are safe to take with your HIV regimen.

Section 29.5

Lipodystrophy

This section includes text excerpted from "HIV and Lipodystrophy," AIDS*info*, U.S. Department of Health and Human Services (HHS), October 10, 2017.

Frequently Asked Questions

What Is Lipodystrophy?

Lipodystrophy refers to the changes in body fat that affect some people with human immunodeficiency virus (HIV). Lipodystrophy can include:

- Buildup of body fat

- Loss of body fat

What Causes Lipodystrophy?

The exact cause of lipodystrophy is unknown. It may be due to HIV infection or medicines used to treat HIV.

Other risk factors for lipodystrophy include:

- Age: Older people are at higher risk.

- Race: Whites have the highest risk.

- Gender: Men are more likely to have fat loss in the arms and legs. Women are more likely to have buildup of breast and abdominal fat.

Length and severity of HIV infection: The risk is higher with longer and more severe HIV infection.

Although more research is needed to prove that there is a link between HIV medicines and lipodystrophy, some HIV medicines have been associated with the condition. While some of the changes caused by lipodystrophy can't be reversed, switching HIV medicines may help reduce the effects. Newer HIV medicines are less likely to cause lipodystrophy than HIV medicines developed in the past.

Many people with HIV never develop lipodystrophy.

What Parts of the Body Are Affected by Lipodystrophy?

Fat buildup (also called lipohypertrophy) can occur:

- Around the organs in the belly (also called the abdomen)
- On the back of the neck between the shoulders (called a buffalo hump)
- In the breasts
- Just under the skin. (The fatty bumps are called lipomas.)

Fat loss (also called lipoatrophy) tends to occur:

- In the arms and legs
- In the buttocks
- In the face

A person with HIV can have fat loss or fat buildup or both. Whether the changes are noticeable or not depends on the degree of fat loss or fat buildup. See images of fat buildup around the neck and fat loss on the face and leg.

Is Lipodystrophy a Serious Health Problem?

It can be. Too much fat gain can increase the risk of heart disease and diabetes.

Fat gain in the breasts can be painful, and some types of fat gain may cause problems with breathing or other body functions.

The changes in appearance caused by lipodystrophy can be upsetting and affect a person's self-esteem. Because of lipodystrophy, a person may decide to stop taking HIV medicines. However, the decision to stop taking HIV medicines (or cut down on the dose of a medicine) should be made only with the help of a healthcare provider. Stopping HIV medicines allows HIV to multiply and damage the immune system, which increases the risk of HIV-related infections and cancer. Stopping HIV medicines also increases the risk of drug resistance.

Can Lipodystrophy Be Cured?

Unfortunately, there isn't a cure for lipodystrophy. More research is needed to understand the cause of lipodystrophy in people with HIV and to find a cure for the condition. However, there are ways to manage lipodystrophy.

In some people, changing HIV medicines may lessen the effects of lipodystrophy. Newer HIV medicines are less likely to cause lipodystrophy than HIV medicines developed in the past.

But, if you are taking HIV medicines, do NOT cut down on, skip, or stop taking your medicines unless your healthcare provider tells you to.

Liposuction (surgical removal of fat) is sometimes used to reduce a buffalo hump. Fat or a fat-like substance can be used as a filler for fat loss in the face. The filler is injected in the cheeks or around the eyes and mouth.

Medicines may help lessen the effects of lipodystrophy. For example, tesamorelin (brand name: Egrifta) is a medicine used to reduce the buildup of abdominal fat due to lipodystrophy.

A healthy diet and daily exercise may help to build muscle and reduce fat buildup.

Section 29.6

Osteoporosis

This section includes text extracted from "HIV and Osteoporosis," AIDS*info*, U.S. Department of Health and Human Services (HHS), October 10, 2017.

Frequently Asked Questions

What Is Osteoporosis?

The human body is made up of more than 200 bones, from the skull to the bones of the toes. We depend on bones to hold us up, help us move, and protect our internal organs, such as the heart, liver, and brain. Osteoporosis is a disease that causes bones to become weak and easy to break. Osteoporosis increases the risk of fractures of the hip, spine, and wrist.

The risk of osteoporosis increases with age. Anyone can get osteoporosis, but it's most common in older women.

Are People with HIV at Risk of Osteoporosis?

Yes. Experts are not sure why, but bone loss occurs faster in people living with human immunodeficiency virus (HIV) than in people without HIV. Factors that increase the rate of bone loss in people with HIV may include:

- HIV infection itself
- Some HIV medicines
- Taking other medicines for a long time (for example, steroids or antacids)
- Older age. HIV medicines are helping people with HIV live longer, and advancing age increases the risk of osteoporosis.

Staying healthy with HIV includes taking steps to prevent osteoporosis.

What Are Other Risk Factors for Osteoporosis?

There are many risk factors for osteoporosis. Some risk factors, such as HIV infection, can't be changed. Other risk factors, such as a poor diet or lack of exercise, can be managed with lifestyle choices.

Risk factors for osteoporosis that can't be changed include:

- Age: The risk of osteoporosis increases as people get older and the bones become thinner and weaker.
- Gender: Compared with men, women have smaller bones, and after menopause, women lose bone more rapidly than men do.
- Race/ethnicity: The risk of osteoporosis is greatest for white and Asian women. However, even though African-American women and Hispanic women tend to have higher bone density than white women, they are still at risk for osteoporosis. Factors that increase the risk of osteoporosis in African-American women include a low-calcium diet, intolerance to lactose (the main sugar in milk), and certain diseases that are more common in African Americans (such as lupus).
- Family history: Reduced bone mass tends to run in families.

The following risk factors for osteoporosis can be controlled by lifestyle choices:

- Poor diet: A diet low in calcium and vitamin D increases the risk of osteoporosis.

- Physical inactivity: Bones become stronger with exercise, so physical inactivity increases the risk of osteoporosis.

- Smoking: Smoking is bad for the bones.

- Drinking: Too much alcohol can cause bone loss and broken bones.

How Does Osteoporosis Develop?

To maintain healthy bones, our body constantly replaces old bone tissue with new bone tissue. Up to about age 30, bone tissue is replaced faster than it is lost. But beyond age 30, the reverse can happen: more bone is broken down than is replaced.

Osteoporosis develops when bone loss is so great that bones can break easily.

There is no cure for osteoporosis. However, once the disease develops, there are medicines that can slow down bone loss or increase bone formation.

What are the Symptoms of Osteoporosis?

Osteoporosis is often called a silent disease because bone loss occurs without symptoms. The first sign of osteoporosis is often a broken bone.

A bone mineral density test is used to measure bone strength and diagnose osteoporosis. The test is quick, safe, painless, and requires no preparation. The U.S. Preventive Services Task Force recommends all women above the age of 65 have a bone mineral density test to screen for osteoporosis. Women who are younger than 65 and are at high risk for fractures should also have a bone mineral density test. The U.S. government currently offers no recommendations for routine screening for osteoporosis in people living with HIV, but individuals with HIV may wish to discuss bone mineral density testing with their healthcare providers.

What Are Steps to Take to Prevent Osteoporosis?

Preventing osteoporosis means making lifestyle choices to reduce the risk of the disease.

- Eat a healthy diet rich in calcium and vitamin D. Foods high in calcium include dairy products, such as milk, yogurt, and cheese. Other foods high in calcium include dark green leafy vegetables (such as collard greens, bok choy, and kale), broccoli, sardines, tofu, and almonds. Milk is fortified with vitamin D. Certain fish and mushrooms are also high in vitamin D. If needed, healthcare providers can offer guidance on taking calcium and vitamin D supplements.

- Stay active. Weight-bearing exercises, such as walking, jogging, and dancing, can make bones stronger and help slow the rate of bone loss.

- Don't smoke.

- Cut down on alcohol. Drinking too much can lead to bone loss and increase the risk of fractures due to both bone loss and falling. If you drink alcohol, drink in moderation—up to one drink a day for women and up to two drinks a day for men. One drink is a bottle of beer, a glass of wine, or a shot of liquor.

Section 29.7

Skin Rash

This section includes text excerpted from "HIV and Rash,"
AIDS*info*, U.S. Department of Health and Human
Services (HHS), October 6, 2017.

Frequently Asked Questions

Why Do People with Human Immunodeficiency Virus (HIV) Develop Rash?

A rash is an irritated area of the skin that is sometimes itchy, red, and painful. Possible causes of rash in people with human immunodeficiency virus (HIV) include:

- HIV infection itself
- Other infections
- HIV medicines
- Other medicines

HIV Infection

Rash may be a symptom of acute HIV infection. Acute HIV infection is the earliest stage of HIV infection, and it generally develops within 2 to 4 weeks after infection with HIV.

A rash may also be a symptom of HIV infection at any stage of the disease.

Other Infections

Rash may be a symptom of other infections. HIV destroys the infection-fighting cells of the immune system. Damage to the immune system puts people with HIV at risk of infections, and rash is a symptom of many infections.

Medicines

Many medicines, including medicines used to treat HIV and other infections, can cause a rash.

Rash is among the most common side effects of HIV medicines. HIV medicines in all HIV drug classes can cause a rash. (HIV medicines are grouped into drug classes according to how they fight HIV.)

Rash due to HIV medicines is often not serious and goes away in several days to weeks without treatment. But sometimes when an HIV medicine is causing a rash, it may be necessary to switch to another HIV medicine.

If you are taking HIV medicines, tell your healthcare provider if you have a rash. In rare cases, a rash caused by an HIV medicine can be a sign of a serious, life-threatening condition.

What Are Serious Rash-Related Conditions?

Rash can be a sign of a serious hypersensitivity reaction. A hypersensitivity reaction is an unusual allergic reaction to a medicine. In addition to rash, signs of a hypersensitivity reaction can include fever, difficulty breathing or swallowing, dizziness or lightheadedness, and kidney damage.

Stevens-Johnson syndrome (SJS) (also called erythema multiforme major) is a rare but life-threatening hypersensitivity reaction reported with use of some HIV medicines. (When SJS affects at least 30 percent of the total surface area of the skin, the condition is called toxic epidermal necrolysis [TEN].) People taking HIV medicines need to know about this condition. It rarely occurs, but when it does, it can cause death.

Symptoms of SJS include fever; pain or itching of the skin; swelling of the tongue and face; blisters that develop on the skin and mucous membranes, especially around the mouth, nose, and eyes; and a rash that starts quickly and may spread.

A severe hypersensitivity reaction can be life-threatening and requires immediate medical attention. SJS must be treated immediately. Go to the emergency room or call 911 if you have symptoms of SJS. However, do NOT cut down on, skip, or stop taking your HIV medicines unless your healthcare provider tells you to.

Chapter 30

Other HIV/AIDS Treatment Complications

Chapter Contents

Section 30.1

Drug Interactions

This section includes text excerpted from "What Is a
Drug Interaction?" AIDS*info*, U.S. Department of
Health and Human Services (HHS), February 6, 2018.

Medicines help us feel better and stay healthy. But sometimes
drug interactions can cause problems. There are three types of drug
interactions:

1. **Drug-drug interaction.** A reaction between two (or more)
   drugs.

2. **Drug-food interaction.** A reaction between a drug and a food
   or beverage.

3. **Drug-condition interaction.** A reaction that occurs when
   taking a drug while having a certain medical condition. For
   example, taking a nasal decongestant if you have high blood
   pressure may cause an unwanted reaction.

Drug interactions can reduce or increase the action of a medicine
or cause adverse (unwanted) side effects.

Human Immunodeficiency Virus (HIV) Medicines and Drug Interactions

Treatment with human immunodeficiency virus (HIV) medicines
(called antiretroviral therapy or ART) helps people with HIV live longer, healthier lives and reduces the risk of HIV transmission. But
drug interactions, especially drug-drug interactions, can complicate
HIV treatment.

Drug-drug interactions between different HIV medicines and
between HIV medicines and other medicines are common. Interactions between medicines may reduce or increase the concentration of
a medicine in the blood. The change in concentration can make the
affected medicine less effective, more effective, or so strong that it
causes dangerous side effects.

Before recommending an HIV regimen, healthcare providers carefully consider potential drug-drug interactions between HIV medicines.
They also ask about other medicines a person may be taking. For
example, a healthcare provider may ask a woman with HIV whether

she is using hormonal birth control. Some HIV medicines may make hormonal birth control less effective, so women using hormonal contraceptives may need to use an additional or different method of birth control to prevent pregnancy.

Drug-Food Interactions and Drug-Condition Interactions Affect People Taking HIV Medicines

The use of HIV medicines can lead to both drug-food interactions and drug-condition interactions. Food or beverages can affect the absorption of some HIV medicines and increase or reduce the concentration of the medicine in the blood. Depending on the HIV medicine, the change in concentration may be helpful or harmful. Directions on how to take HIV medicines specify whether to take the medicine with food, without food, or either way if the HIV medicine isn't affected by food.

Conditions such as kidney disease, hepatitis, and pregnancy can affect how the body processes HIV medicines. For example, because of pregnancy-related changes, dosing of an HIV medicine may change during different stages of pregnancy. But pregnant women should always consult with their healthcare providers before making any changes to their HIV regimens.

Ways to Avoid Drug Interactions

You can take the following steps to avoid drug interactions:

- Tell your healthcare provider about all prescription and nonprescription medicines you are taking or plan to take. Also tell your healthcare provider about any vitamins, nutritional supplements, and herbal products you take.

- Tell your healthcare provider about any other conditions you may have, for example, high blood pressure or diabetes

- Before taking a medicine, ask your healthcare provider or pharmacist the following questions:

  - What is the medicine used for?

  - How should I take the medicine?

  - While taking the medicine, should I avoid any other medicines or certain foods or beverages?

  - Can I take this medicine safely with the other medicines that I am taking? Are there any possible drug interactions

I should know about? What are the signs of those drug interactions?

- In the case of a drug interaction, what should I do?

  - Take medicines according to your healthcare provider's instructions. Always read the information and directions that come with a medicine. Drug labels and package inserts include important information about possible drug interactions.

  - Tell your healthcare provider if you have any side effect that bothers you or that does not go away

Section 30.2

Risk of Muscle Injury

This section includes text excerpted from "Drugs—FDA Drug Safety Communication: Interactions between Certain HIV or Hepatitis C Drugs and Cholesterol-Lowering Statin Drugs Can Increase the Risk of Muscle Injury," U.S. Food and Drug Administration (FDA), January 19, 2016.

The U.S. Food and Drug Administration (FDA) is issuing updated recommendations concerning drug-drug interactions between drugs for human immunodeficiency virus (HIV) or hepatitis C virus (HCV) known as protease inhibitors and certain cholesterol-lowering drugs known as statins. Protease inhibitors and statins are taken together may raise the blood levels of statins and increase the risk for muscle injury (myopathy). The most serious form of myopathy, rhabdomyolysis, can damage the kidneys and lead to kidney failure, which can be fatal.

The labels for both the HIV protease inhibitors and the affected statins have been updated to contain consistent information about the drug-drug interactions. These labels also have been updated to include dosing recommendations for those statins that may safely be coadministered with HIV or HCV protease inhibitors.

Healthcare professionals should refer to the drug labels for protease inhibitors and statins for the recommendations on prescribing these drugs.

Additional Information for Patients

HIV and HCV protease inhibitors can interact with cholesterol-lowering statins to increase the risk of muscle injury. Patients should inform their healthcare professional about all medicines that they are taking or plan to take prior to starting an HIV or HCV protease inhibitor or statin.

HIV and HCV protease inhibitors should never be taken (are contraindicated) with lovastatin (Mevacor) and simvastatin (Zocor).

Patients should contact their healthcare professional if they have any questions or concerns about HIV or HCV protease inhibitors or statins. They should report side effects from the use of HIV or HCV protease inhibitors and/or statins to the FDA MedWatch program.

Data Summary

Atorvastatin

The results from a drug-drug interaction study with atorvastatin and lopinavir/ritonavir that were previously in the atorvastatin label have not yet been validated. Therefore, these results have been removed from the label and the dose cap of atorvastatin 20 mg when coadministered with lopinavir/ritonavir has also been removed. Pending validation of the study, healthcare professionals should use caution when coadministering atorvastatin with lopinavir/ritonavir and use the lowest necessary dose of atorvastatin.

Lovastatin and Simvastatin

Lovastatin and simvastatin are sensitive in vivo cytochrome P450 3A4 (CYP3A4) substrates. Therefore, strong CYP3A4 inhibitors are predicted to significantly increase lovastatin and simvastatin exposures. A literature review indicates that itraconazole, a strong CYP3A4 inhibitor, increases lovastatin exposure up to 20-fold, and the drug interaction appears to result in rhabdomyolysis. Itraconazole increases simvastatin exposure up to 13-fold. Hence, other CYP3A4 inhibitors, including ketoconazole, posaconazole, erythromycin, clarithromycin, telithromycin, nefazodone, HIV protease inhibitors, and the HCV protease inhibitors boceprevir and telaprevir, are also expected to significantly increase lovastatin and simvastatin exposures. Therefore, concomitant administration of lovastatin and simvastatin with HIV protease inhibitors or HCV protease inhibitors (boceprevir and telaprevir) is contraindicated.

Rosuvastatin

The HIV protease inhibitor combinations lopinavir/ritonavir and atazanavir/ritonavir increase rosuvastatin exposure up to 3-fold. For these combinations, the dose of rosuvastatin should be limited to 10 mg.

Table 30.1. Statin Dose Limitations

Statin	Interacting Protease Inhibitor(s)	Prescribing Recommendation
Atorvastatin	• Tipranavir + ritonavir • Telaprevir	Avoid atorvastatin
	• Lopinavir + ritonavir	Use with caution and use with the lowest atorvastatin dose necessary
	• Darunavir + ritonavir • Fosamprenavir • Fosamprenavir + ritonavir • Saquinavir + ritonavir	Do not exceed 20 mg atorvastatin daily
	• Nelfinavir	Do not exceed 40 mg atorvastatin daily
Fluvastatin		No data available
Lovastatin	• HIV protease inhibitors • Boceprevir • Telaprevir	Contraindicated
Pitavastatin	• Atazanavir ± ritonavir • Darunavir + ritonavir • Lopinavir + ritonavir	No dose limitations
Pravastatin	• Darunavir + ritonavir • Lopinavir + ritonavir	No dose limitations
Rosuvastatin	• Atazanavir ± ritonavir • Lopinavir + ritonavir	Limit rosuvastatin dose to 10 mg once daily
Simvastatin	• HIV protease inhibitors • Boceprevir • Telaprevir	Contraindicated

Chapter 31

Antiretroviral Treatment Failure and Its Management

Categories of Treatment Failure

Treatment failure can be categorized as virologic failure, immunologic failure, clinical failure, or some combination of the three. Immunologic failure refers to a suboptimal immunologic response to therapy or an immunologic decline while on therapy, but there is no standardized definition. Clinical failure is defined as the occurrence of new opportunistic infections (excluding immune reconstitution inflammatory syndrome [IRIS]) and/or other clinical evidence of HIV disease progression during therapy. Almost all antiretroviral (ARV) management decisions for treatment failure are based on addressing virologic failure.

Virologic Failure

Virologic failure occurs as an incomplete initial response to therapy or as a viral rebound after virologic suppression is achieved. Virologic suppression is defined as having plasma viral load below the lower level of detection (LLD), as measured by highly sensitive assays with lower limits of quantitation (LLQ) of 20 to 75 copies/mL. Virologic

This chapter includes text excerpted from "Guidelines for the Use of Antiretroviral Agents in Pediatric HIV Infection," AIDS*info*, U.S. Department of Health and Human Services (HHS), May 22, 2018.

failure is defined as a repeated plasma viral load ≥200 copies/mL after 6 months of therapy. Laboratory results must be confirmed with repeat testing before a final assessment of virologic treatment failure is made. Infants with high plasma viral loads at initiation of therapy occasionally take longer than 6 months to achieve virologic suppression. Because of this, some experts continue the treatment regimen for infants receiving lopinavir/ritonavir (LPV/r)-based therapy if viral load is declining but is still ≥200 copies/mL at 6 months and monitor closely for continued decline to virologic suppression. However, ongoing nonsuppression—especially with nonnucleoside reverse transcriptase inhibitor (NNRTI)-based regimens—increases the risk of drug resistance. There is controversy regarding the clinical implications of HIV RNA levels between the LLD and <200 copies/mL in patients on antiretroviral therapy (ART). Adults with HIV who have detectable viral loads and a quantified result <200 copies/mL after 6 months of ART generally achieve virologic suppression without regimen change. However, some studies in adults have found that multiple viral load measurements of 50 to <200 copies/mL may be associated with an increased risk of later virologic failure. "Blips"—defined as isolated episodes of plasma viral load detectable at low levels (i.e., <500 copies/mL) followed by a return to viral suppression—are common and not generally reflective of virologic failure. However, repeated or persistent plasma viral load detection ≥200 copies/mL (especially if >500 copies/mL) after having achieved virologic suppression usually represents virologic failure.

Poor Immunologic Response Despite Virologic Suppression

Poor immunologic response despite virologic suppression is uncommon in children. Patients with baseline severe immunosuppression often take more than 1 year to achieve immune recovery (i.e., CD4 T lymphocyte [CD4] cell count >500 cells/mm^3), even if virologic suppression occurs more promptly. During this early treatment period of persistent immunosuppression, additional clinical disease progression can occur.

In cases of poor immunologic response despite virologic suppression, clinicians should first exclude laboratory error in CD4 or viral load measurements and ensure that CD4 values have been interpreted correctly in relation to the natural decline in CD4 cell count over the first 5 to 6 years of life. Another laboratory consideration is that some viral load assays may not amplify all HIV groups and subtypes (e.g.,

HIV-1 non-M groups or HIV-2), resulting in falsely low or negative viral load results. Once laboratory results are confirmed, evaluation for adverse events, medical conditions, and other factors that can cause CD4 values to decrease is necessary.

Patients who have very low baseline CD4 values before initiating ART are at higher risk of an impaired CD4 response to ART and, based on adult studies, may be at higher risk of death and AIDS-defining illnesses, despite virologic suppression. In a study of 933 children aged ≥5 years who received ART that resulted in virologic suppression, 348 (37%) had CD4 cell counts <500 cells/mm³ at ART initiation, including 92 (9.9%) with CD4 cell counts <200 cells/mm³. After 1 year of virologic suppression, only 7 (1% of the cohort) failed to reach a CD4 cell count ≥200 cells/mm³ and 86% had CD4 cell counts >500 cells/mm³. AIDS-defining events were uncommon overall (1%) but occurred in children who did and did not achieve improved CD4 cell counts.

Several drugs (e.g., corticosteroids, chemotherapeutic agents) and other conditions (e.g., hepatitis C virus, tuberculosis [TB], malnutrition, Sjogren syndrome, sarcoidosis, syphilis, acute viral infections) are independently associated with low CD4 values.

In summary, poor immunologic response to treatment can occur. Management consists of confirming that CD4 and virologic tests are accurate, avoiding drugs associated with low CD4 values, and treating other conditions that could impair CD4 recovery. The Panel on Antiretroviral Therapy and Medical Management of Children Living with HIV does not recommend modifying an ART regimen based on lack of immunologic response if virologic suppression is confirmed.

Poor Clinical Response Despite Adequate Virologic and Immunologic Responses

Clinicians must carefully evaluate patients who experience clinical disease progression despite favorable immunologic and virologic responses to ART. Not all cases represent ART failure. IRIS is one of the most important reasons that new or recurrent opportunistic conditions occur, even in cases where virologic suppression and immunologic restoration/preservation are achieved within the first months of ART. IRIS does not represent ART failure and does not generally require discontinuation of ART. Children who have suffered irreversible damage to their lungs, brain, or other organs—especially during prolonged and profound pretreatment immunosuppression—may continue to have recurrent infections or symptoms in the damaged organs because the immunologic improvement may not reverse damage to the organs.

Such cases do not represent ART failure and, in these instances, children would not benefit from a change in ARV regimen. Before a definitive conclusion of ART clinical failure is reached, a child should also be evaluated to rule out (and, if indicated, treat) other causes or conditions that can occur with or without HIV-related immunosuppression, such as pulmonary TB, malnutrition, and malignancy. Occasionally, however, children will develop new HIV-related opportunistic conditions (e.g., *Pneumocystis jirovecii* pneumonia or esophageal candidiasis occurring more than 6 months after achieving markedly improved CD4 values and virologic suppression) not explained by IRIS, preexisting organ damage, or another reason. Although such cases are rare, they may represent ART clinical failure and suggest that improvement in CD4 values may not necessarily normalize immunologic function. In children who have signs of new or progressive abnormal neurodevelopment, some experts change the ARV regimen, aiming to include agents that are known to achieve higher concentrations in the central nervous system; however, the data supporting this strategy are mixed.

Management of Virologic Treatment Failure

The approach to management and subsequent treatment of virologic treatment failure will differ depending on the etiology of the problem. While the causes of virologic treatment failure may be multifactorial, nonadherence plays a role in most cases. Assessment of a child with suspected virologic treatment failure should include evaluation of therapy adherence and medication intolerance, confirmation that prescribed dosing is correct (and understood by the child and/or caregiver) for all medications in the regimen, consideration of pharmacokinetic (PK) explanations of low drug levels or elevated and potentially toxic levels, and evaluation of suspected drug resistance. The main barrier to long-term maintenance of sustained virologic suppression in adults and children is incomplete adherence to medication regimens, with subsequent emergence of viral mutations conferring partial or complete resistance to one or more of the components of the ART regimen. Please see guidance on assessment of adherence and strategies to improve adherence.

Virologic Treatment Failure with No Viral Drug Resistance Identified

Persistent viremia in the absence of detectable viral resistance to current medications is usually a result of nonadherence, but it is important to exclude other factors such as poor drug absorption, incorrect dosing, and drug interactions. If adequate drug exposure can be ensured, then adherence to the current regimen should result in virologic suppression. Resistance testing should take place while a child is on therapy. After discontinuation of therapy, plasma viral strains may quickly revert to wild-type and reemerge as the predominant viral population, in which case resistance testing would fail to reveal drug-resistant virus. An approach to identifying resistance in this situation is to restart the prior medications while emphasizing adherence; repeat resistance testing in 4 weeks if plasma virus remains detectable. If the HIV plasma viral load becomes undetectable, nonadherence was likely the original cause of virologic treatment failure.

Virologic failure of boosted protease inhibitor (PI)-based regimens (in the absence of prior treatment with full-dose ritonavir) is frequently associated with no detectable major PI resistance mutations. Virologic suppression may be achieved by continuing the PI-based regimen and taking adherence improvement measures.

In some cases, if a new more convenient regimen is available that is anticipated to address the main barrier to adherence, it may be reasonable to change to this new regimen (e.g., a single fixed-dose tablet once daily) with close adherence and viral load monitoring. In most cases, however, when there is evidence of poor adherence to the current regimen and an assessment that good adherence to a new regimen is unlikely, emphasis and effort should be placed on improving adherence before initiating a new regimen.

Virologic Treatment Failure with Viral Drug Resistance Identified

After deciding that a change in therapy is needed, a clinician should attempt to identify at least two, but preferably three, fully active ARV agents from at least two different classes on the basis of all past and recent drug resistance test results, prior ARV exposure, acceptability to the patient, and likelihood of adherence. This often requires using agents from one or more drug classes that are new to the patient. Substitution or addition of a single drug to a failing regimen is not recommended because it is unlikely to lead to durable virologic suppression and will likely result in additional drug resistance. A drug may be new to the patient but have diminished antiviral potency due to the presence of drug-resistance mutations that confer cross-resistance within a drug class.

341

The process of switching a patient to a new regimen must include an extensive discussion of treatment adherence and potential toxicity with the patient and the patient's caregivers. This discussion should be age- and development-appropriate for the patient. Clinicians must recognize that conflicting requirements of some medications with respect to food and concomitant medication restrictions may complicate administration of a regimen. Timing of medication administration is particularly important to ensure adequate ARV drug exposures throughout the day. Palatability, size, and number of pills, and dosing frequency all need to be considered when choosing a new regimen.

Therapeutic Options After Virologic Treatment Failure with Goal of Complete Virologic Suppression

Determination of a new regimen with the best chance for complete virologic suppression in children who have already experienced treatment failure should be made by or in collaboration with a pediatric HIV specialist. ARV regimens should be chosen based on treatment history and drug-resistance testing to optimize ARV drug potency in the new regimen.

If a child experiences failure of initial therapy with an NNRTI-based regimen, a change to a PI-based regimen is generally effective. Studies of adults have found no evidence that a boosted PI regimen that includes raltegravir produces better outcomes than a boosted PI regimen that contains two NRTIs. Therefore, most children who experience treatment failure on an initial NNRTI-based regimen should be changed to a regimen of a boosted PI plus two NRTIs. Limited data support the use of two NRTIs plus an INSTI following failure of an NNRTI-based regimen. Evidence from a trial in adults supports superior outcomes for dolutegravir compared to LPV/r when used in a second-line regimen that includes at least one active NRTI, following failure of an initial NNRTI-based regimen. There is concern about this approach (especially when using INSTIs with a lower barrier to resistance, such as raltegravir) because children who experience treatment failure on NNRTI-based regimens often have substantial NRTI resistance. Resistance to the NNRTI nevirapine results in cross-resistance to the NNRTI efavirenz, and vice versa. The NNRTIs etravirine and rilpivirine can retain activity against nevirapine- or efavirenz-resistant virus in the absence of certain key NNRTI mutations, but etravirine has generally been tested only in regimens that also contain a boosted PI.

If a child experiences initial therapy failure with a PI-based regimen, there is often limited resistance detected,36,37 in which case an alternative PI that is better tolerated and potent can be used. For example, LPV/r-based regimens have been shown to have durable ARV activity in some PI-experienced children. Darunavir/ritonavir-based therapy has also been used. Based on more limited data, a change to an INSTI-based regimen can be effective.

The availability of newer drugs in existing classes and newer classes of drugs increases the likelihood of finding three active drugs, even for children with extensive drug resistance. As discussed, INSTI-based regimens are increasingly used for children who have experienced treatment failure on NNRTI- or PI-based regimens. Raltegravir is the INSTI that has been studied and used most in children, but dolutegravir is increasingly appealing for its once-daily administration, small pill size, and higher barrier to development of drug resistance, including activity in patients who have experienced treatment failure on raltegravir-based therapy. Maraviroc, a CCR5 antagonist, provides a new drug class, but many treatment-experienced children already harbor CXCR4-tropic virus that precludes its use. Regimens including an INSTI and potent, boosted PI plus or minus etravirine have been effective in small studies of extensively ARV-experienced patients with multiclass drug resistance. It is important to review individual drug profiles for information about drug interactions and dose adjustments when devising a regimen for children with multiclass drug resistance.

Previously prescribed drugs that were discontinued because of poor tolerance or poor adherence may sometimes be reintroduced if ARV resistance did not develop and if prior difficulties with tolerance and adherence can be overcome (e.g., by switching from a liquid to a pill formulation or to a new formulation [e.g., ritonavir tablet or a fixed dose combination tablet]). Limited data in adults suggest that continuation of lamivudine can contribute to suppression of HIV replication, despite the presence of lamivudine resistance mutations. Continuation of lamivudine can also maintain lamivudine mutations (184V) that can partially reverse the effect of other mutations, conferring resistance to zidovudine, stavudine, and tenofovir disoproxil fumarate. The use of new drugs that have been evaluated in adults but have not been fully evaluated in children may be justified, and ideally would be done in the framework of a clinical trial. Expanded access programs or clinical trials may be available. New drugs should be used in combination with at least one, and ideally two, additional active agents.

Enfuvirtide has been Food and Drug Administration-approved for use in treatment-experienced children aged ≥6 years, but it must be administered by subcutaneous injection twice daily. PK studies of certain dual-boosted PI regimens (LPV/r with saquinavir) suggest that PK targets for both PIs can be achieved or exceeded when used in combination in children. Multidrug regimens (up to three PIs and/ or two NNRTIs) have shown efficacy in a pediatric case series, but they are complex, often poorly tolerated, and subject to unfavorable drug-drug interactions. Availability of newer PIs (e.g., darunavir for children aged ≥3 years) and new classes of ARV drugs (integrase and CCR5 inhibitors) have lessened the need for use of enfuvirtide, dual-PI regimens, and regimens of four or more drugs.

Studies of NRTI-sparing regimens in adults with virologic failure and multidrug resistance have demonstrated no clear benefit of including NRTIs in the new regimen,58,59 and one of these studies reported higher mortality in adults randomized to a regimen with NRTIs compared to adults randomized to an NRTI-sparing regimen. There are no studies of NRTI-sparing regimens in children with virologic failure and multidrug resistance, but an NRTI-sparing regimen may be a reasonable option for children with extensive NRTI resistance.

When searching for at least two fully active agents in cases of extensive drug resistance, clinicians should consider the potential availability and future use of newer therapeutic agents that may not have been studied or approved in children or may be in clinical development. Information concerning potential clinical trials can be found at the AIDS*info* Clinical Trial Search and through collaboration with a pediatric HIV specialist. Children should be enrolled in clinical trials of new drugs whenever possible.

Pediatric dosing for off-label use of ARV drugs is problematic because of absorption, hepatic metabolism, and excretion change with age. In clinical trials of several ARV agents, direct extrapolation of a pediatric dose from an adult dose, based on a child's body weight or body surface area, was shown to result in an underestimation of the appropriate pediatric dose.

Use of ARV agents that do not have a pediatric indication (i.e., off-label) may be necessary for children with HIV who have limited ARV options. In this circumstance, consultation with a pediatric HIV specialist for advice about potential regimens, assistance with access to unpublished data from clinical trials or other limited off-label pediatric use, and referral to suitable clinical trials is recommended.

Chapter 32

Alternative (Complementary) Therapies for HIV/AIDS

Many people use alternative (sometimes known as complementary) health treatments to go along with the medical care they get from their doctor. These therapies are sometimes called "alternative" because they don't fit into the more mainstream, Western ways of looking at medicine and healthcare. These therapies may not fit in with what you usually think of as "healthcare."

They are called "complementary" therapies because usually they are used alongside the more standard medical care you receive (such as your doctor visits and the anti-HIV (human immunodeficiency virus) drugs you might be taking).

Some common complementary therapies include:

- Physical (body) therapies, such as yoga, massage, and acupuncture

- Relaxation techniques, such as meditation and visualization

- Herbal medicine (from plants)

This chapter includes text excerpted from "Alternative (Complementary) Therapies for HIV/AIDS: Entire Lesson," U.S. Department of Veterans Affairs (VA), February 8, 2018.

With most complementary therapies, your health is looked at from a holistic (or "whole picture") point of view. Think of your body as working as one big system. From a holistic viewpoint, everything you do—from what you eat to what you drink to how stressed you are— affects your health and well-being.

Do Alternative Therapies Work?

Healthy people use these kinds of therapies to try to make their immune systems stronger and to make themselves feel better in general. People who have diseases or illnesses, such as HIV, use these therapies for the same reasons. They also can use these therapies to help deal with symptoms of the disease or side effects from the medicines that treat the disease.

Many people report positive results from using complementary therapies. In most cases, however, there is not enough research to tell if these treatments really help people with HIV.

Here you can read about some of the more common complementary therapies that people with HIV use. Sometimes these are used alone, but often they are used in combination with one another. For example, some people combine yoga with meditation.

Physical (Body) Therapies

Physical, or body, therapies include such activities as yoga, massage, and aromatherapy. These types of therapies focus on using a person's body and senses to promote healing and well-being. Here you can learn about examples of these types of therapies.

Yoga

Yoga is a set of exercises that people use to improve their fitness, reduce stress, and increase flexibility. Yoga can involve breathing exercises, stretching and strengthening poses, and meditation.

Many people, including people with HIV, use yoga to reduce stress and to become more relaxed and calm. Some people think that yoga helps make them healthier in general, because it can make a person's body stronger.

There are many different types of yoga and various classes you can take. You can also try out yoga by following a video program.

Before you begin any kind of exercise program, always talk with your healthcare provider.

Massage

Many people believe that massage therapy is an excellent way to deal with the stress and side effects that go along with having an illness, including HIV.

During massage therapy, a trained therapist moves and rubs your body tissues (such as your muscles). There are many kinds of massage therapy.

You can try massage therapy for reducing muscle and back pain, headaches, and soreness. Massages also can improve your blood flow (your circulation) and reduce tension. Some people think that massages might even make your immune system stronger.

Acupuncture

Acupuncture is part of a whole healing system known as traditional Chinese medicine (TCM). During acupuncture treatment, tiny needles (about as wide as a hair) are inserted into certain areas of a person's body. Most people say that they don't feel any pain at all from the needles.

Many people with HIV use acupuncture. Some people think that acupuncture can help treat symptoms of HIV and side effects from the medicine, like fatigue and nausea.

Some people say that acupuncture can be used to help with neuropathy (body pain caused by nerve damage from HIV or the medicines used to treat HIV).

Others report that acupuncture gives them more energy. If you are interested in trying it out, ask your doctor to recommend an expert.

Aromatherapy

Aromatherapy is based on the idea that certain smells can change the way you feel. The smells used in aromatherapy come from plant oils, and they can be inhaled (breathed in) or used in baths or massages.

People use aromatherapy to help them deal with stress or to help with fatigue. For example, some people report that lavender oil calms them down and helps them sleep better.

Please remember! The oils used in aromatherapy can be very strong and even harmful. Always talk with an expert before using these oils yourself.

Relaxation Techniques

Relaxation therapies, such as meditation and visualization, focus on how a person's mind and imagination can promote overall health and well-being. In this section, you can read about some examples of how you can use relaxation therapies to reduce stress and relax.

Meditation

Meditation is a certain way of concentrating that may allow your mind and body to become very relaxed. Meditation helps people to focus and be quiet.

There are many different forms of meditation. Most involve deep breathing and paying attention to your body and mind.

Sometimes people sit still and close their eyes to meditate. Meditation also can be casual. For instance, you can meditate when you are taking a walk or watching a sunrise.

People with HIV can use meditation to relax. It can help them deal with the stress that comes with any illness. Meditation can help you to calm down and focus if you are feeling overwhelmed.

If you are interested in learning more about meditation, you should ask your healthcare provider. There may be meditation classes you can take.

Visualization

Visualization is another method people use to feel more relaxed and less anxious. People who use visualization imagine that they are in a safe, relaxing place (such as the beach). Most of us use visualization without realizing it—for example, when we daydream or remember a fun, happy time in our lives.

Focusing on a safe, comfortable place can help you to feel less stress, and sometimes it can lessen the pain or side effects from HIV or the medicines you are taking.

You can ask your doctor where you can know more about visualization. There are classes you can take, and there are self-help tapes that you can listen to that lead you through the process.

Herbal Medicine

Herbal medicines are substances that come from plants, and they work like standard medicine. They can be taken from all parts of a plant, including the roots, leaves, berries, and flowers.

People with HIV sometimes take these medicines to help deal with side effects from anti-HIV medicines or with symptoms from the illness.

- It is important to remember to always use herbs carefully. Learn the proper dosage and use. Don't take too much of anything.

- Always ask your doctor before taking anything new. Just because something is "natural" or "nondrug" doesn't mean that it is safe.

- Learn about the possible side effects of an herbal therapy. Remember, some herbs can interfere with your HIV medications.

An important note about St. John's wort. St. John's wort is an herbal medicine that is used by some people to treat depression. It interacts with the liver and can change how some drugs work in your body, including some anti-HIV drugs (for example, protease inhibitors and NNRTIs). If you are taking antiviral drugs for your HIV, you should NOT take St. John's wort. Be sure you tell your provider if you are using St. John's wort. You should also not take St. John's wort if you are taking other antidepressants.

Chapter 33

Medical Marijuana for HIV/AIDS

What Is Medical Marijuana?

The term medical marijuana refers to using the whole, unprocessed marijuana plant or its basic extracts to treat symptoms of illness and other conditions. The U.S. Food and Drug Administration (FDA) has not recognized or approved the marijuana plant as medicine.

However, scientific study of the chemicals in marijuana, called cannabinoids, has led to two FDA-approved medications that contain cannabinoid chemicals in pill form. Continued research may lead to more medications.

Because the marijuana plant contains chemicals that may help treat a range of illnesses and symptoms, many people argue that it should be legal for medical purposes. In fact, a growing number of states have legalized marijuana for medical use.

What Are Cannabinoids?

Cannabinoids are chemicals related to delta-9-tetrahydrocannabinol (THC), marijuana's main mind-altering ingredient that makes people "high." The marijuana plant contains more than 100 cannabinoids. Scientists, as well as illegal manufacturers, have produced many

This chapter includes text excerpted from "Marijuana as Medicine," National Institute on Drug Abuse (NIDA), May 2018.

cannabinoids in the lab. Some of these cannabinoids are extremely powerful and have led to serious health effects when misused.

The body also produces its own cannabinoid chemicals. They play a role in regulating pleasure, memory, thinking, concentration, body movement, awareness of time, appetite, pain, and the senses (taste, touch, smell, hearing, and sight).

How Might Cannabinoids Be Useful as Medicine?

The two main cannabinoids from the marijuana plant that is of medical interest are delta-9-tetrahydrocannabinol (THC) and cannabidiol (CBD).

THC can increase appetite and reduce nausea. THC may also decrease pain, inflammation (swelling and redness), and muscle control problems.

Unlike THC, CBD is a cannabinoid that doesn't make people "high." It may be useful in reducing pain and inflammation, controlling epileptic seizures, and possibly even treating mental illness and addictions.

Many researchers, including those funded by the National Institutes of Health (NIH), are continuing to explore the possible uses of THC, CBD, and other cannabinoids for medical treatment.

For instance, recent animal studies have shown that marijuana extracts may help kill certain cancer cells and reduce the size of others. Evidence from one cell culture study with rodents suggests that purified extracts from whole-plant marijuana can slow the growth of cancer cells from one of the most serious types of brain tumors. Research in mice showed that treatment with purified extracts of THC and CBD, when used with radiation, increased the cancer-killing effects of the radiation.

Scientists are also conducting preclinical and clinical trials with marijuana and its extracts to treat symptoms of illness and other conditions, such as:

- diseases that affect the immune system, including:
  - human immunodeficiency virus/ acquired immunodeficiency syndrome (HIV/AIDS)
  - multiple sclerosis (MS), which causes gradual loss of muscle control
- inflammation
- pain
- seizures

- substance use disorders

- mental disorders

Are People with Health- and Age-Related Problems More Vulnerable to Marijuana's Risks?

State-approved medicinal use of marijuana is a fairly new practice. For that reason, marijuana's effects on people who are weakened because of age or illness are still relatively unknown. Older people and those suffering from diseases such as cancer or AIDS could be more vulnerable to the drug's harmful effects, but more research is needed.

What Medications Contain Cannabinoids?

Two FDA-approved drugs, dronabinol, and nabilone, contain THC. They treat nausea caused by chemotherapy and increase appetite in patients with extreme weight loss caused by AIDS. Continued research might lead to more medications.

The United Kingdom, Canada, and several European countries have approved nabiximols (Sativex®), a mouth spray containing THC and CBD. It treats muscle control problems caused by MS, but it isn't FDA-approved.

Epidiolex, a CBD-based liquid drug to treat certain forms of childhood epilepsy, is being tested in clinical trials but isn't yet FDA-approved.

Chapter 34

HIV/AIDS Treatments in Development

Chapter Contents

Section 34.1

Antiretroviral Drug Discovery and Development

This section includes text excerpted from "Antiretroviral Drug Discovery and Development," National Institute of Allergy and Infectious Diseases (NIAID), May 3, 2017.

For more than three decades, the National Institute of Allergy and Infectious Diseases (NIAID) has fostered and promoted development of antiretroviral therapies (ARTs) that have transformed human immunodeficiency virus (HIV) infection from an almost uniformly fatal infection into a manageable chronic condition. In the 1980s, the average life expectancy following an acquired immunodeficiency syndrome (AIDS) diagnosis was approximately one year. At present, with combination ART drug treatments started early in the course of HIV infection, people living with HIV can expect a near-normal lifespan.

Azidothymidine (AZT)—The First Drug to Treat Human Immunodeficiency Virus (HIV) Infection

Scientists funded by the National Institutes of Health's (NIH) National Cancer Institute (NCI) first developed azidothymidine (AZT) in 1964 as a potential cancer therapy. AZT proved ineffective against cancer and was shelved, but in the 1980s it was included in an NCI screening program to identify drugs to treat HIV/AIDS. In the laboratory, AZT suppressed HIV replication without damaging normal cells, and the British pharmaceutical company Burroughs Wellcome funded a clinical trial to evaluate the drug in people with advanced AIDS. AZT decreased deaths and opportunistic infections, albeit with serious adverse effects. In March 1987, AZT became the first drug to gain approval from the U.S. Food and Drug Administration (FDA) for treating AIDS. AZT, also referred to as zidovudine, belongs to a class of drugs known as nucleoside reverse transcriptase inhibitors, or NRTIs.

The ACTG, established in 1987, quickly began work to build on this discovery. The ACTG 016 clinical trial established a lower therapeutic dosage of AZT, helping to reduce some of the drug's serious side effects. The pivotal ACTG 019 trial investigated whether it was beneficial to put people living with HIV on AZT before they progressed to AIDS. ACTG 019 showed that AZT effectively delayed the onset of AIDS in asymptomatic people with HIV, marking the first demonstration of a treatment for HIV infection.

Accelerating Antiretroviral Drug Development

Established in the early years of the HIV/AIDS pandemic, the NIAID-supported National Cooperative Drug Discovery Group program for the treatment of AIDS (NCDDG-AIDS) provided a framework for scientists from academia, industry, and government to collaborate on research related to identification and development of drugs. The NIAID-supported researchers developed cell culture and biochemical test systems that allowed researchers to more easily screen drug candidates, and NIAID also played a key role in development of animal models for preclinical testing.

In the early 1990s, additional nucleoside analog reverse-transcriptase inhibitors (NRTI) drugs gained FDA approval. Development of AZT and other NRTIs showed that treating HIV was possible, and these drugs paved the way for discovery and development of new generations of antiretroviral drugs.

While the earliest ART agents were developed before HIV diagnostics were available in the clinic, the development of laboratory tests to measure viral load and cluster of differentiation 4+ (CD4+) cell count greatly accelerated progress in drug development. Viral load describes the amount of HIV in the blood. The higher the viral load, the faster the CD4+ cell count—an indicator of how well the immune system is working—will fall. These advances made it possible for researchers to use lab test results, viral load measurements in particular, to assess how well an investigational antiretroviral agent worked. This approach requires drug trials to last roughly 6 months, whereas relying solely on clinical indicators such as progression to AIDS or death ordinarily requires trials to last years before a result is available.

The Advent of Combination Therapy

The limitations of single-drug treatment regimens quickly became apparent. HIV replicates swiftly and is prone to errors each time it does. These errors, or mutations, cause small changes in the virus. HIV variants with mutations that confer resistance to an antiretroviral drug can evolve rapidly. In some people taking AZT, drug resistance developed in a matter of days. Scientists thus tested whether combining drugs would make it difficult for the virus to become resistant to all the drugs simultaneously.

In the early 1990s, data from an NIAID-funded study of AZT in combination with ddC showed that this two-drug therapy was more effective than AZT alone, raising hopes about the use of combination therapy in treating AIDS.

Results from the ACTG 175 trial, announced in 1995, showed that two-drug combinations were superior to AZT alone in preventing decline in CD4+ cell count or death. The trial also showed that ART reduced the risk of death in people with asymptomatic, intermediate-stage disease.

Around the same time, another NIAID-supported trial called CPCRA 007 assessed combination therapy for HIV-infected people with more advanced disease, the majority of whom had previously been treated with AZT. This study was conducted by the NIAID-supported Terry Beirn Community Programs for Clinical Research on AIDS (CPRCA), a network of community-based healthcare providers who integrated scientific research into primary care that later became part of the INSIGHT network.

CPCRA investigators found that two-drug therapy had no significant benefit over AZT alone in slowing disease progression or death in this patient group. However, among CPCRA 007 participants with little or no prior AZT use, combination therapy was more effective than AZT alone.

The results of ACTG 175 and CPCRA 007, as well as other studies, indicated that prior antiretroviral experience can profoundly influence the effectiveness of some treatments, underscoring the importance of careful planning in the use of antiretroviral drugs.

Durable HIV Suppression with Triple-Drug Therapy

While the effects of two-NRTI therapy were better than those of single-drug therapy for many people with HIV, they were of limited duration. A major advance came in 1996, when researchers found that triple-drug therapy could durably suppress HIV replication to minimal levels, while creating a high genetic barrier against development of drug resistance.

The possibility and success of triple-drug therapy, also called highly active antiretroviral therapy or HAART, was partially due to the appearance of a new antiretroviral drug class—the protease inhibitors. In December 1995, saquinavir became the first protease inhibitor to receive FDA approval. In 1996, results from an NIAID-sponsored trial showed that a three-drug regimen of saquinavir, (2'-3'-dideoxycytidine, ddC), also called dideoxycytidine, and AZT was more effective than two-drug therapy with ddC and AZT.

One of the key studies demonstrating the efficacy of triple-drug therapy was ACTG 320, also supported by NIAID. This study found that a three-drug combination of the protease inhibitor indinavir and two NRTIs reduced the viral load to very low levels for up to one year in people who had previously been taking single-drug therapy. ACTG 320 also showed that adding at least two new drugs when switching therapy is more effective than adding single new drugs.

With HAART, which combines drugs from at least two different classes, many patients saw the amount of HIV in their blood drop to undetectable levels. But while HAART was lifesaving, the early regimens were far from perfect. The side effects were burdensome, and the daily dosing was complex. Certain drugs had to be taken in combination at different intervals throughout the day, some with food and some without. The complexity made it difficult for people to adhere to the regimens long-term.

Identifying New Classes of Antiretroviral Drugs

To address the complexity of antiretroviral regimens, drug toxicities, and the issue of drug resistance, NIAID supports research aimed at novel formulations and development of drugs that work by different mechanisms and target various steps in the HIV replication process. As of now, more than 30 ART drugs are available, including several fixed-dose combinations, which contain two or more medications from one or more drug classes in a single tablet. At present, some people control their HIV by taking as little as one pill once a day.

The mid-1990s marked the emergence of another class of ART drugs called nonnucleoside reverse transcriptase inhibitors (NNRTIs). Because they are cheaper and easier to produce than protease inhibitors, they helped scale up ART in resource-limited settings.

Identification of novel drug targets has played a key role in discovery and development of antiretroviral drug classes. For example, since the 1980s, scientists have known that a molecule called CD4 is the primary receptor for HIV on immune system cells. In the mid-1990s, NIAID scientists reported the discovery of a coreceptor called C-X-C chemokine receptor type 4 (CXCR4), which is required for entry of certain HIV strains into immune cells. This discovery inspired researchers to look other coreceptors. A number of research groups, including the NIAID scientists, determined that a different receptor called C-C chemokine receptor type 5 (CCR5) is actually the primary coreceptor used by HIV to infect immune cells. This work laid the foundation for the development of the CCR5-blocking drug maraviroc, which received FDA approval in 2007.

Another major ART drug class emerged in 2007, with FDA approval of the integrase inhibitor raltegravir. Raltegravir quickly became a valued component for combination antiretroviral therapy, but HIV can follow several pathways to develop resistance to the drug. HIV variants resistant to raltegravir may also be resistant to elvitegravir, another first-generation integrase inhibitor.

Dolutegravir, which received the FDA approval in 2013, is a second-generation integrase inhibitor that appears to have a high barrier to development of HIV drug resistance. In clinical trials, dolutegravir was effective both for people living with HIV who had not previously taken HIV therapy and for people who were treatment-experienced, including those for whom first-generation integrase inhibitors were ineffective. Additional advantages of dolutegravir include convenient once-daily dosing, a good safety profile, and a relatively low production cost. Dolutegravir now is included in two of the first-line regimens that the U.S. Department of Health and Human Services (HHS) medical practice guidelines recommend for adults with HIV, and it was added to the World Health Organization (WHO) guidelines as an alternative first-line agent for adults. Experts consider it likely that dolutegravir will be used globally with increasing frequency in the future.

Section 34.2

Therapeutic HIV Vaccines

This section includes text excerpted from "What Is a Therapeutic HIV Vaccine?" AIDS*info*, U.S. Department of Health and Human Services (HHS), August 16, 2017.

A therapeutic human immunodeficiency virus (HIV) vaccine is a vaccine that's designed to improve the body's immune response to HIV in a person who already has HIV. Researchers are developing and testing therapeutic HIV vaccines to slow down the progression of

HIV infection and ideally result in undetectable levels of HIV without the need for regular antiretroviral therapy (ART). ART is the recommended treatment for HIV infection and involves using a combination of different HIV medicines to prevent HIV from replicating. At present, a person with HIV must remain on ART to keep HIV at undetectable levels.

A therapeutic HIV vaccine may also slow a person's progression to acquired immunodeficiency syndrome (AIDS) and may make it less likely that a person could transmit HIV to others.

Researchers are also evaluating therapeutic HIV vaccines as part of a larger strategy to eliminate all HIV from the body and cure people of HIV. This kind of strategy may involve using other drugs and therapies in addition to a therapeutic HIV vaccine. HIV cure research is still in early exploratory stages, and it is not known what strategies may or may not work.

Therapeutic HIV Vaccine Is Different from a Preventive HIV Vaccine

A preventive HIV vaccine is given to people who do not have HIV, with the goal of preventing HIV infection in the future. The vaccine would teach the person's immune system to recognize and effectively fight HIV in case the virus ever enters the person's body.

A therapeutic HIV vaccine is given to people who already have HIV. The goal of a therapeutic HIV vaccine is to strengthen a person's immune response to the HIV that is already in the person's body.

Availability of the U.S. Food and Drug Administration (FDA)-Approved Therapeutic HIV Vaccines

There are no FDA-approved therapeutic HIV vaccines available as of now, but research is underway.

Chapter 35

Investigational HIV Drug and Its Role in HIV Treatment

What Is an Investigational Human Immunodeficiency Virus (HIV) Drug?

An investigational HIV drug is a drug that is being tested to treat or prevent HIV infection and is not approved by the U.S. Food and Drug Administration (FDA) for general use or sale in the United States. Medical research studies—also called clinical trials—are done to evaluate the safety and effectiveness of an investigational HIV drug.

What Types of Investigational HIV Drugs Are Being Studied?

Currently, there are investigational drugs for treating HIV and preventing HIV. There are also investigational drugs for treating HIV-related opportunistic infections. (Opportunistic infections are infections and infection-related cancers that occur more frequently or are more severe in people with weakened immune systems than in people with healthy immune systems.)

This chapter includes text excerpted from "What is an Investigational HIV Drug?" AIDS*info*, U.S. Department of Health and Human Services (HHS), August 25, 2017.

363

Although no HIV vaccines exist yet, researchers are studying investigational preventive vaccines and treatment vaccines. The goal of a preventive HIV vaccine is to prevent HIV in people who don't have HIV but who may be exposed to the virus. The goal of an HIV treatment vaccine also called a therapeutic vaccine, is to slow the progression of HIV infection or delay the onset of Acquired Immunodeficiency Syndrome (AIDS) in people with HIV.

How Are Clinical Trials of Investigational Drugs Conducted?

Clinical trials, which are medical research studies, are conducted in phases. Each phase has a different purpose and helps researchers answer different questions about the investigational drug.

- **Phase 1 trials:** Researchers test the investigational drug in a small group of people (20–80) for the first time. The purpose is to evaluate its safety and identify side effects.

- **Phase 2 trials:** The investigational drug is administered to a larger group of people (100–300) to determine its effectiveness and to further evaluate its safety.

- **Phase 3 trials:** The investigational drug is administered to large groups of people (1,000–3,000) to confirm its effectiveness, monitor side effects, compare it with standard or equivalent treatments, and collect information that will allow the investigational drug to be used safely.

  - In most cases, an investigational drug must be proven effective and must show continued safety in Phase 3 clinical trial to be considered for approval by the Food and Drug Administration (FDA) for sale in the United States. (Some drugs go through FDA's accelerated approval process and are approved before a Phase 3 clinical trial is complete.) After a drug is approved by FDA and made available to the public, researchers track its safety in Phase 4 trials to seek more information about the drug's risks, benefits, and optimal use.

How Can I Get Access to an Investigational HIV Drug?

One way to get access to an investigational HIV drug is by enrolling in a clinical trial that is studying the drug. Another way is through

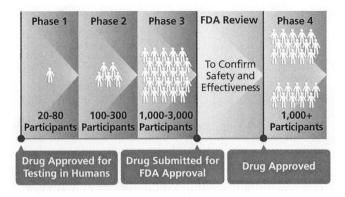

Figure 35.1. *Phases of Clinical Trials*

an expanded access program. Expanded access involves using an investigational drug outside of a clinical trial to treat a person who has a serious or immediately life-threatening disease and who has no FDA-approved treatment options. Drug companies must have permission from FDA to make an investigational drug available for expanded access. Talk to your healthcare provider to see if you may qualify to take part in an expanded access program.

How Can I Find a Clinical Trial on an Investigational HIV Drug?

To find an HIV/AIDS clinical trial on an investigational HIV drug, use the AIDS*info* clinical trial search. For help with your search, call an AIDS*info* health information specialist at 800-448-0440 or email ContactUs@aidsinfo.nih.gov.

You can also join ResearchMatch, which is a free, secure online tool that makes it easier for the public to become involved in clinical trials.

Is It Safe to Use an Investigational HIV Drug?

One goal of HIV research is to identify new drugs that are less toxic and have fewer side effects. Researchers also try to make HIV/AIDS clinical trials as safe as possible. But investigational HIV drugs may have side effects that are not well known yet. Although this risk of poorly understood side effects is explained to you before you start taking the investigational drug, this makes it hard to know your actual risk. As testing of an investigational HIV drug continues, additional information on possible side effects is collected.

Chapter 36

HIV/AIDS Clinical Trials and Research

Chapter Contents

Section 36.1

Basics of Clinical Trials

This section includes text excerpted from "HIV/AIDS—
Clinical Trials and HIV," U.S. Department of Veterans
Affairs (VA), February 9, 2018.

Frequently Asked Questions on Clinical Trial

What Is a Clinical Trial?

A clinical trial is a research study that tests a new medicine to see if it is safe and works well. When a new medicine (or drug) is first developed, you cannot get it by prescription. Researchers must first test it in a laboratory with animals. Then, they must do a clinical trial in a hospital or clinic to test it in people. They test it to see if it is safe and to see how much of the medicine (or what dose) is enough to work.

The U.S. Food and Drug Administration (FDA) is a government agency that decides if a drug is safe enough to give to patients by prescription. It looks at the results of the clinical trials to make this decision. Testing drugs for HIV is very important, and clinical trials are a way to find new and better medicines. All medicines that you can now get to treat human immunodeficiency virus (HIV) were first tested in clinical trials.

Clinical trials follow a set of rules called a protocol. The protocol says who can participate, how long the study is, and which tests need to be done.

Clinical trials are managed by doctors and are usually run by nurses or other healthcare professionals. The clinical trial staff will follow your progress closely and can help tell your regular doctor what is happening with your treatment.

Trials are also checked by an institutional review board (IRB). This is a group of people who reviews the clinical trial regularly to protect your rights, safety, and well-being.

When you are in a clinical trial, you may need to see the study doctor more often. This is because they want to check the effects of the medicine carefully. Because clinical trials are research, they will often test the real drug against a placebo (or sugar pill). You will be told if the trial involves one group of participants taking a placebo, but you may not know if you are taking the medicine or the placebo until the clinical trial is over.

How Do Clinical Trials Work?

Before you start a clinical trial, you will go through a screening process. This is to make sure that it is safe for you to start taking the medicine. The staff will ask you about your health history, and you may have a blood test, urine test, or others (such as a physical exam or a heart test).

Who Can Join a Clinical Trial?

There are many types of clinical trials. For example, some trials are for people who have never been on anti-HIV medicines, others are for people whose treatment isn't working and who need a new medication. Not everyone can join a trial, though. Most clinical trials have eligibility criteria. These are rules about who can participate, based on health, age, and maybe other things. For example, some trials take only people who have a particular viral load or cluster of differentiation 4 (CD4) count. Usually, you can't participate in a clinical trial if you have any conditions are using medicines that might make it hard to measure how well the test treatment is working. You also cannot participate if the test treatment might harm you.

If you do qualify for a trial and decide to participate, you should be willing to follow the guidelines of the study.

What Is Informed Consent?

You will also go through a process called informed consent. The doctors and nurses will explain exactly what will happen during the clinical trial. They will answer your questions and tell you about the risks and benefits of the clinical trial. They will ask you to sign a document called a consent form. When you sign this form, you are saying that you understand what is going to happen and that you agree to participate. Even after you have started a clinical trial, you are free to quit at any time for any reason. Quitting early will not affect your medical care in the future.

Does It Cost Anything to Participate?

No. It will not cost you anything because you are helping the researchers to test a medicine. Sometimes you may even get extra money to pay for your time or travel.

Who Pays for Clinical Trials?

Trials are paid for by government agencies, pharmaceutical (or drug) companies, individual doctors, and hospitals, or clinics. The doctors and nurses will tell you who is paying for the study before you begin a trial.

How Long Do Clinical Trials Last?

Clinical trials can last from a few weeks to several years. After the treatment is over, they will usually ask you to come back for some follow-up visits. The follow-up period may be as short as a few weeks or as long as 6 months and helps to make sure that you are safe.

Are There Different Types of Clinical Trials?

There are four different types of clinical trials: Phase I, Phase II, Phase III, and Phase IV.

Phase I

- is the first time they have tried the drug in people
- tests for the drug's safety and helps find the right dose
- may ask for frequent tests or a stay in the hospital to check for safety and effectiveness
- lasts a fairly short time
- has a small number of patient volunteers

Phase II

- happens when early studies show that the drug may work well to fight HIV
- tests for safety and effective dose level
- lasts longer than Phase I trials
- tries to find out what kind of side effects people may get with this medicine
- has several hundred patients

Phase III

- happens if the drug worked well in Phase I and II

- compares standard treatments (medicines that you can already get by prescription) or sugar pills (placebos) with the new medicine
- may last longer than Phases I and II
- looks for ways to reduce the side effects and improve the quality of your life while you are taking the medicine
- is the last phase of study before a drug is sent to the FDA for consideration for approval
- has many patients (sometimes thousands)

Phase IV

- happens when the drug is already available by prescription
- happens less often than other phases
- checks other safety issues and long-term side effects
- may be used to check higher or lower amounts (doses) of the medicine

What Are the Benefits and Risks?

Before you start a clinical trial, you should think about the positive and negative things that may happen.

Benefits:

- You may get frequent free checkups from specialists
- You can get free medicine
- You can get new medicine that is not yet available from your regular doctor and may work better than the old medicine
- You may learn a lot about your condition and how to take care of yourself
- You may help medical researchers to find better treatments for all patients with HIV

Risks:

- You may have side effects from the medicine that you did not expect
- You may have to have frequent office visits, blood tests, and other medical exams
- You may not get better from the treatment

371

How Long Does the U.S. Food and Drug Administration (FDA) Take to Approve a Drug?

It usually takes about 10 years for a drug to be developed and approved for prescription. Many people would like to take the newest medicine as soon as it is proven to work. However, even after a drug has been successful in a Phase III trial, it still may take 6–12 months before that drug is approved for prescription.

Section 36.2

Clinical Trials for HIV Treatment in Pregnant Women

This section includes text excerpted from "NIH Begins Large HIV Treatment Study in Pregnant Women," National Institutes of Health (NIH), January 24, 2018.

The National Institutes of Health (NIH) has launched a large international study to compare the safety and efficacy of three antiretroviral treatment regimens for pregnant women living with human immunodeficiency virus (HIV) and the safety of these regimens for their infants. The study will evaluate the current preferred first-line regimen for pregnant women recommended by the World Health Organization (WHO) and two regimens containing newer antiretroviral drugs that are becoming more widely used. It will provide data on the use of these newer drugs during pregnancy, helping to ensure that women living with HIV and their infants receive the best available treatments.

Each year worldwide, an estimated 1.5 million women living with HIV give birth. Previous research has clearly demonstrated that antiretroviral therapy to suppress HIV prevents perinatal HIV transmission and benefits the health of both mother and child. In this study, investigators will compare the virologic efficacy of the three regimens by measuring the mother's viral load (amount of HIV in the blood) at delivery. The study also will compare how the regimens affect rates of adverse pregnancy outcomes, such as preterm delivery and low infant birth weight; maternal adverse events; and infant adverse events.

"Women should have access to the best available HIV medications throughout their lives," said Anthony S. Fauci, M.D., director of the NIH's National Institute of Allergy and Infectious Diseases (NIAID). "Our priority is to evaluate newer, improved antiretroviral drugs during pregnancy to identify the optimal regimens for women living with HIV and their infants."

The first participants in the clinical trial have begun receiving treatment at research sites in Zimbabwe. Clinical trial sites in the United States and Zimbabwe are now open for enrollment, with additional sites in Botswana, Brazil, Haiti, India, Malawi, South Africa, Tanzania, Thailand, Uganda, the United States and Zimbabwe expected to open in the coming months. The trial is supported by NIAID, the *Eunice Kennedy Shriver* National Institute of Child Health and Human Development (NICHD) and the National Institute of Mental Health (NIMH), all part of NIH. It is being conducted by the International Maternal Pediatric Adolescent AIDS Clinical Trials (IMPAACT) network.

As of day, WHO recommends a regimen of three antiretroviral drugs—efavirenz (EFV), lamivudine (3TC) or emtricitabine (FTC), and tenofovir disoproxil fumarate (TDF)—for pregnant women living with HIV in resource-limited settings. However, this regimen is not well-tolerated by or otherwise appropriate for all women. EFV has been linked to neuropsychiatric symptoms, including suicidal thoughts, as well as liver problems. TDF can cause kidney problems and loss of bone mineral density in adults, and some evidence suggests that prenatal exposure to TDF could cause bone loss in infants.

The new study will compare maternal EFV/FTC/TDF with regimens containing a newer drug, dolutegravir (DTG), and either tenofovir alafenamide (TAF), an alternative formulation of tenofovir, or TDF. The study, known as IMPAACT 2010 or VESTED (Virologic Efficacy and Safety of Antiretroviral Therapy Combinations with TAF/TDF, EFV, and DTG), is co-chaired by Shahin Lockman, M.D., M.Sc., of Brigham and Women's Hospital (BWH) in the United States, and Lameck Chinula, M.B.B.S., M.Med., of the University of North Carolina (UNC) Project at Kamuzu Central Hospital in Malawi.

DTG is included in two of the preferred first-line regimens recommended for adults living with HIV in the United States, and was included in the WHO guidelines as an alternative first-line agent in nonpregnant adults. Advantages of DTG include once-daily dosing, a good safety profile, a high barrier to development of drug resistance and a relatively low production cost. Research so far indicates that TAF is as effective as TDF but appears to cause fewer kidney and bone side effects. Only a few studies have assessed the use of DTG in pregnancy, and minimal data are available on the safety and efficacy of TAF in pregnant women.

"Therapies for pregnant women and new mothers should be based on the best available evidence, always keeping in mind the health of the woman, her developing fetus and her newborn," said Nahida Chakhtoura, M.D., of the Maternal and Pediatric Infectious Disease Branch (MPIDB) at the NICHD. "The results of this study will help inform optimal treatment of pregnant women living with HIV in both resource-limited and well-resourced settings."

The International Maternal Pediatric Adolescent AIDS (acquired immunodeficiency syndrome) Clinical Trials Network (IMPAACT 2010), a Phase 3 study, aims to enroll 639 women who are 14–28 weeks into their pregnancies, are living with HIV and are not currently on antiretroviral treatment. The women will be randomly assigned to treatment with EFV/FTC/TDF, DTG/FTC/TAF or DTG/FTC/TDF. Their infants also will be enrolled in the study and will receive local standard-of-care interventions for HIV prophylaxis after birth. Mothers will be counseled on infant feeding options consistent with local standards of care, which may include breastfeeding or formula feeding.

The investigators will monitor both mother and infant for 50 weeks after delivery. Study staff will provide women with counseling on antiretroviral medication adherence, which is essential to keep HIV suppressed. The mothers' viral loads will be closely monitored, and infants also will be tested for HIV. If an infant becomes infected with HIV during the study, investigators will provide referrals to local sources of HIV care and treatment. Throughout the study, investigators will closely monitor the health of mother and infant, including assessing the mother's liver and kidney function and screening for anxiety and depression. Investigators also will conduct bone density scans of a subset of infants at 26 weeks of age and their mothers at 50 weeks postpartum. The study is expected to last for approximately three years.

"Limited pregnancy data for newer, better antiretroviral drugs— such as DTG and TAF—can mean that pregnant women may not receive the most effective and safest medications, and can delay the general adoption of better regimens in low-resource settings with high HIV prevalence," said Dr. Lockman. "We hope that the VESTED trial will provide urgently needed information regarding the safety and efficacy of these newer drugs in pregnant women and their babies, so that optimal antiretroviral regimens can be offered to pregnant women and recommended for first-line treatment of adults living with HIV throughout the world."

The NIAID and the NICHD provide funding to the IMPAACT 2010 (VESTED) clinical research sites. Gilead Sciences, Mylan, and ViiV Healthcare Ltd. are providing antiretroviral drugs for the study. ViiV also is providing funding to IMPAACT for nonparticipant costs.

The NIAID conducts and supports research—at NIH, throughout the United States, and worldwide—to study the causes of infectious and immune-mediated diseases, and to develop better means of preventing, diagnosing and treating these illnesses.

The NICHD conducts and supports research in the United States and throughout the world on fetal, infant and child development; maternal, child and family health; reproductive biology and population issues; and medical rehabilitation.

Section 36.3

Combination HIV Prevention Reduces New Infections

This section includes text excerpted from "Combination HIV Prevention Reduces New Infections by 42 Percent in Ugandan District," National Institutes of Health (NIH), November 29, 2017.

A study published in the *New England Journal of Medicine (NEJM)* provides real-world evidence that implementing a combination of proven human immunodeficiency virus (HIV) prevention measures across communities can substantially reduce new HIV infections in a population.

Investigators found that HIV incidence dropped by 42 percent among nearly 18,000 people in Rakai District, Uganda, during a seven-year period in which the rates of HIV treatment and voluntary medical male circumcision increased significantly.

The HIV prevention strategy whose impact was observed in the study is based on earlier findings by the National Institutes of Health (NIH) and others demonstrating the protective effect of voluntary medical male circumcision for HIV-uninfected men and of HIV-suppressing antiretroviral therapy (ART) for halting sexual transmission of the virus to uninfected partners. The strategy is also based on studies showing that changes in sexual behavior, such as having only one sexual partner, can help prevent HIV infection.

"Before this study, we knew that these HIV prevention measures worked at an individual level, yet it was not clear that they would substantially reduce HIV incidence in a population—or even if it would be possible to get large numbers of people to adopt them," said Anthony S. Fauci, M.D., director of the National Institute of Allergy and Infectious Diseases (NIAID), part of the NIH. "This new analysis demonstrates that scaling up combination HIV prevention is possible and can turn the tide of the epidemic."

The NIAID cofunded the research, and NIAID investigators oversaw all laboratory operations. The President's Emergency Plan for AIDS (acquired immunodeficiency syndrome) Relief (PEPFAR) funded the provision of combination HIV prevention, including ART and circumcision services, during the period observed in the study.

The reported research involved nearly 34,000 people ages 15–49 years residing in 30 communities that participate in the Rakai Community Cohort Study (RCCS) conducted by the Rakai Health Sciences Program in Uganda. With funding from the NIH and others, this program promoted HIV testing, ART, and voluntary medical male circumcision to study participants. Every one or two years from April 1999 until September 2016, participants were tested for HIV and surveyed about their sexual behavior, use of HIV treatment, and male circumcision status. The authors analyzed these survey data under the leadership of M. Kate Grabowski, Ph.D., an assistant professor of pathology at the Johns Hopkins University School of Medicine (JHUSOM) in Baltimore and of epidemiology at the Johns Hopkins University Bloomberg School of Public Health (JHSPH), and an epidemiologist with the Rakai Health Sciences Program (RHSP).

The investigators found that the proportion of study participants living with HIV who reported taking ART climbed from zero in 2003 to 69 percent in 2016. The proportion of male study participants who were voluntarily circumcised grew from 15 percent in 1999 to 59 percent in 2016. While levels of condom use with casual partners and the proportion of people reporting multiple sexual partners remained largely unchanged, the proportion of adolescents ages 15–19 who reported never having sex rose from 30 percent in 1999 to 55 percent in 2016.

As an apparent consequence of these increases, particularly in ART use and voluntary male circumcision, the annual number of new HIV infections in the cohort fell from 1.17 per 100 person-years in 2009 to 0.66 per 100 person-years in 2016, a 42 percent decrease. Person-years are the sum of the number of years that each cohort member participated in the study. The researchers calculated the annual number of addition in HIV infections using data from nearly 18,000 of the almost 34,000 total participants.

In addition, the proportion of cohort members living with HIV whose treatment suppressed the virus increased from 42 percent in 2009 to 75 percent in 2016, showing the feasibility of meeting the goal of the Joint United Nations Programme on HIV/AIDS (UNAIDS) 90-90-90 initiative to achieve 73 percent viral suppression.

"These findings are extremely encouraging and suggest that with sustained commitment to increase the number of people who use combination HIV prevention, it may be possible to achieve epidemic control and eventual elimination of HIV," said David Serwadda, M.B.Ch.B., M.Med., M.P.H., co-founder of the RHSP and professor at Makerere University School of Public Health (MUSPH) in Kampala, Uganda.

HIV incidence dropped the most—by 57 percent—among circumcised men, likely because both their own circumcision and ART taken by their female sexual partners living with HIV protected these men from the virus. HIV incidence declined by 54 percent among all men but by only 32 percent among all women. According to the investigators, this difference probably occurred because a greater percentage of women living with HIV than men living with HIV took ART, and because nearly two-thirds of men chose the extra preventive benefit of circumcision. The researchers suggest addressing this gender imbalance by influencing more men living with HIV to take ART and by giving HIV-uninfected women HIV prevention tools that they can control unilaterally, such as preexposure prophylaxis (PrEP). The scientists anticipate that the RCCS will add PrEP to its combination HIV prevention package as the study continues.

"We expect that this multifaceted approach to HIV prevention will work as well in other populations as it has in rural Uganda," said Dr. Grabowski. "Our results make a strong case for further expanding ART and male circumcision for HIV prevention in Rakai District and beyond. Additional proven HIV prevention interventions, such as PrEP, should be added to the mix to reduce HIV infections in women and other high-risk groups."

Section 36.4

HIV Research Activities

This section includes text excerpted from "Supporting Research
to Effectively Prevent, Diagnose, and Treat HIV," HIV.gov, U.S.
Department of Health and Human Services (HHS), May 20, 2017.

In the three decades since the first cases of acquired immunodeficiency virus (AIDS) were reported, federal investments in basic, biomedical, behavioral, and social science research have led to numerous
human immunodeficiency virus (HIV) prevention interventions and
life-saving treatment.

Leading the Way in Human Immunodeficiency Virus (HIV) Research

The National Institutes of Health (NIH) is the global leader in
research to understand, prevent, diagnose, and treat HIV infection
and its many associated conditions. The NIH-funded researchers—in
partnership with academia and the biotechnology and pharmaceutical
industries—have helped develop, test, and demonstrate the efficacy of
more than 30 life-saving antiretroviral drugs and drug combinations
for treating HIV infection. These antiretroviral drugs have transformed life with HIV infection for those who have access to and can
tolerate treatment.

The NIH has also supported other ground-breaking research,
including the HIV Prevention Trials Network (HPTN) 052 study—
called the scientific breakthrough of 2011 by Science magazine—which
demonstrated that early treatment for HIV reduces the risk of HIV
transmission to uninfected sexual partners by 96 percent while simultaneously improving health outcomes for people living with HIV. In
addition, the NIH-supported the Strategic Timing of Anti-Retroviral
Treatment (START) study demonstrated that those with HIV who
received immediate treatment significantly reduced their risk of illness and death.

Other key areas of NIH-supported research include studies to
better understand the basic biology of HIV and the body's immune
response to HIV infection; design, develop, and test potential drugs
for the prevention and treatment of HIV and its associated coinfections, comorbidities, and other complications; develop HIV cure
strategies to control and eliminate the viral reservoir; and advanced

HIV testing strategies and diagnostic tools. The NIH also conducts and supports research on the development of effective and affordable biomedical prevention strategies, such as the use of antiretroviral drugs and other agents for prevention; the development of safe, effective, and affordable HIV vaccines that can be used in combination with other prevention strategies; and strategies to better understand and address the risk behaviors and social contexts that can facilitate HIV transmission, acquisition, and disease progression.

Seeking a Cure for HIV

Research to find a cure for HIV/AIDS is also one of NIH's overarching HIV/AIDS research priorities. In 2013, President Obama announced that NIH would redirect $100 million to launch an HIV Cure Initiative to further advance HIV/AIDS research with the hope of catalyzing a new generation of therapies aimed at curing HIV or inducing lifelong remission. HIV cure research includes studies to identify the precise locations where HIV hides in the body (known as viral reservoirs), to determine how those reservoirs are established and maintained, and to develop strategies to minimize or deplete them. It also includes studies to develop a functional cure whereby the virus would not eliminated, but controlled and suppressed.

Research to Prevent HIV Infection and Transmission

With the ultimate goal of ending the HIV/AIDS pandemic as we know it, NIH continually develops and supports the research infrastructure and scientific expertise needed to enable innovative approaches aimed at halting the spread of HIV through effective and acceptable prevention strategies and a safe and effective vaccine.

The Centers for Disease Control and Prevention (CDC) also provides national leadership for HIV prevention research, including the development of biomedical and behavioral interventions to prevent HIV transmission and reduce disease progression in the United States and internationally. The CDC's research efforts include identifying scientifically proven, cost-effective, and scalable interventions and prevention strategies to be implemented as part of a high-impact prevention approach for maximal impact on the HIV epidemic.

Advancing the National HIV Priorities through Research

The National HIV/AIDS Strategy

Updated to 2020 calls for numerous ongoing research efforts, including the prioritization and promotion of research to fill in gaps in prevention science among the highest risk populations and communities; the promotion and prioritization of research to fill in gaps in knowledge along the HIV care continuum; the scaling up of effective, evidence-based programs that address social determinants of health; support for research to better understand the scope of the intersection of HIV and violence against women and girls, as well as the development of effective interventions; and the strengthening of the timely availability and use of data. Across the federal government, agencies and programs are engaged in these efforts.

Section 36.5

Drug Combination Reduces Risk of HIV Infection among Teen Males

This section includes text excerpted from "Drug Combination Reduces Risk of HIV Infection among Teen Males," National Institutes of Health (NIH), September 5, 2017.

A National Institutes of Health (NIH) network study has confirmed that a combination of two drugs taken daily to reduce the chances of human immunodeficiency virus (HIV) infection among high-risk adults also works well and appears safe in males ages 15–17 years.

Truvada, a single pill containing the drugs tenofovir and emtricitabine (TDF/FTC), is currently approved for daily use in adults. The drug is the cornerstone of preexposure prophylaxis (PrEP), a strategy in which healthy people at risk for HIV infection take one or more anti-HIV drugs to reduce this risk.

The study published in *Journal of the American Medical Association (JAMA) Pediatrics*, was funded by NIH's *Eunice Kennedy Shriver*

National Institute of Child Health and Human Development (NICHD), the National Institute on Drug Abuse (NIDA), and the National Institute of Mental Health (NIMH).

"Several studies have shown that daily oral PrEP is effective in preventing HIV among people at high risk of becoming infected, but none of them included adolescents under age 18," said study author Bill Kapogiannis, M.D., of NICHD's Maternal and Pediatric Infectious Diseases Branch (MPIDB). "Our study suggests that this therapy can safely reduce HIV risk for those under 18."

The study was conducted by researchers in the NICHD-funded Adolescent Medicine Trials Network for HIV/AIDS Interventions (ATN). When the study began, participants ranging in age from 15–17 years old were not infected with HIV, and were considered at-risk for HIV because of factors such as having unprotected sex with a male partner who had HIV or whose HIV status was unknown, having at least three male partners, or having a sexually transmitted infection (STI) other than HIV. Youth with poor kidney function and a history of bone fractures were excluded from the study because the drug combination may sometimes stress the kidneys and cause bone loss.

Study participants received periodic tests for HIV and other sexually transmitted diseases (STDs), counseling, and other interventions to help them avoid risky behaviors. The 72 youth who took part in the study also received daily oral TDF/FTC for 48 weeks.

As the study progressed, many participants skipped doses of their medication. Levels of the drug sufficient to prevent HIV infection were found in 54 percent of participants by week four, 49 percent by week 12, 28 percent by week 24, and 22 percent by week 48. The principal reason participants gave for skipping the medications was worry that "others will see me taking pills and think I am HIV-positive." Other reasons for missing doses included being away from home (32 percent), being too busy (28 percent), forgetting (26 percent), and experiencing changes in routine (19 percent).

In general, study participants tolerated the drug well, and there were no reports of effects on the kidneys or bones. Three participants were diagnosed with HIV during the study: one at weeks 32, 36, and 48. All three had no detectable blood levels of TDF/FTC at the visit before their HIV infection was first diagnosed, indicating that they likely were missing doses or not taking the medicine at all.

The authors concluded that the lack of significant adverse health events during the study indicates that the drug is safe for males under age 18. Similarly, the lack of HIV infection among participants who had sufficiently high blood levels of medication is consistent with studies in adults and suggests that the drug can be effective in this population when taken appropriately. The researchers added that the tendency of youth to skip medications demonstrates the need for more contact with clinical staff during therapy, and for the development of strategies to ensure that at-risk youth take the drug as prescribed.

The NIH also is funding studies of PrEP therapy for girls and young women. In an upcoming NIH-funded study in several African countries, adolescent females ages 16–21 will use a vaginal ring for six months, oral PrEP for six months, then choose which method they want to use for the final six months of the study.

Section 36.6

Potential Source of HIV Persistence Confirmed

This section includes text excerpted from "Potential Source of HIV Persistence Confirmed," National Institute of Mental Health (NIMH), April 18, 2017.

Research with a unique animal model provides evidence that a class of immune cells not thought to be a primary reservoir for human immunodeficiency virus (HIV) can harbor the virus even following antiretroviral treatment. While earlier work has reported persistence of HIV in these cells—macrophages—investigators in this work developed a mouse model with an immune system generated from human cells but lacking T cells, which are a primary target of and reservoir for HIV. The absence of T cells enabled the team to establish definitively the persistence of HIV in macrophages.

Jenna Honeycutt, Ph.D., and J. Victor Garcia, Ph.D., at the University of North Carolina at Chapel Hill, along with scientists at several collaborating centers, conducted this work. The persistence of HIV in this type of cell—macrophages—means that treatment to eradicate HIV will have to target these cells in addition to those already demonstrated to have a role in the rebounding of HIV if ART is stopped.

The study is reported in the journal *Nature Medicine*, online April 17; it was funded by the National Institute of Mental Health (NIMH) and the National Institute of Allergy and Infectious Diseases (NIAID). NIMH's Division of acquired immunodeficiency virus (AIDS) Research supports a broad range of studies on HIV/AIDS, including research aimed at understanding and alleviating the consequences of HIV infection of the central nervous system.

Section 36.7

Biomarker Tracks Accelerated HIV-Associated Aging

This section includes text excerpted from "Biomarker Tracks Accelerated HIV-Associated Aging," National Institute of Mental Health (NIMH), April 21, 2016.

By measuring a molecular signature of aging, researchers have found that human immunodeficiency virus (HIV) infection accelerates aging, adding an average of five years to someone's biological age. The more rapid aging is occurring in people receiving antiretroviral treatment, so that even though treatment enables them to live for many decades, they remain at higher risk of aging-related chronic disease.

Studies of people with HIV infection have noted a higher risk of diseases associated with aging, such as liver and kidney failure, cancer, and heart disease. While the observations have suggested that HIV infection causes accelerated aging, there hasn't been a biologically based marker of aging with which scientists could clarify and quantify the impact of HIV on aging.

In search of such a marker, scientists at the University of Nebraska Medical Center (UNMC), led by Howard Fox, M.D., Ph.D., in collaboration with scientists at the University of California, San Diego (UCSD) School of Medicine, led by Trey Ideker, Ph.D., turned to epigenetics, a term for changes to deoxyribonucleic acid (DNA) that affect its function without altering the sequence of bases that make up DNA. Through epigenetic processes, experience can alter the genome, silencing or activating genes.

Previous research by Ideker's group had found that aging is associated with an epigenetic change called methylation, the addition of a chemical (methyl) group to specific sites on the DNA chain. In this work, analysis of the "methylomes" in the blood cells of 137 HIV-positive individuals found marked differences in methylation in comparison with 44 matched but HIV-negative individuals. The investigators controlled for factors besides HIV infection that might alter methylation, such as other health conditions and differences in the methylation levels of different types of cells, given that HIV can alter cell populations. Building on information from previous research on methylation and aging, the team found that methylation tracked well with chronological age in those without HIV. In HIV-positive individuals, however, the changes in methylation were accelerated, adding an average of five years to "epigenetic" age. This fast-forward occurred even in those who had had HIV for short duration, less than five years. Previous models found that aging-related changes in methylation parallel increases in mortality; the changes found here in HIV positive patients suggest a 19 percent increase in mortality.

"The medical issues in treating people with HIV have changed," says Fox. "We're no longer as worried about infections that come from being immunocompromised. Now we worry about diseases related to aging, like cardiovascular disease, neurocognitive impairment, and liver problems."

The team also found that one region of the genome was particularly rich in HIV-associated changes in methylation: this region, the human leukocyte antigen locus, encompasses genes that encode molecules that are central to immune responses. The authors suggest that epigenetic processes may contribute to the changes in regulation of this region of the genome and thus the progression, or control, of HIV.

The work provides an objective method of assessing the impact in individuals of HIV on biological age. It provides insight into the mechanisms behind the accelerated aging, and may offer a means of identifying individuals vulnerable to aging-related chronic disease, and who may benefit from more careful attention to monitoring and preventive treatments. Given epigenetic changes observed in the human leukocyte antigen (HLA) region, it may provide clues to future approaches to controlling infection.

"Among the areas that NIH has identified as high priority for HIV research in the next three to five years are studies on the impact of HIV-associated comorbidities such as premature aging associated with long-term HIV disease and antiretroviral therapy (ART)," said National Institute of Mental Health's (NIMH) Division of AIDS (acquired immunodeficiency syndrome) Research (DAR) Director Dianne M. Rausch, Ph.D. "This work is important for the insight it provides into the mechanism of HIV-associated accelerated aging and the potential it offers in terms of a biomarker for identifying individuals with HIV infection who are at greatest risk of aging-related disease as well as the development of targeted interventions."

Section 36.8

Experimental Combination Surprises with Anti-HIV Effectiveness

This section includes text excerpted from "Experimental Combination Surprises with Anti-HIV Effectiveness," National Institute of Mental Health (NIMH), January 20, 2016.

A compound developed to protect the nervous system from human immunodeficiency virus (HIV) surprised researchers by augmenting the effectiveness of an investigational antiretroviral drug beyond anything expected. The potency of the combination treatment, tested so far in mice, suggests that it would be possible to rid the body of HIV for months, reducing the frequency with which patients must take these medications from daily to several times a year.

Even when people with HIV infection take antiretroviral drugs, more than 50 percent have HIV-associated neurocognitive disorders (HAND), which can result in any of a variety of symptoms, including confusion and problems with memory. The National Institutes of Health (NIH)-supported scientists led by Harris A. Gelbard, M.D., Ph.D., at the University of Rochester School of Medicine and Dentistry developed the compound University of Rochester Medical Center (URMC-099) to protect against HIV-associated neurologic damage. This and similar compounds would always be administered with an antiretroviral medication; the objective of this research was to test URMC-099 as such an adjunct.

The antiretroviral medication used is in a class of antiretroviral drugs (protease inhibitors) commonly used to treat HIV, but in this case, the NIH-supported researchers at the University of Nebraska Medical Center (UNMC), led by Howard E. Gendelman, M.D., used nanotechnology to reconstitute the compound in an effort to enhance its ability to reach and remain in target tissues. (Nanotechnology involves use or creation of materials in very small dimensions—billionths of a meter.) The process renders the drug into crystal form and adds a protective coat. The small scale formulation of nano-antiretroviral therapy (nanoART) enables it to penetrate and endure in immune cells, forming reservoirs of antiretroviral activity.

Previous work had shown that URMC-099 was anti-inflammatory and protected neuronal tissue. Used alone it is not antiviral, but it was possible, the researchers reasoned, that its anti-inflammatory effects could enhance the beneficial effects of an antiviral. They tested the combination therapy in HIV-infected mice that have what is essentially a human immune system; human immune stem cells are introduced in mice that are born lacking components of a normal immune system. On a number of measures, URMC-099 enhanced the effects of nanoART beyond expectations. It reduced HIV levels beyond what nanoART could achieve alone and below what is detectable. It increased the ability of nanoART to form persistent antiretroviral "depots" in immune cells which are thought to be central to these drugs' ability to inhibit HIV replication.

"Our ultimate hope is that we're able to create a therapy that could be given less frequently than the daily therapy that is required," said Gelbard. "If a drug could be given once every six months or longer, that would greatly increase compliance, reduce side effects, and help people manage the disease, because they won't have to think about taking medication every day."

"The NIH Office of AIDS (acquired immunodeficiency syndrome) Research (OAR) has identified the development of long-acting HIV therapies and research towards a cure as high priority topics for research support," said Dianne M. Rausch, Ph.D., director of the National Institute of Mental Health's (NIMH) Division of AIDS Research (DAR). "The nanoformulation strategies reported here could facilitate targeting HIV anatomic reservoirs such as lymph nodes and brain which are currently difficult to reach because of limited penetration of antiretroviral drugs into tissue compartments."

Section 36.9

HIV Can Spread Early, Evolve in Patients' Brains

This section includes text excerpted from "HIV Can
Spread Early, Evolve in Patients' Brains," National Institute
of Mental Health (NIMH), March 26, 2015.

The acquired immunodeficiency virus (AIDS) virus can genetically evolve and independently replicate in patients' brains early in the illness process, researchers funded by the National Institutes of Health (NIH) have discovered. An analysis of cerebral spinal fluid (CSF), a window into brain chemical activity, revealed that for a subset of patients human immunodeficiency virus (HIV) had started replicating within the brain within the first four months of infection. CSF in 30 percent of HIV-infected patients tracked showed at least transient signs of inflammation—suggesting an active infectious process—or viral replication within the first two years of infection. There was also evidence that the mutating virus can evolve a genome in the central nervous system that is distinct from that in the periphery.

"These results underscore the importance of early diagnosis and treatment with antiretroviral therapy," said Dianne Rausch, Ph.D., director of the Division of AIDS Research (DAR) of the NIH's National Institute of Mental Health (NIMH). "Any delay runs the risk that the virus could find refuge and cause damage in the brain, where some medications are less effective—potentially enabling it to re-emerge, even after it is suppressed in the periphery."

The National Institute of Mental Health (NIMH) grantees Serena Spudich, M.D., of Yale University, New Haven, Connecticut; Ronald Swanstrom, Ph.D., of the University of North Carolina (UNC), Chapel Hill; Richard Price, M.D., University of California, San Francisco; and Christa Buckheit Sturdevant, Ph.D., UNC (now at Duke), and colleagues, report on their findings in the March 2015 issue of the journal *PLoS Pathogens*.

Prior to the study, it was known that HIV readily penetrates the brain and can trigger neurological problems and eventually cause dementia over the course of the infection. Yet there was little evidence about how quickly it can take hold and thrive there. Nor was it clear to what extent the brain serves as a hard-to-reach hideout from which the virus might re-infect the body—even if it is eliminated from peripheral blood and lymph node tissue by treatment.

To know more, the researchers compared evidence of HIV activity in CSF versus blood from 72 untreated HIV-infected patients over the first two years of their infection. Overall, 10–22 percent of the patients showed evidence of HIV replication or inflammation in the brain at the different time points analyzed within the first two years—and the signs persisted over time in about 16 percent of the participants.

The evidence suggests that in most patients peripheral forms of the virus infect immune cells that spread to the brain via blood. Yet in some patients, genetic versions of the virus not found in blood evolve in the brain environment. So it could become an independent, compartmentalized viral reservoir, capable of generating treatment-resistant mutant forms that could break out and re-infect the rest of the body after seemingly successful treatment, explained Rausch.

Whether the potential brain damage caused by early HIV replication and inflammation might be reversible with antiviral therapy awaits further research, said Swanstrom.

Section 36.10

Starting Antiretroviral Treatment Early Improves Outcomes for HIV-Infected Individuals

This section includes text excerpted from "Starting Antiretroviral Treatment Early Improves Outcomes for HIV-Infected Individuals," National Institutes of Health (NIH), May 27, 2015.

A major international randomized clinical trial has found that human immunodeficiency virus (HIV)-infected individuals have a considerably lower risk of developing acquired immunodeficiency syndrome (AIDS) or other serious illnesses if they start taking antiretroviral drugs sooner, when their cluster of differentiation 4+ (CD4+) T-cell count—a key measure of immune system health—is higher, instead of waiting until the CD4+ cell count drops to lower levels. Together with data from previous studies showing that antiretroviral treatment reduced the risk of HIV transmission to uninfected sexual partners, these findings support offering treatment to everyone with HIV.

The finding is from the Strategic Timing of AntiRetroviral Treatment (START) study, the first large-scale randomized clinical trial to establish that earlier antiretroviral treatment benefits all HIV-infected individuals. The National Institute of Allergy and Infectious Diseases (NIAID), part of the National Institutes of Health (NIH), provided primary funding for the START trial. Though the study was expected to conclude at the end of 2016, an interim review of the study data by an independent data and safety monitoring board (DSMB) recommended that results be released early.

"We now have clear-cut proof that it is of significantly greater health benefit to an HIV-infected person to start antiretroviral therapy sooner rather than later," said NIAID Director Anthony S. Fauci, M.D. "Moreover, early therapy conveys a double benefit, not only improving the health of individuals but at the same time, by lowering their viral load, reducing the risk they will transmit HIV to others. These findings have global implications for the treatment of HIV."

"This is an important milestone in HIV research," said Jens Lundgren, M.D., of the University of Copenhagen and one of the co-chairs of the START study. "We now have strong evidence that early treatment is beneficial to the HIV-positive person. These results support treating everyone irrespective of CD4+ T-cell count."

The START study, which opened widely in March 2011, was conducted by the International Network for Strategic Initiatives in Global HIV Trials (INSIGHT) at 215 sites in 35 countries. The trial enrolled 4,685 HIV-infected men and women ages 18 and older, with a median age of 36. Participants had never taken antiretroviral therapy (ART) and were enrolled with CD4+ cell counts in the normal range—above 500 cells per cubic millimeter (cells/mm^3). Approximately half of the study participants were randomized to initiate antiretroviral treatment immediately (early treatment), and the other half were randomized to defer treatment until their CD4+ cell count declined to 350 cells/mm^3. On average, participants in the study were followed for three years.

The study measured a combination of outcomes that included serious AIDS events (such as AIDS-related cancer), serious non-AIDS events (major cardiovascular, renal and liver disease and cancer), and death. Based on data from March 2015, the DSMB found 41 instances of AIDS, serious non-AIDS events or death among those enrolled in the study's early treatment group compared to 86 events in the deferred treatment group. The DSMB's interim analysis found risk of developing serious illness or death was reduced by 53 percent among those in the early treatment group, compared to those in the deferred group.

Rates of serious AIDS-related events and serious non-AIDS-related events were both lower in the early treatment group than the deferred treatment group. The risk reduction was more pronounced for the AIDS-related events. Findings were consistent across geographic regions, and the benefits of early treatment were similar for participants from low- and middle-income countries and participants from high-income countries.

"The study was rigorous and the results are clear," said INSIGHT principal investigator James D. Neaton, Ph.D., a professor of biostatistics at the University of Minnesota, Minneapolis. "The definitive findings from a randomized trial like START are likely to influence how care is delivered to millions of HIV-positive individuals around the world." The University of Minnesota served as the trial's regulatory sponsor and statistical and data management center.

Prior to the START trial, there was no randomized controlled trial evidence to guide initiating treatment for individuals with higher CD4+ cell counts. Previous evidence to support early treatment among HIV-positive people with CD4+ cell counts above 350 was limited to data from nonrandomized trials or observational cohort studies, and on expert opinion.

START is the first large-scale randomized clinical trial to offer concrete scientific evidence to support the current U.S. HIV treatment guidelines, which recommend that all asymptomatic HIV-infected individuals take antiretrovirals, regardless of CD4+ cell count. Current World Health Organization (WHO) HIV treatment guidelines recommend that HIV-infected individuals begin ART when CD4+ cell counts fall to 500 cells/mm^3 or less.

In light of the DSMB findings, study investigators are informing all participants of the interim results. Participants will be offered treatment if they are not already on antiretroviral therapy, and they will continue to be followed through 2016.

The HIV medicines used in the trial are approved medications donated by AbbVie, Inc., Bristol-Myers Squibb, Gilead Sciences, GlaxoSmithKline (GSK)/ViiV Healthcare, Janssen Scientific Affairs, LLC, and Merck Sharp and Dohme Corp.

In addition to NIAID, funding for the START trial came from other NIH entities, including the National Cancer Institute (NCI), the National Heart, Lung and Blood Institute (NHLBI); the National Institute of Mental Health (NIMH); the National Institute of Neurological

Disorders and Stroke (NINDS); the *Eunice Kennedy Shriver* National Institute of Child Health and Human Development (NICHD); the NIH Clinical Center (CC); and the National Institute of Arthritis and Musculoskeletal and Skin Diseases (NIAMS). Funding was also provided by the National Agency for Research on AIDS and Viral Hepatitis (ANRS) in France, the Federal Ministry of Education and Research (BMBF) in Germany, the European AIDS Treatment Network (EATG) and government organizations based in Australia, Denmark, and the United Kingdom.

Chapter 37

Treatment Recommendations for Pediatric HIV Infection

Since the introduction of potent combination antiretroviral (ARV) drug regimens in the mid-1990s, the treatment of pediatric human immunodeficiency virus (HIV) infection has steadily improved. These potent regimens have the ability to suppress viral replication thus lowering the risk of virologic failure due to the development of drug resistance. Antiretroviral therapy (ART) regimens including at least 3 drugs from at least 2 drug classes are recommended; such regimens have been associated with enhanced survival, reduction in opportunistic infections and other complications of HIV infection, improved growth and neurocognitive function, and improved quality of life in children. In the United States and the United Kingdom, significant declines in morbidity, mortality, and hospitalizations have been reported in children living with HIV, concomitant with increased use of highly active combination regimens. As a result, children with perinatal HIV infection are now living in the third and fourth decades of life, and likely beyond.

The increased survival of children with HIV is associated with challenges in selecting successive new ARV drug regimens. In addition,

This chapter includes text excerpted from "Treatment Recommendations," AIDS*info*, U.S. Department of Health and Human Services (HHS), April 27, 2017.

therapy is associated with short- and long-term toxicities, which can be recognized in childhood or adolescence.

ARV drug-resistant virus can develop during ART when viral replication occurs in the presence of subtherapeutic ARV levels associated with poor adherence, poor absorption, a regimen that is not potent, or a combination of these factors. In addition, primary drug resistance may be seen in ARV-naive children who have become infected with a resistant virus. Thus, decisions about what drugs to choose in ARV-naive children and how to best treat ARV-experienced children remain complex. Whenever possible, decisions regarding the management of pediatric HIV infection should be directed by or made in consultation with a specialist in pediatric and adolescent HIV infection.

In addition to trials demonstrating benefits of ART in symptomatic adults and those with lower cluster of differentiation 4 (CD4)-T lymphocyte cell counts,15 a randomized clinical trial has provided evidence of benefit with initiation of ART in asymptomatic adults with CD4 cell counts >500 cells/mm^3.16 Similarly, improved outcomes have been shown with initiation of ART in asymptomatic infants between 6–12 weeks of age. Although there are fewer available data on the risks and benefits of immediate therapy in asymptomatic children with HIV than in adults, this Panel recommends ART for all children with HIV, with differing strengths of recommendation based on age and CD4-cell counts. Several factors need to be considered in making decisions about the urgency of initiating and changing ART in children, including:

- The severity of HIV disease and risk of disease progression, as determined by age, presence or history of HIV-related illnesses, the degree of CD4 immunosuppression,

- Availability of appropriate (and palatable) drug formulations and pharmacokinetic (PK) information on appropriate dosing in a child's age/weight group;

- Potency, complexity (e.g., dosing frequency, and food requirements), and potential short- and long-term adverse effects of the ART regimen;

- Effect of initial regimen choice on later therapeutic options;

- A child's ART history;

- Presence of ARV drug-resistant virus;

- Presence of comorbidities, such as tuberculosis (TB), hepatitis B or C virus infection, or chronic renal or liver disease, that could affect decisions about drug choice and the timing of initiation of therapy;

- Potential ARV drug interactions with other prescribed, over-the-counter (OTC), or complementary/alternative medications taken by a child; and

- The anticipated ability of the caregiver and child to adhere to the regimen.

The following recommendations provide general guidance for decisions related to the treatment of children living with HIV, and flexibility should be exercised according to a child's individual circumstances. Guidelines for treatment of children living with HIV are evolving as new data from clinical trials become available. Although prospective, randomized, controlled clinical trials offer the best evidence for the formulation of guidelines, most ARV drugs are approved for use in pediatric patients based on efficacy data from clinical trials in adults, with supporting PK and safety data from Phase I/II trials in children. In addition, efficacy has been defined in most adult trials based on surrogate marker data, as opposed to clinical endpoints. For the development of these guidelines, the Panel reviewed relevant clinical trials published in peer-reviewed journals or in abstract form, with attention to data from pediatric populations when available.

Goals of Antiretroviral Treatment (ART)

Present available ART has not been shown to eradicate HIV infection in infants with perinatally acquired HIV due to the persistence of HIV in CD4 lymphocytes and other cells. This was demonstrated when a child with HIV treated with ART at 30 hours of age experienced viremic rebound after more than 2 years of undetectable HIV ribonucleic acid (RNA) levels while off ART. Some data suggest that the half-life of intracellular HIV proviral DNA is even longer in children with HIV infection than in adults (median 14 months versus 5–10 months, respectively). Thus, based on available data, HIV causes a chronic infection likely requiring treatment for life once a child starts therapy. The goals of ART for children and adolescents living with HIV include:

- Preventing and reducing HIV-related morbidity and mortality;

- Restoring and/or preserving immune function as reflected by CD4-cell measures;

- Maximally and durably suppressing viral replication;

- Preventing emergence of viral drug-resistance mutations;

- Minimizing drug-related toxicity;

- Maintaining normal physical growth and neurocognitive development; and

- Improving the quality of life.

Strategies to achieve these goals require a complex balance of potentially competing considerations.

Use and Selection of Combination ART

The treatment of choice for children with HIV infection is a regimen containing at least 3 drugs from at least 2 classes of ARV drugs. The Panel has recommended several preferred and alternative regimens. The most appropriate regimen for an individual child depends on multiple factors as noted above. A regimen that is characterized as an alternative choice may be a preferred regimen for some patients.

Drug Sequencing and Preservation of Future Treatment Option

The choice of ARV treatment regimens should include consideration of future treatment options, such as the presence of or potential for drug resistance. Multiple changes in ARV drug regimens can rapidly exhaust treatment options and should be avoided. Appropriate sequencing of drugs for use in initial and second-line therapy can preserve future treatment options and is another strategy to maximize long-term benefit from therapy. Present recommendations for initial therapy are to use 2 classes of drugs), thereby sparing 3 classes of drugs for later use.

Maximizing Adherence

Poor adherence to prescribed regimens can lead to subtherapeutic levels of ARV medications, which increases the risk of development of drug resistance and the likelihood of virologic failure. Outside of the very young age group (<1 year) and children with significant immunologic impairment or clinical HIV symptoms (where therapy should be initiated within 1–2 weeks of diagnosis, with an expedited discussion on adherence and close follow up), the risk of rapid disease progression is low and more time can be taken to fully assess, identify, discuss, and address issues associated with potential adherence problems with the caregivers and the child (when age-appropriate) prior to initiating therapy. Participation by the caregiver and child in the decision-making process is crucial. In addition, frequent follow-up is important to assess virologic response to therapy, drug intolerance, viral resistance, and adherence. Finally, in patients who experience virologic failure, it is critical to fully assess adherence and possible viral resistance before making changes to the ART regimen.

Chapter 38

HIV and AIDS Treatment for Pregnant Women

Human Immunodeficiency Virus (HIV) Medicines during Pregnancy

All pregnant women with human immunodeficiency virus (HIV) should take HIV medicines during pregnancy to prevent mother-to-child transmission of HIV. HIV medicines work by preventing HIV from multiplying, which reduces the amount of HIV in the body (also called the viral load). A low viral load during pregnancy reduces the chances that any HIV will pass from mother to child during pregnancy and childbirth. Having less HIV in the body also helps keep the mother-to-be healthy.

Safety Concerns Regarding Use of HIV Medicines during Pregnancy

Most HIV medicines are safe to use during pregnancy. In general, HIV medicines don't increase the risk of birth defects. When recommending HIV medicines for pregnant women with HIV, healthcare providers carefully consider the benefits and risks of specific HIV medicines.

This chapter includes text excerpted from "HIV Medicines during Pregnancy and Childbirth," AIDS*info*, U.S. Department of Health and Human Services (HHS), November 28, 2017.

When Pregnant Women with HIV Should Start Taking HIV Medicines

All pregnant women with HIV should start taking HIV medicines as soon as possible during pregnancy. In general, women who are already taking HIV medicines when they become pregnant should continue taking those HIV medicines throughout their pregnancies.

HIV Medicines a Pregnant Woman with HIV Should Take

The choice of an HIV regimen to use during pregnancy depends on several factors, including a woman's current or past use of HIV medicines, other medical conditions she may have, and the results of drug resistance testing. In general, pregnant women with HIV can use the same HIV regimens recommended for nonpregnant adults—unless the risk of any known side effects to a pregnant woman or her baby outweighs the benefit of a regimen. Also, the regimen must be able to control a woman's HIV even with pregnancy-related changes that can affect how the body processes medicine.

In most cases, women who are already on an effective HIV regimen should continue on the same regimen throughout their pregnancies. But sometimes a woman's HIV regimen may change during pregnancy. For example, a change in HIV medicines may be needed to avoid the increased risk of a side effect during pregnancy. Sometimes, changing the dose of an HIV medicine can help offset pregnancy-related changes that make it harder for the body to absorb the medicine. But before making any changes to an HIV regimen, women should always talk to their healthcare providers.

Intake of HIV Medicines during Childbirth

The risk of mother-to-child transmission of HIV is greatest during a vaginal delivery when a baby passes through the birth canal and is exposed to any HIV in the mother's blood and other fluids. During childbirth, HIV medicines that pass from mother to baby across the placenta prevent mother-to-child transmission of HIV, especially near delivery.

Women who are already taking HIV medicines when they go into labor should continue taking their HIV medicines on schedule as much as possible during childbirth. Women with a high viral load (more than 1,000 copies/mL) or an unknown viral load near the time of delivery should receive an HIV medicine called zidovudine (brand name: Retrovir) by intravenous (IV) injection.

Zidovudine passes easily from a pregnant woman to her unborn baby across the placenta. Once in a baby's system, zidovudine protects the baby from any HIV that passes from mother to child during childbirth. For this reason, the use of zidovudine during childbirth prevents mother-to-child transmission of HIV even in women with high viral loads near the time of delivery.

Cesarean Delivery and the Risk of Mother-to-Child Transmission of HIV

A scheduled cesarean delivery (sometimes called a C-section) can reduce the risk of mother-to-child transmission of HIV in women who have a high viral load (more than 1,000 copies/mL) or an unknown viral load near the time of delivery. A cesarean delivery to reduce the risk of mother-to-child transmission of HIV is scheduled for the 38th week of pregnancy, 2 weeks before a woman's expected due date.

It's unclear whether a scheduled C-section can reduce the risk of mother-to-child transmission of HIV in pregnant women with a viral load of less than 1,000 copies/mL. Of course, regardless of her viral load, a woman with HIV may have a C-section for other medical reasons.

With the help of their healthcare providers, women can decide which HIV medicines to use during childbirth and whether they should schedule a C-section to prevent mother-to-child transmission of HIV.

Intake of HIV Medicines after Childbirth

Prenatal care for women with HIV includes counseling on the benefits of continuing HIV medicines after childbirth. Life-long use of HIV medicines prevents HIV from advancing to acquired immunodeficiency syndrome (AIDS) and reduces the risk of transmitting HIV. Together with their healthcare providers, women with HIV make decisions about continuing or changing their HIV medicines after childbirth.

In general, babies born to women with HIV receive zidovudine for 4–6 weeks after birth. (In certain situations, a baby may receive other HIV medicines in addition to zidovudine.) The HIV medicine protects the babies from infection by any HIV that may have passed from mother to child during childbirth.

Chapter 39

Paying for HIV Care and Treatment

Human immunodeficiency virus (HIV) care and treatment involves taking antiretroviral therapy (ART) and having regular checkups with your healthcare provider who will monitor your health status on an ongoing basis.

These things are important because, with the proper care and treatment, you can reduce your viral load, protect your health, enjoy a long and healthy life, and reduce the potential of transmitting the virus to others.

But you might have concerns about how to pay for this. There are resources that can help you pay for the care you need.

Private Insurance

Job-Based and Individual Insurance

Many people have private health insurance through their employer (or a family member's employer), or they have individual insurance they have purchased. Under the Affordable Care Act (ACA), most job-based and individual plans are required to offer benefits and protections. For example, plans can't drop you or deny you coverage just

This chapter includes text excerpted from "Paying for HIV Care," HIV.gov, U.S. Department of Health and Human Services (HHS), May 15, 2017.

because you have a preexisting health condition, like HIV. And insurers can't impose lifetime caps on your insurance benefits. However, you'll still need to pay any deductibles, copayments, and coinsurance your plan requires. Make sure you read your plan carefully so that you know what your plan will (and won't) cover.

When you leave a job, you may be able to keep your job-based health insurance for a period, usually up to 18 months. This is called the Consolidated Omnibus Budget Reconciliation Act (COBRA) continuation coverage. With COBRA coverage, you usually have to pay the entire monthly premium yourself, plus a small administrative fee. Your former employer no longer pays any of your insurance costs.

The Health Insurance Marketplace

Established under the ACA, the Health Insurance Marketplace helps uninsured people find and apply for quality, affordable health coverage. Private plans in the Marketplace are required to cover a set of essential health benefits. And, low and middle-income people may qualify for lower costs, based on their household size and income. In 2017, the Administration and Congress proposed changes to ACA. At this time, the final outcome of these efforts was not known.

Federal Resources

If you do not have private health insurance—or you need help because your insurance doesn't pay for the HIV care and treatment you need—there are federal resources that may help you.

Getting Help

Figuring out which programs and services you qualify for can be confusing. But don't worry! There are case managers and benefits counselors who can help you. They know what services are available and can help you get care. Their services are free. You can find one near you by contacting a local HIV/acquired immunodeficiency syndrome (AIDS) service organization. Toll-free state HIV/AIDS hotlines will help put you in touch with agencies that can determine what programs and services you may be eligible for and help you access them.

Here are federal resources that are available:

Medicaid

A state and federal partnership, Medicaid provides coverage for people with lower incomes, older people, people with disabilities, and some families and children. It is a critical source of coverage for many people living with HIV/AIDS. States establish and administer their own Medicaid programs and determine the type, amount, duration, and scope of services within broad federal guidelines. States are required to cover certain "mandatory benefits" and can choose to provide other "optional benefits," including prescription drugs. The eligibility rules for Medicaid are different in each state, but most states offer coverage for adults with children at some income level. And, under the ACA, states have the option, which is fully federally funded for the first three years, to expand Medicaid eligibility to generally include people below certain income levels, including low-income childless adults who were previously not generally eligible for Medicaid. As a result, in states that opt for Medicaid expansion, people living with HIV who meet the income threshold no longer have to wait for an AIDS diagnosis in order to become eligible for Medicaid. You can apply for and enroll in Medicaid at any time. There is no limited enrollment period. If you qualify, your coverage can begin immediately. Even if your state hasn't expanded Medicaid, you should still apply for coverage to see if you qualify under your state's existing rules. See if you qualify to save in your state.

The Ryan White HIV/AIDS Program

The Ryan White HIV/AIDS Program works with cities, states, and local community-based organizations to provide HIV-related services to more than half a million people living with HIV/AIDS each year. The program is for those who do not have sufficient healthcare coverage or financial resources to cope with HIV disease. Ryan White fills gaps in care not covered by these other sources. The program is divided into several "parts" to meet the needs of different communities and populations and includes support for an AIDS Drug Assistance Program (ADAP). To find a Ryan White clinic near you, use the HIV.gov HIV Testing and Care Services Locator.

The Health Center Program

Health centers provide high quality preventive and primary healthcare services, including HIV testing and medical care, to patients regardless of their ability to pay. Some patients receive services directly at the health center itself, while others are referred to an HIV specialist in the community. Major investments in the network of community health centers over the past several years have created

405

more opportunities for HIV care delivery. You can find a health center near you by going to the HIV Testing and Care Services Locator.

Medicare

Medicare is health insurance for people age 65 or older, people under 65 with certain disabilities, and people of all ages with end-stage renal disease. Medicare coverage for eligible individuals includes outpatient care, prescription drugs, and inpatient hospital care.

Federal Programs for Women and Children

There are several federal programs to help low-income women and children access healthcare. The Children's Health Insurance Program (CHIP) provides free or low-cost health insurance coverage for children up to age 19. Each state has its own rules about who qualifies for CHIP. You can apply for and enroll a child in CHIP at any time. There is no limited enrollment period. If the child qualifies, his/her coverage can begin immediately. In addition, programs supported by the Maternal and Child Health Services Block Grant, authorized by Title V of the Social Security Act (SSA), serve low-income women, children, and youth with limited access to healthcare, including children with special needs. Specifically, the Title V Maternal and Child Health program seeks to assure access to quality care, especially for those with low-incomes or limited availability of care.

American Indian and Alaska Native Programs

The Indian Health Service (IHS) provides healthcare services — including HIV services — for members and descendants of federally-recognized American Indian and Alaska Native Tribes.

Veterans Programs

The Veterans Administration (VA) is the largest single provider of medical care to people living with HIV in the United States, supporting over 24,000 veterans living with HIV. If you are eligible, you may be able to receive HIV care through the Veterans Health Administration (VHA). The VA offers an online benefits website where veterans, service members, and their families can know about their healthcare benefits.

Part Five

Common Co-Occurring Infections and Complications of HIV/AIDS

Chapter 40

Opportunistic Infections and Their Relationship to HIV/AIDS

What Is an Opportunistic Infection (OI)?

Opportunistic infections (OIs) are infections that occur more often or are more severe in people with weakened immune systems than in people with healthy immune systems. People with weakened immune systems include people living with human immunodeficiency virus (HIV) or people receiving chemotherapy.

OIs are caused by a variety of germs (viruses, bacteria, fungi, and parasites). OI-causing germs can spread in the air; in saliva, semen, blood, urine, or feces (poop); or in contaminated food and water. Here are examples of common HIV-related OIs:

- Herpes simplex virus 1 (HSV-1) infection—a viral infection that can cause lesions (sores) on the mouth and face.

This chapter contains text excerpted from the following sources: Text beginning with the heading "What Is an Opportunistic Infection (OI)?" is excerpted from "HIV and Opportunistic Infections, Coinfections, and Conditions," AIDS*info*, U.S. Department of Health and Human Services (HHS), July 24, 2017; Text beginning with the heading "Most Common Opportunistic Infections" is excerpted from "HIV/AIDS—Opportunistic Infections," Centers for Disease Control and Prevention (CDC), May 30, 2017.

- Salmonella infection—a bacterial infection that affects the intestines (the gut).

- Candidiasis (or thrush)—a fungal infection of the mouth, esophagus, or vagina.

- Toxoplasmosis—a parasitic infection that can affect the brain.

Why Do People with HIV Get Opportunistic Infection?

Once a person is infected with HIV, the virus begins to multiply and to damage the immune system. A weakened immune system makes it harder for the body to fight off HIV-related OIs.

HIV medicines prevent HIV from damaging the immune system. But if a person with HIV does not take HIV medicines, HIV infection can gradually destroy the immune system and advance to acquired immunodeficiency syndrome (AIDS). Many OIs, for example, certain forms of pneumonia and tuberculosis (TB), are considered AIDS-defining conditions. AIDS-defining conditions are infections and cancers that are life-threatening in people with HIV.

Are Opportunistic Infection Common in People with HIV?

Before HIV medicines were available to treat HIV infection, OIs were the main cause of illness and death in people with HIV. HIV medicines are now widely used in the United States so fewer people with HIV get OIs. By preventing HIV from damaging the immune system, HIV medicines reduce the risk of OIs.

However, OIs are still a problem for many people with HIV. Some people with HIV get OIs for the following reasons:

- About 20 percent of people who have HIV don't know that they are infected. An OI may be the first sign that they have HIV.

- Some people who know they have HIV aren't getting treatment with HIV medicines. Without HIV treatment, they are more likely to get an OI.

- Some people may be taking HIV medicines, but the medicines aren't controlling their HIV. Poorly controlled HIV can be due to many factors, including lack of healthcare, poor medication adherence, or incomplete absorption of HIV medicines. People with poorly controlled HIV have an increased risk of getting an OI.

Most Common Opportunistic Infections

When a person living with HIV gets certain infections (called opportunistic infections, or OIs), he or she will get the diagnosis of AIDS, the most serious stage of HIV infection. AIDS is also diagnosed if a type of blood cell that fights infection (known as CD4 cells) falls below a certain level in persons with HIV. These blood cells are a critical part of a person's immune system.

The Centers for Disease Control and Prevention (CDC) has developed a list of OIs that indicate a person has AIDS. It does not matter how many CD4 cells a person has, receiving a diagnosis with any of these OIs means HIV infection has progressed to AIDS. HIV treatment can help restore the person's immune system.

Table 40.1. Common Opportunistic Infections

Candidiasis of bronchi, trachea, esophagus, or lungs	This illness is caused by infection with a common (and usually harmless) type of fungus called Candida. Candidiasis, or infection with Candida, can affect the skin, nails, and mucous membranes throughout the body. Persons with HIV infection often have trouble with Candida, especially in the mouth and vagina. However, candidiasis is only considered an OI when it infects the esophagus (swallowing tube) or lower respiratory tract, such as the trachea and bronchi (breathing tube), or deeper lung tissue.
Invasive cervical cancer	This is cancer that starts within the cervix, which is the lower part of the uterus at the top of the vagina, and then spreads (becomes invasive) to other parts of the body. This cancer can be prevented by having your care provider perform regular examinations of the cervix
Coccidioidomycosis	This illness is caused by the fungus *Coccidioides* immitis. It most commonly acquired by inhaling fungal spores, which can lead to pneumonia that is sometimes called desert fever, San Joaquin Valley fever, or valley fever. The disease is especially common in hot, dry regions of the southwestern United States, Central America, and South America.
Cryptococcosis	This illness is caused by infection with the fungus Cryptococcus neoformans. The fungus typically enters the body through the lungs and can cause pneumonia. It can also spread to the brain, causing swelling of the brain. It can infect any part of the body, but (after the brain and lungs) infections of skin, bones, or urinary tract are most common.

411

Table 40.1. Continued

Cryptosporidiosis, chronic intestinal (greater than one month's duration)	This diarrheal disease is caused by the protozoan parasite *Cryptosporidium*. Symptoms include abdominal cramps and severe, chronic, watery diarrhea.
Cytomegalovirus diseases (particularly retinitis) (CMV)	This virus can infect multiple parts of the body and cause pneumonia, gastroenteritis (especially abdominal pain caused by infection of the colon), encephalitis (infection) of the brain, and sight-threatening retinitis (infection of the retina at the back of the eye). People with CMV retinitis have difficulty with a vision that worsens ever time. CMV retinitis is a medical emergency because it can cause blindness if not treated promptly.
Encephalopathy, HIV-related	This brain disorder is a result of HIV infection. It can occur as part of acute HIV infection or can result from chronic HIV infection. Its exact cause is unknown but it is thought to be related to infection of the brain with HIV and the resulting inflammation.
Herpes simplex (HSV): chronic ulcer(s) (greater than one month's duration); or bronchitis, pneumonitis, or esophagitis	Herpes simplex virus (HSV) is a very common virus that for most people never causes any major problems. HSV is usually acquired sexually or from an infected mother during birth. In most people with healthy immune systems, HSV is usually latent (inactive). However, stress, trauma, other infections, or suppression of the immune system, (such as by HIV), can reactivate the latent virus and symptoms can return. HSV can cause painful cold sores (sometimes called fever blisters) in or around the mouth or painful ulcers on or around the genitals or anus. In people with severely damaged immune systems, HSV can also cause infection of the bronchus (breathing tube), pneumonia (infection of the lungs) and esophagitis (infection of the esophagus, or swallowing tube).
Histoplasmosis	This illness is caused by the fungus Histoplasma capsulatum. Histoplasma most often infects the lungs and produces symptoms that are similar to those of influenza or pneumonia. People with severely damaged immune systems can get a very serious form of the disease called progressive disseminated histoplasmosis. This form of histoplasmosis can last a long time and involves organs other than the lungs.
Isosporiasis, chronic intestinal (greater than one month's duration)	This infection is caused by the parasite Isospora belli, which can enter the body through contaminated food or water. Symptoms include diarrhea, fever, headache, abdominal pain, vomiting, and weight loss.

Table 40.1. Continued

Kaposi's sarcoma (KS)	This cancer, also known as KS, is caused by a virus called Kaposi's sarcoma herpesvirus (KSHV) or human herpesvirus 8 (HHV-8). KS causes small blood vessels, called capillaries, to grow abnormally. Because capillaries are located throughout the body, KS can occur anywhere. KS appears as firm pink or purple spots on the skin that can be raised or flat. KS can be life-threatening when it affects organs inside the body, such as the lung, lymph nodes or intestines.
Lymphoma, multiple forms	Lymphoma refers to cancer of the lymph nodes and other lymphoid tissues in the body. There are many different kinds of lymphomas. Some types, such as non-Hodgkin lymphoma and Hodgkin lymphoma, are associated with HIV infection.
Tuberculosis (TB)	Tuberculosis (TB) infection is caused by the bacteria *Mycobacterium tuberculosis*. TB can be spread through the air when a person with active TB coughs, sneezes or speaks. Breathing in the bacteria can lead to infection in the lungs. Symptoms of TB in the lungs include a cough, tiredness, weight loss, fever, and night sweats. Although the disease usually occurs in the lungs, it may also affect other parts of the body, most often the larynx, lymph nodes, brain, kidneys, or bones.
Mycobacterium avium complex (MAC) or Mycobacterium kansasii, disseminated or extrapulmonary. Other Mycobacterium, disseminated or extrapulmonary.	MAC is caused by infection with different types of Mycobacterium: *Mycobacterium avium*, Mycobacterium intracellulare, or Mycobacterium kansasii. These mycobacteria live in our environment, including in soil and dust particles. They rarely cause problems for persons with healthy immune systems. In people with severely damaged immune systems, infections with these bacteria spread throughout the body and can be life-threatening.
Pneumocystis carinii pneumonia (PCP)	This lung infection, also called PCP, is caused by a fungus, which used to be called *Pneumocystis carinii*, but now is named *Pneumocystis jirovecii*. PCP occurs in people with weakened immune systems, including people with HIV. The first signs of infection are difficulty breathing, high fever, and dry cough.

Table 40.1. Continued

Pneumonia, recurrent	Pneumonia is an infection in one or both of the lungs. Many germs, including bacteria, viruses, and fungi can cause pneumonia, with symptoms such as a cough (with mucus), fever, chills, and trouble breathing. In people with immune systems severely damaged by HIV, one of the most common and life-threatening causes of pneumonia is infection with the bacteria *Streptococcus pneumoniae*, also called Pneumococcus. There are now effective vaccines that can prevent infection with *Streptococcus pneumoniae* and all persons with HIV infection should be vaccinated.
Progressive multifocal leukoencephalopathy	This rare brain and spinal cord disease is caused by the JC virus. It is seen almost exclusively in persons whose immune systems have been severely damaged by HIV. Symptoms may include loss of muscle control, paralysis, blindness, speech problems, and an altered mental state. This disease often progresses rapidly and may be fatal.
Salmonella septicemia, recurrent	*Salmonella* is a kind of bacteria that typically enter the body through ingestion of contaminated food or water. Infection with *salmonella* (called salmonellosis) can affect anyone and usually causes a self-limited illness with nausea, vomiting, and diarrhea. Salmonella septicemia is a severe form of infection in which the bacteria circulate through the whole body and exceeds the immune system's ability to control it.
Toxoplasmosis of brain	This infection, often called toxo, is caused by the parasite *Toxoplasma gondii*. The parasite is carried by warm-blooded animals including cats, rodents, and birds and is excreted by these animals in their feces. Humans can become infected with it by inhaling dust or eating food contaminated with the parasite. Toxoplasma can also occur in commercial meats, especially red meats and pork, but rarely poultry. Infection with toxo can occur in the lungs, retina of the eye, heart, pancreas, liver, colon, testes, and brain. Although cats can transmit toxoplasmosis, litter boxes can be changed safely by wearing gloves and washing hands thoroughly with soap and water afterward. All raw red meats that have not been frozen for at least 24 hours should be cooked through to an internal temperature of at least 150oF.
Wasting syndrome due to HIV	Wasting is defined as the involuntary loss of more than 10% of one's body weight while having experienced diarrhea or weakness and fever for more than 30 days. Wasting refers to the loss of muscle mass, although part of the weight loss may also be due to loss of fat.

Preventing Opportunistic Infections

The best ways to prevent getting an OI are to get into and stay on medical care and to take HIV medications as prescribed. Sometimes, your healthcare provider will also prescribe medications specifically to prevent certain OIs. By staying on HIV medications, you can keep the amount of HIV in your body as low as possible and keep your immune system healthy. It is especially important that you get regular check-ups and take all of your medications as prescribed by your caregiver. Taking HIV medications is a life-long commitment.

In addition to taking HIV medications to keep your immune system strong, there are other steps you can take to prevent getting an OI.

- Use condoms consistently and correctly to prevent exposure to sexually transmitted infections.

- Don't share drug injection equipment. Blood with hepatitis C in it can remain in syringes and needles after use and the infection can be transmitted to the next user.

- Get vaccinated—your doctor can tell you what vaccines you need. If he or she doesn't, you should ask.

- Understand what germs you are exposed to (such as tuberculosis or germs found in the stools, saliva, or on the skin of animals) and limit your exposure to them.

- Don't consume certain foods, including undercooked eggs, unpasteurized (raw) milk and cheeses, unpasteurized fruit juices, or raw seed sprouts.

- Don't drink untreated water such as water directly from lakes or rivers. Tap water in foreign countries is also often not safe. Use bottled water or water filters.

- Ask your doctor to review with you the other things you do at work, at home, and on vacation to make sure you aren't exposed to an OI.

Treating Opportunistic Infections

If you do develop an OI, there are treatments available, such as antibiotics or antifungal drugs. Having an OI may be a very serious medical situation and its treatment can be challenging. The development of an OI likely means that your immune system is weakened and that your HIV is not under control. That is why it is so important to be on medication, take it as prescribed, see your care provider regularly, and undergo the routine monitoring he or she recommends to ensure your viral load is reduced and your immune system is healthy.

Chapter 41

Preventing Opportunistic Infections

Opportunistic infections can be caused by viruses, bacteria, and fungus, even parasites. One way to avoid these infections is to reduce your risk of exposure to these germs. Here are some practical suggestions.

Sexual Exposures

- Use condoms every time you have sex.

- Avoid oral-anal sex.

- Use waterproof gloves if you're going to insert your finger into your partner's anus.

- Frequently wash hands and genitals with warm soapy water after any sex play that brings them in contact with feces.

Injection Drug Use

- Do not inject drugs.

- If you cannot stop using, avoid sharing needles and other equipment.

This chapter includes text excerpted from "HIV/AIDS—Preventing Opportunistic Infections (OIs)," U.S. Department of Veterans Affairs (VA), February 8, 2018.

- Get vaccinated against hepatitis A and hepatitis B.

Job Exposure

Certain type of jobs or facilities can put an human immunodeficiency virus (HIV)-positive person at risk of OIs. These include work in:

- healthcare facilities
- homeless shelters
- day-care centers
- prisons
- places that involved work with animals (such as farms, veterinary clinics, pet stores)

Pet Exposure

Pets can carry diseases that don't affect a healthy person but can pose a serious risk to someone with HIV. For that reason, if you have a pet, follow these suggestions.

General

- Wash your hands after handling your pet (especially before eating).
- Avoid contact with your pet's feces. If your pet has diarrhea, ask a friend or family member to take care of it.
- If you are getting a new pet, try not to get one that is younger than a year old, especially if it has diarrhea. (Young animals are more likely to carry certain germs like *Salmonella*.) Avoid stray animals.

Cat

- Keep your cat indoors. It should not be allowed to hunt, and should not be fed raw or undercooked meat.
- Clean the litter box daily. If you do it yourself, wash your hands thoroughly afterward.
- Control fleas (ask your vet how to do this).
- Avoid playing with your cat in ways that may result in scratches or bites. If you do get scratched or bitten, wash the area right away. Don't let your cat lick your cuts or wounds.

Birds

- Avoid areas where there are bird droppings. Do not disturb soil underneath bird-roosting sites.

Others

- Avoid touching reptiles, such as snakes, lizards, iguanas, and turtles.
- Wear gloves if you are cleaning an aquarium.

Cautions about Food and Water

- Avoid raw or undercooked eggs (including hollandaise sauce, Caesar salad dressing, some mayonnaise, eggnog, cake and cookie batter).
- Avoid raw or undercooked poultry, meat, and seafood (especially raw seafood). Use a meat thermometer. Cook poultry to 180°F, and other meats to 165°F. If you don't have a meat thermometer, cook meat until no traces of pink remain.
- Avoid unpasteurized dairy products and fruit juice.
- Avoid raw seed sprouts (such as alfalfa, mung beans).
- Thoroughly wash fruits and vegetables before eating.
- Don't let uncooked meats come into contact with other uncooked foods. (Wash thoroughly hands, cutting boards, counters, knives, and other utensils after contact with uncooked meats.)
- Do not drink water directly from lakes or rivers. Filtered water is preferable, particularly if your immune system is weak.

People with HIV whose immune systems are severely weakened may want to:

- Avoid soft cheeses (feta, brie, camembert, blue-veined, and Mexican-style cheeses, such as queso fresco)
- Cook leftover foods or ready-to-eat foods, such as hot dogs, until they are steaming hot
- Avoid food from delicatessens, such as prepared meats, salads, and cheeses—or heat these foods until steaming before eating

Cautions about Travel

Before you travel to other countries, particularly developing countries, talk to your doctor about ways you can avoid getting sick on your trip.

When traveling in developing countries, people who have HIV should be especially cautious of food and water that may be contaminated. It is best to avoid:

- raw fruits and vegetables (unless you peel them first)

- raw or undercooked seafood or meat

- tap water (or ice made with tap water)

- unpasteurized milk or dairy products

- swallowing water when swimming

Talk to your healthcare provider about whether you need to get vaccinated before your trip and whether you need to take drugs to prevent diseases that are common in the country you are going to visit.

Chapter 42

HIV/AIDS and Co-Occurring Bacterial Infections

Chapter Contents

Section 42.1

Mycobacterium avium *Complex*

This section includes text excerpted from "*Mycobacterium avium* Complex," Genetic and Rare Diseases Information Center (GARD), National Center for Advancing Translational Sciences (NCATS), December 21, 2015.

Mycobacterium avium complex (MAC) refers to infections caused by two types of bacteria: *Mycobacterium avium* and *Mycobacterium intracellulare*. MAC primarily affects people with compromised immune systems (for example from acquired immunodeficiency syndrome (AIDS), hairy cell leukemia, or immunosuppressive chemotherapy) or underlying lung disease. Symptoms can be nonspecific and may include fever, sweats, weight loss, abdominal pain, fatigue, chronic diarrhea, and anemia. It may cause local disease affecting the central nervous system (CNS), lymph nodes, soft tissue, or bones; or, it may cause multi-system disease also affecting other organs and systems. MAC is spread when the bacteria, found in water, soil and dust particles, are inhaled or ingested. Treatment for MAC varies depending on the type and may include antibiotics, antituberculosis drugs, and/or surgery.

Symptoms

Mycobacterium avium complex is associated with several different conditions including pulmonary MAC, which affects the lungs; disseminated MAC, which affects many different parts of the body; and MAC lymphadenitis, which causes swollen lymph nodes.

Pulmonary MAC is the most common type of MAC infection. The onset is usually gradual and symptoms may be present for weeks to months. Affected people may experience cough, weight loss, fever, fatigue, and night sweats.

Disseminated MAC is generally only found in people who have human immunodeficiency virus (HIV)/AIDS. Usual signs and symptoms include:

- Fever
- Sweating
- Weight loss
- Fatigue

- Diarrhea

- Shortness of breath

- Abdominal pain

- Anemia

Less common features of MAC infection in people with HIV/AIDS include mastitis (an infection of the breast tissue); pyomyositis (an infection of the skeletal muscle); abscesses of the skin or brain; and gastrointestinal problems.

MAC lymphadenitis generally affects children aged 1–4 years. Swollen lymph nodes, primarily on a single side of the neck, are generally the only symptom of this form.

Cause

Mycobacterium avium complex (MAC) refers to infections caused by two types of bacteria: *Mycobacterium avium* and *Mycobacterium intracellulare*. To become infected, a person must be exposed to one of these bacteria, which are found in many places including water (fresh or salt), household dust, and soil. MAC is usually spread when the bacteria are inhaled into the respiratory tract or ingested into the gastrointestinal tract. Although these infections can affect anyone, MAC primarily affects people who have compromised immune systems or underlying lung disease.

Inheritance

Mycobacterium avium complex (MAC) is an infection, not an inherited condition. To become infected with MAC, a person must be exposed to one of the associated types of bacteria.

There have been a couple of reports in the literature describing familial cases of MAC. While no single gene is thought to be responsible for MAC, it is possible that variations in a gene (or genes) may contribute to susceptibility. However, to our knowledge, no such genes have been identified.

Diagnosis

A diagnosis of pulmonary *mycobacterium avium* (MAC) is usually based on a physical examination that reveals concerning signs and symptoms; laboratory tests performed on mucus samples; imaging studies of the chest and lungs (X-ray or computed tomography (CT) scan); and the exclusion of other conditions that affect the lungs. If disseminated MAC is suspected testing should also be performed on blood, urine, and/or stool. A lymph node biopsy is usually necessary to confirm a diagnosis of MAC lymphadenitis.

Treatment

Mycobacterium avium complex is associated with several different conditions including pulmonary MAC, which affects the lungs; disseminated MAC, which affects many different parts of the body; and MAC lymphadenitis, which causes swollen lymph nodes. The best treatment options vary by condition. Pulmonary MAC and disseminated MAC are usually treated with a combination of antibiotics and/ or antituberculosis medications. Care must be taken in choosing the appropriate combination of medications as some of the disease-causing bacteria can be resistant to many types of antibiotics and antituberculosis drugs. Surgical treatment may be considered in people with a poor response to drug therapy, drug-resistant MAC or the presence of many condition-related complications if the infection only affects one lung and the procedure is thought to be well-tolerated.

Treatment of MAC lymphadenitis usually involves surgical removal of affected lymph nodes. Affected people may also be prescribed antibiotics depending on the severity of condition and their response to surgery.

Prognosis

The long-term outlook (prognosis) for people with *mycobacterium avium* complex varies. Without treatment, pulmonary MAC often leads to respiratory failure, which can result in severe disability or death. In HIV-negative people with pulmonary MAC, the treatment success rates range from 20–90 percent in various studies, with an average rate of 50–60 percent. People with certain types of lung disease (fibrocavitary), body mass index (BMI) less than 18.5 kg/m², and anemia are more likely to have a poor prognosis than other HIV-negative people affected by MAC.

Prior to the availability of newer antibiotics, HIV-positive people with disseminated MAC had an average life expectancy of 4 months. Although MAC in this population is still associated with a shortened lifespan, those receiving antiretroviral therapy and MAC treatment have a relatively better prognosis.

MAC lymphadenitis in children generally has a benign course. In some cases, the condition may resolve spontaneously even without surgery.

Section 42.2

Tuberculosis

This section includes text excerpted from "HIV and Opportunistic Infections, Coinfections, and Conditions," AIDS*info*, U.S. Department of Health and Human Services (HHS), July 26, 2017.

What Is Tuberculosis?

Tuberculosis (TB) is a contagious disease that can spread from person to person. TB is caused by bacteria called Mycobacterium tuberculosis. The TB bacteria spread in the air.

TB usually affects the lungs. But TB causing bacteria can attack any part of the body, including the kidneys, spine, or brain. If not treated, TB can cause death.

How Does TB Spread from Person to Person?

A person with TB disease of the lungs or throat can spread droplets of TB bacteria in the air, particularly when they cough or sneeze. People who breathe in the TB bacteria can get TB.

Once in the body, TB can be inactive or active. Inactive TB is called latent TB. Active TB is called TB disease.

What Is the Connection between Human Immunodeficiency Virus (HIV) and TB?

TB is an opportunistic infection (OI). OIs are infections that occur more often or are more severe in people with weakened immune systems than in people with healthy immune systems. The human immunodeficiency virus (HIV) weakens the immune system, increasing the risk of TB in people with HIV.

Infection with both HIV and TB is called HIV/TB coinfection. Latent TB is more likely to advance to TB disease in people with HIV than in people without HIV. TB disease may also cause HIV to worsen.

Treatment with HIV medicines is called antiretroviral therapy (ART). ART protects the immune system and prevents HIV infection from advancing to AIDS.

ART also has TB-related benefits:

- ART reduces the risk of TB infection in people with HIV.

- ART reduces the chances that latent TB will advance to TB disease in people with HIV/TB coinfection.

How Common Is HIV/TB Coinfection?

Worldwide, TB disease is one of the leading causes of death among people with HIV. In the United States, where HIV medicines are widely used, fewer people with HIV get TB than in many other countries. But TB still affects many people with HIV in the United States, especially those born outside the United States.

Should People with HIV Get Tested for TB?

Yes, people with HIV should get tested for TB infection. If test results show that a person has latent TB, additional testing is needed. More testing will determine whether the person has TB disease.

What Are the Symptoms of TB?

People with latent TB don't have any signs of the disease. But if latent TB advances to TB disease, there will usually be signs of the disease. Common symptoms of TB disease include:

- A persistent cough that may bring up blood or sputum

- Fatigue

- Weight loss

- Fever

- Night sweats

Other symptoms of TB disease depend on the part of the body affected. For example, signs of TB infection of the kidneys may include blood in the urine, and signs of TB infection of the spine may include back pain.

What Is the Treatment for TB?

In general, TB treatment is the same for people with HIV and people without HIV. TB medicines are used to prevent latent TB from advancing to TB disease and to treat TB disease. The choice of TB medicines and the length of treatment depend on whether a person has latent TB or TB disease.

People with HIV/TB coinfection should be treated for both diseases. In most cases, HIV and TB can be treated at the same time. Taking HIV and TB medicines at the same time can increase the risk of drug-drug interactions and side effects. People being treated for HIV/TB coinfection are carefully monitored by their healthcare providers.

The choice of medicines to treat HIV/TB coinfection depends on a person's individual circumstances. For example, some medicines can't be safely used during pregnancy. If you have HIV/TB coinfection, talk to your healthcare provider about the best medicines for you.

Chapter 43

HIV/AIDS and Co-Occurring Fungal Infections

Chapter Contents

Section 43.1

Risk of Fungal Infections among People with HIV/AIDS

This section includes text excerpted from "Fungal Diseases—People Living with HIV/AIDS," Centers for Disease Control and Prevention (CDC), January 25, 2017.

As a person living with human immunodeficiency virus (HIV) / acquired immunodeficiency syndrome (AIDS), you have many opportunities for a healthy and full life. You may also have some health challenges. One of those challenges is avoiding infections.

Many fungal infections are called opportunistic infections, which means that they usually affect people with weak immune systems. Because HIV weakens the immune system, you have a greater chance of getting some types of fungal infections, like cryptococcosis, coccidioidomycosis, histoplasmosis, and *pneumocystis* pneumonia (PCP).

HIV/AIDS and Fungal Infections

One of the first signs that the HIV/AIDS epidemic was beginning in the United States was a cluster of five cases of a type of fungal pneumonia called PCP in California in 1981. Before antiretroviral therapy was discovered, fungal and other opportunistic infections were a major problem for people with HIV/AIDS. Since then, the numbers of fungal infections and deaths due to fungal infections in people living with HIV/AIDS have decreased substantially. For example, one study showed that the incidence of cryptococcosis in AIDS patients decreased by approximately 90 percent in the 1990s. The decrease in opportunistic infections is primarily because antiretroviral therapy (ART) helps keep people with HIV from reaching the stage where their immune systems are most vulnerable to fungal infections and other infections. However, fungal diseases are still a concern for people living with HIV/AIDS in the United States. Awareness is your best protection, and learning about the different fungal diseases will help you safeguard your health.

What You Need to Know about Fungal Infections

Your CD4 count is important. You're at greatest risk for fungal infection when your CD4 count is less than 200. Keeping your CD4 count above 200 may help you avoid serious illness.

Antiretroviral therapy (ART) is important. Starting ART helps slow the progress of HIV and can reduce your chances of getting a fungal infection.

Fungal infections can range from mild to life-threatening. Some fungal infections are mild skin rashes, but others can be deadly, like fungal meningitis. Because of this, it's important to seek treatment as soon as possible to try to avoid serious infection.

Fungal infections can look like bacterial or viral infections. If you're taking medicine to fight an infection and you aren't getting better, ask your doctor about testing you for a fungal infection.

Where you live (geography) matters. Some disease-causing fungi are more common in certain parts of the world. If you have HIV/AIDS and live in or visit these areas, you're more likely to get these infections than the general population.

Your activities matter. Disease-causing fungi can be found in air, dust, and soil, especially soil that contains bird or bat droppings. Doing activities that disturb the soil, like gardening, cleaning chicken coops, construction, demolition, and visiting caves can cause you to inhale more fungi and increases your chance of infection.

Some fungal infections can interfere with taking your medications. Thrush, an infection in the mouth and throat, is sometimes seen among people living with HIV/AIDS. This infection is not usually life-threatening but can be painful, make it difficult to eat, or interfere with taking your medications. Your nutrition is an important part of staying healthy, so it's important to seek care for this infection.

Preventing fungal infections in people Living with HIV/AIDS

Fungi are difficult to avoid because they are a natural part of the environment. Fungi live outdoors in soil, on plants, trees, and other vegetation. They are also on many indoor surfaces and on your skin. However, there may be some ways for you to lower your chances of getting a serious fungal infection.

Learn about fungal infections. There are different types of fungal infections. Learning about them can help you and your healthcare provider recognize the symptoms early, which may prevent serious illness.

Find out about your risk. The danger of getting a fungal infection can change depending on your location and your CD4 count. Learning what things can put you at risk may prevent serious illness.

Get additional medical care if necessary. Fungal infections often resemble other illnesses. Visiting your healthcare provider may help with faster diagnosis and may prevent serious illness.

Antifungal medication. Your healthcare provider may prescribe medication to prevent fungal infections. For example, they may recommend medication (TMP-SMX, also called Bactrim, Septra, or Cotrim) to prevent a type of fungal pneumonia called *Pneumocystis jirovecii* pneumonia (PCP).

Protect yourself from the environment. There may be some ways to lower your chances of getting a serious fungal infection by trying to avoid disease-causing fungi in the environment. It's important to note that although these actions are recommended, they have not been proven to prevent fungal infections.

- Try to avoid areas with a lot of dust like construction or excavation sites.
- Stay inside during dust storms.
- Stay away from areas with bird and bat droppings. This includes places like chicken coops and caves.
- Wear gloves when handling materials such as soil, moss, or manure.
- Wear shoes, long pants, and a long-sleeved shirt when doing outdoor activities such as gardening, yard work, or visiting wooded areas.

Section 43.2

Candidiasis

This section includes text excerpted from "Fungal Diseases—Candidiasis," Centers for Disease Control and Prevention (CDC), June 12, 2015.

Candidiasis is a fungal infection caused by yeasts that belong to the genus *Candida*. There are over 20 species of *Candida* yeasts that can cause infection in humans, the most common of which is *Candida albicans*. *Candida* yeasts normally reside in the intestinal tract and can be found on mucous membranes and skin without causing infection; however, overgrowth of these organisms can cause symptoms to develop. Symptoms of candidiasis vary depending on the area of the body that is infected.

Types of Candidiasis

Candida *Infections of the Mouth, Throat, and Esophagus*

Candidiasis in the mouth and throat is also called "thrush" or oropharyngeal candidiasis. Candidiasis in the esophagus (the tube that connects the throat to the stomach) is called esophageal candidiasis or *Candida esophagitis*. Esophageal candidiasis is one of the most common infections in people living with human immunodeficiency virus (HIV) / acquired immunodeficiency syndrome (AIDS).

Symptoms

Candidiasis in the mouth and throat can have many different symptoms, including:

- White patches on the inner cheeks, tongue, the roof of the mouth, and throat (photo showing candidiasis in the mouth)

- Redness or soreness

- The cottony feeling in the mouth

- Loss of taste

- Pain while eating or swallowing

- Cracking and redness at the corners of the mouth

Symptoms of candidiasis in the esophagus usually include pain when swallowing and difficulty swallowing. Contact your healthcare provider if you have symptoms that you think are related to candidiasis in the mouth, throat, or esophagus.

Risk and Prevention

Who Gets Candidiasis in the Mouth, Throat, or Esophagus?

Candidiasis in the mouth, throat, or esophagus is uncommon in healthy adults. People who are at higher risk for getting candidiasis in the mouth and throat include babies, especially those younger than one month old, and people who:

- Wear dentures

- Have diabetes

- Have cancer

- Have HIV/AIDS

- Take antibiotics or corticosteroids, including inhaled corticosteroids for conditions like asthma

- Take medications that cause dry mouth or have medical conditions that cause dry mouth

- Smoke

Most people who get candidiasis in the esophagus have weakened immune systems, meaning that their bodies don't fight infections well. This includes people living with HIV/AIDS and people who have blood cancers such as leukemia and lymphoma. People who get candidiasis in the esophagus often also have candidiasis in the mouth and throat.

How can I prevent candidiasis in the mouth, throat, or esophagus? Ways to help prevent candidiasis in the mouth and throat include:

- Maintain good oral health

- Rinse your mouth or brush your teeth after using inhaled corticosteroids

- Some studies have shown that chlorhexidine mouthwash may help to prevent oral candidiasis in people undergoing cancer treatment

Sources

Candida normally lives in the mouth, throat, and the rest of the digestive tract without causing any problems. Sometimes, it can multiply and cause an infection if the environment inside the mouth, throat, or esophagus changes in a way that encourages its growth. This can happen when a person's immune system becomes weakened if antibiotics affect the natural balance of microbes in the body, or for a variety of other reasons in other groups of people.

Diagnosis and Testing

Healthcare providers can usually diagnose candidiasis in the mouth or throat simply by looking inside. Sometimes a healthcare provider will take a small sample from the mouth or throat. The sample is sent to a laboratory for testing, usually to be examined under a microscope.

Healthcare providers usually diagnose candidiasis in the esophagus by doing an endoscopy. An endoscopy is a procedure to examine the digestive tract using a tube with a light and a camera. A healthcare provider might prescribe antifungal medication without doing an endoscopy to see if the patient's symptoms get better.

Treatment

Candidiasis in the mouth, throat, or esophagus is usually treated with antifungal medicine. The treatment for mild to moderate infections in the mouth or throat is usually an antifungal medicine applied to the inside of the mouth for 7–14 days. These medications include clotrimazole, miconazole, or nystatin. For severe infections, the treatment is usually fluconazole or another type of antifungal medicine given by mouth or through a vein for people who don't get better after taking fluconazole. The treatment for candidiasis in the esophagus is usually fluconazole. Other types of prescription antifungal medicines can also be used for people who can't take fluconazole or who don't get better after taking fluconazole.

Vaginal Candidiasis

Candida can multiply and cause an infection if the environment inside the vagina changes in a way that encourages its growth. Candidiasis in the vagina is commonly called a "vaginal yeast infection." Other names for this infection are "vaginal candidiasis," "vulvovaginal candidiasis," or "candidal vaginitis."

Symptoms

The symptoms of vaginal candidiasis include:

- Vaginal itching or soreness

- Pain during sexual intercourse

- Pain or discomfort when urinating

- Abnormal vaginal discharge

Although most vaginal candidiasis is mild, some women can develop severe infections involving redness, swelling, and cracks in the wall of the vagina.

Contact your healthcare provider if you have any of these symptoms. These symptoms are similar to those of other types of vaginal infections, which are treated with different types of medicines. A healthcare provider can tell you if you have vaginal candidiasis and how to treat it.

Risk and Prevention

Who Gets Vaginal Candidiasis?

Vaginal candidiasis is common, though more research is needed to understand how many women are affected. Women who are more likely to get vaginal candidiasis include those who:

- Are pregnant

- Use hormonal contraceptives (for example, birth control pills)

- Have diabetes

- Have a weakened immune system (for example, due to HIV infection or medicines that weaken the immune system, such as steroids and chemotherapy)

- Are taking or have taken antibiotics

How Can I Prevent Vaginal Candidiasis?

Wearing cotton underwear might help reduce the chances of getting a yeast infection. Because taking antibiotics can lead to vaginal candidiasis, take these medicines only when prescribed and exactly as your healthcare provider tells you. Learn more about when antibiotics work and when they should be avoided.

Sources

Candida normally lives inside the body (in places such as the mouth, throat, gut, and vagina) and on skin without causing any problems. Scientists estimate that about 20 percent of women normally have *Candida* in the vagina without having any symptoms. Sometimes, *Candida* can multiply and cause an infection if the environment inside the vagina changes in a way that encourages its growth. This can happen because of hormones, medicines, or changes in the immune system.

Diagnosis and Testing

A laboratory test is usually needed to diagnose vaginal candidiasis because the symptoms are similar to those of other types of vaginal infections. A healthcare provider will usually diagnose vaginal candidiasis by taking a small sample of vaginal discharge to be examined under a microscope or sent to a laboratory for a fungal culture. However, a positive fungal culture does not always mean that *Candida* is causing the symptoms because some women can have *Candida* in the vagina without having any symptoms.

Treatment

Vaginal candidiasis is usually treated with antifungal medicine. For most infections, the treatment is an antifungal medicine applied inside the vagina or a single dose of fluconazole taken by mouth. For more severe infections, infections that don't get better, or keep coming back after getting better, other treatments might be needed. These treatments include more doses of fluconazole taken by mouth or other medicines applied inside the vagina such as boric acid, nystatin, or flucytosine.

Invasive Candidiasis

Invasive candidiasis is an infection caused by a yeast (a type of fungus) called *Candida*. Unlike *Candida* infections in the mouth and throat (also called "thrush") or vaginal "yeast infections," invasive candidiasis is a serious infection that can affect the blood, heart, brain, eyes, bones, and other parts of the body. Candidemia, a bloodstream infection with *Candida,* is a common infection in hospitalized patients and it often results in long hospital stays, high medical costs, and poor outcomes.

Invasive candidiasis can be treated with antifungal medication, and antifungal medication is often given to prevent the infection from developing in certain patient groups.

Symptoms

People who develop invasive candidiasis are often already sick from other medical conditions, so it can be difficult to know which symptoms are related to a *Candida* infection. However, the most common symptoms of invasive candidiasis are fever and chills that don't improve after antibiotic treatment for suspected bacterial infections. Other symptoms can develop if the infection spreads to other parts of the body, such as the heart, brain, eyes, bones, or joints.

Risk and Prevention

Who Gets Invasive Candidiasis?

Most cases of invasive candidiasis occur in people who have been admitted to a hospital or been in contact with other healthcare settings such as nursing homes. People who are at high risk for developing invasive candidiasis include:

- Patients who have a central venous catheter

- Patients in the intensive care unit (ICU)

- People who have weakened immune systems (for example, people who have had an organ transplant, have HIV/AIDS, or are on cancer chemotherapy)

- People who have taken broad-spectrum antibiotics

- People who have a very low neutrophil (a type of white blood cell) count (neutropenia)

- People who have kidney failure or are on hemodialysis

- Patients who have had surgery, especially gastrointestinal surgery

- Patients who have diabetes

Is Invasive Candidiasis Contagious?

Invasive candidiasis doesn't spread directly from person to person. However, some species of the fungus that causes invasive candidiasis normally live on skin, so it's possible that *Candida* can be passed from one person to another and possibly cause an infection in someone who is at high risk.

How Can Invasive Candidiasis Be Prevented?

- **Antifungal medication.** If you're at high risk for developing invasive candidiasis, your healthcare provider may prescribe an antifungal medication to prevent the infection. This is called "antifungal prophylaxis," and it is typically recommended for:

  - Some organ transplant patients

  - High-risk ICU patients

  - Chemotherapy patients who have neutropenia

  - Stem cell transplant patients who have neutropenia

- Some doctors may also consider giving antifungal prophylaxis to very low birth weight infants (less than 2.2 pounds) in nurseries with high rates of invasive candidiasis.

- **Be a safe patient.** There are some actions that you can take to help protect yourself from infections, including:

  - Speak up. Patients and caregivers can ask how long a central venous catheter (central line) is needed, and if so, how long it should stay in place. Tell your doctor if the skin around the catheter becomes red or painful.

  - Keep hands clean. Be sure everyone cleans their hands before touching you. Washing hands can prevent the spread of germs.

- **Healthcare providers** can follow CDC-recommended infection control practices every time they work with a central line.

Diagnosis and Testing

How Is Invasive Candidiasis Diagnosed?

Healthcare providers rely on your medical history, symptoms, physical examinations, and laboratory tests to diagnose invasive candidiasis. The most common way that healthcare providers test for invasive candidiasis is by taking a blood sample and sending it to a laboratory to see if it will grow *Candida* in a culture.

How Long Will It Take to Get My Test Results?

Results from a blood test will usually be available in a few days.

Sources of Invasive Candidiasis

Candida lives in and on the body

Candida, the fungus that causes invasive candidiasis, normally lives in the gastrointestinal tract and on skin without causing any problems. In people who are at higher risk for the infection, invasive candidiasis may occur when a person's own *Candida* yeasts enter the bloodstream, for example, where an intravenous (IV) catheter was inserted or during surgery. Medical equipment or devices, particularly intravenous catheters, can also become contaminated with *Candida* and allow the fungus to enter the bloodstream. Healthcare workers can also carry *Candida* on their hands. There have been a few outbreaks of candidemia linked to healthcare workers' hands, so hand hygiene in healthcare settings is important for preventing the spread of infections.

Types of *Candida*

There are over 150 species of *Candida,* but only about 15 of these are known to cause infections. The most common species that cause infections are *C. albicans, C. glabrata, C. parapsilosis, C. tropicalis,* and *C. krusei.*

Treatment for Invasive Candidiasis

How Is Invasive Candidiasis Treated?

The specific type and dose of antifungal medication used to treat invasive candidiasis usually depend on the patient's age, immune status, and location and severity of the infection. For most adults, the initial recommended antifungal treatment is an echinocandin (caspofungin, micafungin, or anidulafungin) given through the vein (intravenous or IV). Fluconazole, amphotericin B, and other antifungal medications may also be appropriate in certain situations.

How Long Does the Treatment Last?

For candidemia, treatment should continue for 2 weeks after signs and symptoms have resolved and *Candida* yeasts are no longer in the bloodstream. Other forms of invasive candidiasis, such as infections in the bones, joints, heart, or central nervous system, usually need to be treated for a longer period of time.

Section 43.3

Cryptococcus neoformans

This section includes text excerpted from "Fungal Diseases—*C. neoformans* Infection," Centers for Disease Control and Prevention (CDC), November 28, 2015.

Cryptococcus neoformans is a fungus that lives in the environment throughout the world. People can become infected with *C. neoformans* after breathing in the microscopic fungus, although most people who are exposed to the fungus never get sick from it. *C. neoformans* infections are extremely rare in people who are otherwise healthy; most cases occur in people who have weakened immune systems, particularly those who have advanced human immunodeficiency virus (HIV) / acquired immunodeficiency syndrome (AIDS).

Symptoms of C. neoformans *Infection*

C. neoformans usually infects the lungs or the central nervous system (CNS; the brain and spinal cord), but it can also affect other parts of the body. The symptoms of the infection depend on the parts of the body that are affected.

In the Lungs

A *C. neoformans* infection in the lungs can cause a pneumonia-like illness. The symptoms are often similar to those of many other illnesses, and can include:

- Cough
- Shortness of breath
- Chest pain
- Fever

In the Brain (Cryptococcal Meningitis)

Cryptococcal meningitis is an infection caused by the fungus Cryptococcus after it spreads from the lungs to the brain. The symptoms of cryptococcal meningitis include:

- Headache
- Fever

- Neck pain

- Nausea and vomiting

- Sensitivity to light

- Confusion or changes in behavior

If you have symptoms that you think may be due to a *C. neoformans* infection, please contact your healthcare provider.

Risk and Prevention

Who Gets **C. neoformans** *Infections?*

C. neoformans infections are extremely rare among people who are otherwise healthy. Most cases of *C. neoformans* infection occur in people who have weakened immune systems, such as people who:

- Have advanced HIV/AIDS,

- Have had an organ transplant, or

- Are taking corticosteroids, medications to treat rheumatoid arthritis or other medications that weaken the immune system.

Is **C. neoformans** *Infection Contagious?*

No. The infection can't spread between people or between people and animals.

Can Pets Get **C. neoformans** *Infections?*

Yes. Pets can get *C. neoformans* infections, but it is very rare, and the infection cannot spread between animals and people. If you're concerned about your pet's risk of getting a *C. neoformans* infection, or if you think that your pet has the infection, please talk to a veterinarian.

How Can I Prevent a **C. neoformans** *Infection?*

It's difficult to avoid breathing in *C. neoformans* because it's thought to be common in the environment. Most people who breathe in *C. neoformans* never get sick from it. However, in people who have weakened immune systems, *C. neoformans* can stay hidden in the body and cause infection later when the immune system becomes too weak to fight it off. This leaves a window of time when the silent infection can be detected and treated early before symptoms develop (see "Detecting silent cryptococcal infection in people who have HIV/AIDS").

Detecting Silent Cryptococcal Infections in People Who Have HIV/AIDS

One approach to prevent cryptococcal meningitis is called "targeted screening." Research suggests that *C.* neoformans are able to live in the body undetected, especially when a person's immune system is weaker than normal. In a targeted screening program, a simple blood test is used to detect a cryptococcal antigen (an indicator of cryptococcal infection) in HIV-infected patients before they begin taking antiretroviral treatment (ART). A patient who tests positive for a cryptococcal antigen can take fluconazole, an antifungal medication, to fight off the silent fungal infection and prevent it from developing into life-threatening meningitis.

Sources of C. neoformans

Where Does C. neoformans Live?

C. neoformans lives in the environment throughout the world. The fungus is typically found in soil, on decaying wood, in tree hollows, or in bird droppings.

How Does Someone Get a C. neoformans Infection?

C. neoformans infections are not contagious. Humans and animals can get the infection after inhaling the microscopic fungus from the environment. Some research suggests that people may be exposed to *C. neoformans* in the environment when they are children. Most people who breathe in *C. neoformans* never get sick from it. However, in people who have weakened immune systems, *C. neoformans* can stay hidden in the body and cause infection later when the immune system becomes too weak to fight it off.

Diagnosis and Testing

How Is a C. neoformans Infection Diagnosed?

Healthcare providers rely on your medical history, symptoms, physical examinations, and laboratory tests to diagnose a *C. neoformans* infection.

Your healthcare provider will take a sample of tissue or body fluid (such as blood, cerebrospinal fluid, or sputum) and send the sample to a laboratory to be examined under a microscope, tested with an antigen test, or cultured. Your healthcare provider may also perform tests such as a chest X-ray or computed tomography (CT) scan of your lungs, brain, or other parts of the body.

Treatment

How Are C. neoformans *Infections Treated?*

People who have *C. neoformans* infection need to take prescription antifungal medication for at least 6 months, often longer. The type of treatment usually depends on the severity of the infection and the parts of the body that are affected.

- For people who have *asymptomatic infections (e.g., diagnosed via targeted screening) or mild-to-moderate pulmonary infections*, the treatment is usually fluconazole.

- For people who have *severe lung infections or infections in the central nervous system (CNS)* (brain and spinal cord), the recommended initial treatment is amphotericin B in combination with flucytosine. After that, patients usually need to take fluconazole for an extended time to clear the infection.

The type, dose, and duration of antifungal treatment may differ for certain groups of people, such as pregnant women, children, and people in resource-limited settings. Some people may also need surgery to remove fungal growths (cryptococcomas).

Section 43.4

Coccidioidomycosis

This section includes text excerpted from "Fungal Diseases—Valley Fever (Coccidioidomycosis)," Centers for Disease Control and Prevention (CDC), January 30, 2017.

Valley fever, also called coccidioidomycosis, is an infection caused by the fungus *Coccidioides*. The fungus is known to live in the soil in the southwestern United States and parts of Mexico and Central and South America. The fungus was also found in south-central Washington. People can get valley fever by breathing in the microscopic fungal spores from the air, although most people who breathe in the spores don't get sick. Usually, people who get sick with valley fever will get better on their own within weeks to months, but some people will need antifungal medication. Certain groups of people are at higher risk for becoming severely ill. It's difficult to prevent exposure to *Coccidioides* in areas where it's common in the environment, but people who are at higher risk for severe valley fever should try to avoid breathing in large amounts of dust if they're in these areas.

Symptoms of Valley Fever (Coccidioidomycosis)

Many people who are exposed to the fungus *Coccidioides* never have symptoms. Other people may have flu-like symptoms that go usually away on their own after weeks to months. If your symptoms last for more than a week, contact your healthcare provider.

Symptoms of valley fever include:

- Fatigue (tiredness)
- Cough
- Fever
- Shortness of breath
- Headache
- Night Sweats
- Muscle aches or joint pain
- Rash on upper body or legs

In extremely rare cases, the fungal spores can enter the skin through a cut, wound, or splinter and cause a skin infection.

How Soon Do the Symptoms Appear?

Symptoms of valley fever may appear between 1 and 3 weeks after a person breathes in the fungal spores.

How Long Do the Symptoms Last?

The symptoms of valley fever usually last for a few weeks to a few months. However, some patients have symptoms that last longer than this, especially if the infection becomes severe.

Severe Valley Fever

Approximately 5–10 percent of people who get valley fever will develop serious or long-term problems in their lungs. In an even smaller percentage of people (about 1%), the infection spreads from the lungs to other parts of the body, such as the central nervous system (brain and spinal cord), skin, or bones and joints.

Valley Fever (Coccidioidomycosis) Risk and Prevention

Who Gets Valley Fever?

Anyone who lives in or travels to the southwestern United States (Arizona, California, Nevada, New Mexico, Texas, or Utah), or parts of Mexico, or Central or South America can get valley fever. Valley fever can affect people of any age, but it's most common in adults aged 60 and older. Certain groups of people may be at higher risk for developing the severe forms of valley fever, such as:

- People who have weakened immune systems, for example, people who:
  - Have human immunodeficiency virus (HIV) / acquired immunodeficiency syndrome (AIDS)
  - Have had an organ transplant
  - Are taking medications such as corticosteroids or tumor necrosis factor (TNF)-inhibitors
- Pregnant women
- People who have diabetes
- People who are Black or Filipino

Is Valley Fever Contagious?

No. The fungus that causes valley fever, *Coccidioides,* can't spread from the lungs between people or between people and animals. However, in **extremely** rare instances, a wound infection with *Coccidioides* can spread valley fever to someone else, or the infection can be spread through an organ transplant with an infected organ.

Traveling to an Endemic Area

Should I Worry about Valley Fever If I'm Traveling to an Area Where the Fungus Is Common?

The risk of getting valley fever is low when traveling to an area where *Coccidioides* lives in the environment, such as the southwestern United States, Mexico, or Central or South America. Your risk for infection could increase if you will be in a very dusty setting, but even then the risk is still low. If you have questions about your risk of getting valley fever while traveling, talk to your healthcare provider.

I've Had It Before; Could I Get It Again?

Usually not. If you've already had valley fever, your immune system will most likely protect you from getting it again. Some people can have the infection come back again (a relapse) after getting better the first time, but this is very rare.

Can My Pets Get Valley Fever?

Yes. Pets, particularly dogs, can get valley fever, but it is **not** contagious between animals and people. Valley fever in dogs is similar to valley fever in humans. Like humans, many dogs that are exposed to *Coccidioides* never get sick. Dogs that do develop symptoms often have symptoms that include coughing, lack of energy, and weight loss. If you're concerned about your pet's risk of getting valley fever or if you think that your pet has valley fever, please talk to a veterinarian.

Coccidioides *at My Workplace*

What Should I Do If I Think I've Been Exposed to Coccidioides *at My Workplace or in a Laboratory?*

If you think you've been exposed to *Coccidioides* at work or in a laboratory, you should contact your Occupational Health (OH), Infection

Control (IC), Risk Management (RM), or Safety/Security Department (SSD). If your workplace or laboratory doesn't have these services, you should contact your local city, county, or state health department. Recommendations about what to do in the event of a laboratory exposure have been published. There is no evidence showing that antifungal medication (i.e., prophylaxis) prevents people from getting sick with valley fever after a workplace exposure to *Coccidioides*. If you develop symptoms of valley fever, contact your healthcare provider.

How Can I prevent Valley Fever?

It's very difficult to avoid breathing in the fungus *Coccidioides* in areas where it's common in the environment. People who live in these areas can try to avoid spending time in dusty places as much as possible. People who are at risk for severe valley fever (such as people who have weakened immune systems, pregnant women, people who have diabetes, or people who are Black or Filipino) may be able to lower their chances of developing the infection by trying to avoid breathing in the fungal spores.

The following are some common-sense methods that may be helpful to avoid getting valley fever. It's important to know that although these steps are recommended, they haven't been proven to prevent valley fever.

- Try to avoid areas with a lot of dust like construction or excavation sites. If you can't avoid these areas, wear an N95 respirator (a type of face mask) while you're there.

- Stay inside during dust storms and close your windows.

- Avoid activities that involve close contact with dirt or dust, including yard work, gardening, and digging.

- Use air filtration measures indoors.

- Clean skin injuries well with soap and water to reduce the chances of developing a skin infection, especially if the wound was exposed to dirt or dust.

- Take preventive antifungal medication if your healthcare provider says you need it.

Is There a Vaccine for Valley Fever?

No. Currently, there is no vaccine to prevent valley fever, but scientists have been trying to make one since the 1960s. Because people who've had valley fever are usually protected from getting it again, a vaccine could make the body's immune system think that it's already had valley fever, which would likely prevent a person from being able to get the infection.

Scientists have tried several different ways to make a valley fever vaccine. When one version of the vaccine was tested on humans in the 1980s, it didn't provide good protection, and it also caused people to develop side effects such as swelling at the injection site. Since then, scientists have been looking at ways to make a vaccine with different ingredients that will provide better protection against valley fever and won't cause side effects. Studies of these new vaccines are ongoing, so it's possible that a vaccine to prevent valley fever could become available in the future.

Sources of Valley Fever (Coccidioidomycosis)

Where Does Coccidioides Live?

Coccidioides lives in dust and soil in some areas in the southwestern United States, Mexico, and South America. In the United States, *Coccidioides* lives in Arizona, California, Nevada, New Mexico, Texas, and Utah. The fungus was also found in south-central Washington.

Life Cycle of Coccidioides

Coccidioides spores circulate in the air after contaminated soil and dust are disturbed by humans, animals, or the weather. The spores are too small to see without a microscope. When people breathe in the spores, they are at risk for developing valley fever. After the spores enter the lungs, the person's body temperature allows the spores to change shape and grow into spherules. When the spherules get large enough, they break open and releases smaller pieces (called endospores) which can then potentially spread within the lungs or to other organs and grow into new spherules.

Uncommon Sources of Valley Fever

The most common way for someone to get valley fever is by inhaling *Coccidioides* spores that are in the air. In extremely rare cases, people can get the infection from other sources, such as:

- From an organ transplant if the organ donor had valley fever

- From inhaling spores from a wound infected with *Coccidioides*

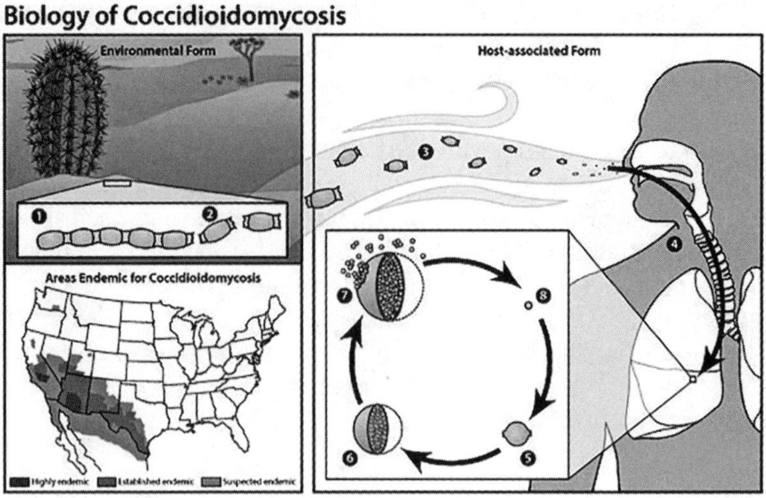

Biology of Coccidioidomycosis

Figure 43.1. *Biology of Coccidioidomycosis*

- From contact with objects (such as rocks or shoes) that have been contaminated with *Coccidioides*

Testing Soil

I'm Worried That Coccidioides Is in the Soil near My Home. Can Someone Test the Soil to Find out If the Fungus Is There?

No, in this situation, testing soil for *Coccidioides* isn't likely to be useful because the fungus is thought to be common in the soil in certain areas. A soil sample that tests positive for *Coccidioides* doesn't necessarily mean that the soil will release the fungus into the air and cause infection. Also, there are no commercially-available tests to detect *Coccidioides* in soil. Testing soil for *Coccidioides* is currently only done for scientific research.

Testing Soil for Research

Scientists sometimes test soil or other environmental samples for *Coccidioides* to understand more about its habitat and how weather or climate patterns may affect its growth. The available methods to detect *Coccidioides* in the soil don't always detect *Coccidioides* spores even if they are present. However, new tests are being developed so that researchers can better detect *Coccidioides* in the environment.

Valley Fever and the Weather

Scientists continue to study how weather and climate patterns affect the habitat of the fungus that causes valley fever. *Coccidioides* is thought to grow best in the soil after heavy rainfall and then disperse into the air most effectively during hot, dry conditions. For example, hot and dry weather conditions have been shown to correlate with an increase in the number of valley fever cases in Arizona and in California (but to a lesser extent). The ways in which climate change may be affecting the number of valley fever infections, as well as the geographic range of *Coccidioides,* isn't known yet but is a subject for further research.

Diagnosis and Testing

How Is Valley Fever Diagnosed?

Healthcare providers rely on your medical and travel history, symptoms, physical examinations, and laboratory tests to diagnose valley fever. The most common way that healthcare providers test for valley fever is by taking a blood sample and sending it to a laboratory to look for *Coccidioides* antibodies or antigens.

Healthcare providers may do imaging tests such as chest X-rays or computed tomography (CT) scans of your lungs to look for valley fever pneumonia. They may also perform a tissue biopsy, in which a small sample of tissue is taken from the body and examined under a microscope. Laboratories may also see if *Coccidioides* will grow from body fluids or tissues (this is called a culture).

Where Can I Get Tested for Valley Fever?

Any healthcare provider can order a test for valley fever.

How Long Will It Take to Get My Test Results?

It depends on the type of test. Results from a blood test will usually be available in a few days. If your healthcare provider sends a sample to a laboratory to be cultured, the results could take a few days to a couple of weeks.

Skin Testing

A skin test can detect whether you have developed an immune response to the fungus *Coccidioides,* the cause of valley fever. This test became available again in the United States in 2014 for the first time since the late 1990s. Your healthcare provider might do this test if you have a history of valley fever.

The test involves getting a small injection on the inside of your forearm, similar to a skin test for tuberculosis. If the test is positive, a bump will appear at the injection site. A healthcare provider must examine the injection site two days (48 hours) after the test was given to measure the size of the bump.

A positive test result means that you have an immune response to *Coccidioides* because of a past or current *Coccidioides* infection. Some people with a positive test result have been sick with valley fever, which can cause a flu-like illness and other symptoms, but many people with a positive test have not had symptoms from the infection. A positive skin test generally means that you are immune to *Coccidioides* and will not get valley fever in the future.

A negative skin test can mean that you have not been exposed to *Coccidioides* and have not had valley fever. However, some people may not react to the skin test even though they have had a *Coccidioides* infection. This is called a false-negative result. False-negative results occur more commonly in people who:

- Have had a *Coccidioides* infection that is recent or severe

- Have a condition or illness that interferes with the skin test results

- Are taking a medication that interferes with the skin test results

Treatment

How Is Valley Fever Treated?

For many people, the symptoms of valley fever will go away within a few months without any treatment. Healthcare providers choose to prescribe an antifungal medication for some people to try to reduce the severity of symptoms or to prevent the infection from getting worse. Antifungal medication is typically given to people who are at higher risk for developing severe valley fever. The treatment is usually 3 to 6 months of fluconazole or another type of antifungal medication. There are no over-the-counter (OTC) medications to treat valley fever. If you have valley fever, you should talk to your healthcare provider about whether you need treatment. The healthcare provider who diagnoses you with valley fever may suggest that you see other healthcare providers who specialize in treating valley fever.

People who have severe lung infections or infections that have spread to other parts of the body always need antifungal treatment and may need to stay in the hospital. For these types of infections, the course of treatment is usually longer than 6 months. Valley fever that develops into meningitis is fatal if it's not treated, so lifelong antifungal treatment is necessary for those cases.

If I Have Valley Fever, Should I Stay at Home?

Valley fever isn't contagious, so you don't need to stay at home to avoid spreading the infection to other people. However, your health-care provider may recommend that you rest at home to help your body fight off the infection.

Does Valley Fever Have Any Long-Term Effects?

Most people who have valley fever will make a full recovery. A small percentage of people develop long-term lung infections that can take several years to get better. In very severe cases of valley fever, the nervous system can be affected and there may be long-term damage, but this is very rare.

Section 43.5

Histoplasmosis

This section includes text excerpted from "Fungal Diseases—Definition of Histoplasmosis," Centers for Disease Control and Prevention (CDC), November 21, 2015.

Symptoms of Histoplasmosis

Histoplasmosis is an infection caused by the fungus *Histoplasma*. The fungus lives in the environment, particularly in soil that contains large amounts of bird or bat droppings. In the United States, *Histoplasma* mainly lives in soil in the central and eastern states, especially areas around the Ohio and Mississippi River valleys. The fungus also lives in parts of Central and South America, Africa, Asia, and Australia.

People can get histoplasmosis after breathing in the microscopic fungal spores from the air, often after participating in activities that disturb the soil. Although most people who breathe in the spores don't get sick, those who do may have a fever, cough, and fatigue. Many people who get sick will get better on their own without medication. In some people, such as those who have weakened immune systems, the infection can become severe, especially if it spreads from the lungs to other organs.

Risk and Prevention

Most people who are exposed to the fungus never have symptoms. Other people may have flu-like symptoms that usually go away on their own.

Symptoms of histoplasmosis include:

- Fever

- A cough

- Fatigue (extreme tiredness)

- Chills

- A headache

- Chest pain

- Body aches

How Soon Do the Symptoms of Histoplasmosis Appear?

Symptoms of histoplasmosis may appear between 3 and 17 days after a person breathes in the fungal spores.

How Long Do the Symptoms of Histoplasmosis Last?

For most people, the symptoms of histoplasmosis will go away within a few weeks to a month. However, some people have symptoms that last longer than this, especially if the infection becomes severe.

Severe Histoplasmosis

In some people, usually those who have weakened immune systems, histoplasmosis can develop into a long-term lung infection, or it can spread from the lungs to other parts of the body, such as the central nervous system (the brain and spinal cord).

Who Gets Histoplasmosis?

Anyone can get histoplasmosis if they've been in an area where Histoplasma lives in the environment. Histoplasmosis is often associated with activities that disturb the soil, particularly soil that contains bird or bat droppings. Certain groups of people are at higher risk for developing the severe forms of histoplasmosis:

People who have weakened immune systems, for example, people who:

- Have HIV/AIDS

- Have had an organ transplant

- Are taking medications such as corticosteroids or TNF-inhibitors

- Infants

- Adults aged 55 and older

Is Histoplasmosis Contagious?

No. Histoplasmosis can't spread from the lungs between people or between people and animals. However, in extremely rare cases, the infection can be passed through an organ transplant with an infected organ.

If I've Already Had Histoplasmosis, Could I Get It Again?

It's possible for someone who's already had histoplasmosis to get it again, but the body's immune system usually provides some partial protection so that the infection is less severe the second time. In people who have weakened immune systems, histoplasmosis can remain hidden in the body for months or years and then cause symptoms later (also called a relapse of infection).

Can My Pets Get Histoplasmosis?

Yes. Pets, particularly cats, can get histoplasmosis, but it is not contagious between animals and people. Histoplasmosis in cats and dogs is similar to histoplasmosis in humans. Like humans, many cats and dogs that are exposed to Histoplasma never get sick. Cats and dogs that do develop symptoms often have symptoms that include coughing, lack of energy, and weight loss. The fungus that causes histoplasmosis grows well in soil that contains bird droppings, but birds don't appear to be able to get histoplasmosis. If you're concerned about your pet's risk of getting histoplasmosis or if you think that your pet has histoplasmosis, please talk to a veterinarian.

How Can I Prevent Histoplasmosis?

It can be difficult to avoid breathing in Histoplasma in areas where it's common in the environment. In areas where Histoplasma is known to live, people who have weakened immune systems (for example, by HIV/AIDS, an organ transplant, or medications such as corticosteroids or TNF-inhibitors) should avoid doing activities that are known to be associated with getting histoplasmosis, including:

- Disturbing material (for example, digging in soil or chopping wood) where there are bird or bat droppings
- Cleaning chicken coops
- Exploring Caves
- Cleaning, remodeling, or tearing down old buildings
- Large amounts of bird or bat droppings should be cleaned up by professional companies that specialize in the removal of hazardous waste.

What Are Public Health Agencies Doing about Histoplasmosis?

- **Surveillance.** In some states, healthcare providers and laboratories are required to report histoplasmosis cases to public health authorities. Disease reporting helps government officials and healthcare providers understand how and why outbreaks occur and allow them to monitor trends in the number of histoplasmosis cases.

- **Developing better diagnostic tools.** The symptoms of histoplasmosis can be similar to those of other respiratory diseases. Faster, more reliable methods to diagnosis histoplasmosis are in development, which could help minimize delays in treatment, save money and resources looking for other diagnoses, and reduce unnecessary treatment for other suspected illnesses.

- **Building laboratory capacity.** Equipping laboratories in Latin America to be able to diagnose histoplasmosis and perform laboratory-based surveillance will help reduce the burden of HIV-associated histoplasmosis in these areas.

Histoplasmosis of Sources

Where Does Histoplasma Live?

Histoplasma, the fungus that causes histoplasmosis, lives throughout the world, but it's most common in North America and Central America. In the United States, *Histoplasma* mainly lives in soil in the central and eastern states, particular areas around the Ohio and Mississippi River Valleys, but it can likely live in other parts of the U.S. as well. The fungus also lives in parts of Central and South America, Africa, Asia, and Australia.

Histoplasma grows best in soil that contains bird or bat droppings. Bats can get histoplasmosis and spread the fungus in their droppings.

Life Cycle of Histoplasma

Histoplasma spores circulate in the air after contaminated soil is disturbed. The spores are too small to see without a microscope. When people breathe in the spores, they are at risk for developing histoplasmosis. After the spores enter the lungs, the person's body temperature allows the spores to transform into yeast. The yeast can then travel to lymph nodes and can spread to other parts of the body through the bloodstream.

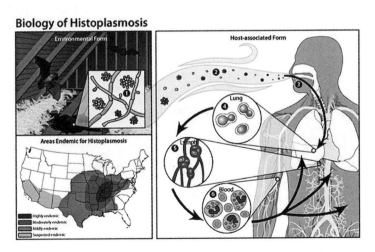

Figure 43.2. *Biology of Histoplasmosis*

I'm Worried That **Histoplasma** *Is in the Soil or in Bird / Bat Droppings Near My Home. Can Someone Test the Environment to Find out If the Fungus Is There?*

No, in this situation, testing the environment for *Histoplasma* isn't likely to be useful because the fungus is thought to be common in the environment in certain areas. A soil sample that tests positive for *Histoplasma* doesn't necessarily mean that it's a source of infection, and a sample that tests negative doesn't necessarily mean that the fungus isn't there. Also, there are no commercially-available tests to detect *Histoplasma* in the environment. Testing environmental samples for *Histoplasma* is currently only done for scientific research. If there are bird or bat droppings near your home, you should have it cleaned up, if possible. If it's not possible to clean up, try not to disturb it.

Diagnosis and Testing

How Is Histoplasmosis Diagnosed?

Healthcare providers rely on your medical and travel history, symptoms, physical examinations, and laboratory tests to diagnose histoplasmosis. The most common way that healthcare providers test for histoplasmosis is by taking a blood sample or a urine sample and sending it to a laboratory.

Healthcare providers may do imaging tests such as chest X-rays or CT scans of your lungs. They may also collect a sample of fluid from your respiratory tract or perform a tissue biopsy, in which a small sample of affected tissue is taken from the body and examined under a microscope. Laboratories may also see if *Histoplasma* will grow from body fluids or tissues (this is called a culture).

Where Can I Get Tested for Histoplasmosis?

Most healthcare providers can order a test for histoplasmosis.

How Long Will It Take to Get My Test Results?

It depends on the type of test. Results from a blood test or a urine test will usually be available in a few days. If your healthcare provider sends a sample to a laboratory to be cultured, the results could take a couple of weeks.

Treatment

How Is Histoplasmosis Treated?

For some people, the symptoms of histoplasmosis will go away without treatment. However, prescription antifungal medication is needed to treat severe histoplasmosis in the lungs, chronic histoplasmosis, and infections that have spread from the lungs to other parts of the body (disseminated histoplasmosis). Itraconazole is one type of antifungal medication that's commonly used to treat histoplasmosis. Depending on the severity of the infection and the person's immune status, the course of treatment can range from 3 months to 1 year.

Section 43.6

Pneumocystis *Pneumonia*

This section includes text excerpted from "Fungal Diseases—
Pneumocystis pneumonia," Centers for Disease Control and
Prevention (CDC), April 26, 2017.

Pneumocystis pneumonia (PCP) is a serious infection caused by the fungus *Pneumocystis jirovecii.*

Most people who get PCP have a medical condition that weakens their immune system, like human immunodeficiency virus (HIV) / acquired immunodeficiency syndrome (AIDS) or takes medicines that lower the body's ability to fight germs and sickness. In the United States, people with HIV/AIDS are less likely to get PCP today than before the availability of antiretroviral therapy (ART). However, PCP is still a substantial public health problem. Much of the information about PCP and its treatment comes from caring for patients with HIV/AIDS.

Scientists have changed both the classification and the name of this organism since it first appeared in patients with HIV in the 1980s. *Pneumocystis jirovecii* used to be classified as a protozoan but is now considered a fungus. *Pneumocystis jirovecii* used to be called *Pneumocystis carinii.* When scientists renamed P. carinii to P. jirovecii, some

459

people considered using the abbreviation "PJP," but to avoid confusion, *Pneumocystis jirovecii* pneumonia is still abbreviated "PCP."

Symptoms

The symptoms of PCP include:

- Fever
- A cough
- Difficulty breathing
- Chest pain
- Chills
- Fatigue (tiredness)

In people with HIV/AIDS, PCP symptoms usually develop over several weeks and include a mild fever. In people who have weakened immune systems for reasons other than HIV/AIDS, PCP symptoms usually develop over a few days, often with a high fever. Contact your healthcare provider if you have symptoms that you think are related to PCP.

Risk and Prevention

Who Gets PCP?

PCP is extremely rare in healthy people, but the fungus that causes this disease can live in their lungs without causing symptoms. In fact, up to 20 percent of adults might carry this fungus at any given time, and the immune system removes the fungus after several months.

Most people who get PCP have weakened immune systems, meaning that their bodies don't fight infections well. About 40 percent of people who get PCP have HIV/AIDS. The other 60 percent of people who get PCP are usually taking medicine that lowers the body's ability to fight germs or sickness or have other medical conditions, such as:

- Solid organ transplant
- Blood cancer
- Inflammatory diseases or autoimmune diseases (for example, lupus or rheumatoid arthritis)
- Stem cell transplant

How Can I Prevent PCP?

There is no vaccine to prevent PCP. A healthcare provider might prescribe medicine to prevent PCP for people who are more likely to develop the disease. The medicine most commonly used to prevent PCP is called trimethoprim/sulfamethoxazole (TMP/SMX), which is also known as co-trimoxazole and by several different brand names, including Bactrim, Septra, and Cotrim. Other medicines are available for people who cannot take TMP/SMX.

Medicine to prevent PCP is recommended for some people infected with HIV, stem cell transplant patients, and some solid organ transplant patients. Healthcare providers might also prescribe medicine to prevent PCP in other patients, such as people who are taking long-term, high-dose corticosteroids.

Sources

PCP spreads from person to person through the air. Some healthy adults can carry the Pneumocystis fungus in their lungs without having symptoms, and it can spread to other people, including those with weakened immune systems.

Many people are exposed to Pneumocystis as children, but they likely do not get sick because their immune systems prevent the fungus from causing an infection. In the past, scientists believed that people who had been exposed to Pneumocystis as children could later develop PCP from that childhood infection if their immune systems become weakened. However, it is more likely that people get PCP after being exposed to someone else who has PCP or who is carrying the fungus in their lungs without having symptoms.

Diagnosis and Testing

PCP is diagnosed using a sample from a patient's lungs. The sample is usually mucus that is either coughed up by the patient (called sputum) or collected by a procedure called bronchoalveolar lavage. Sometimes, a small sample of lung tissue (a biopsy) is used to diagnose PCP. The patient's sample is sent to a laboratory, usually to be examined under a microscope. Polymerase chain reaction (PCR) can also be used to detect Pneumocystis DNA in different types of samples. A blood test to detect β-D-glucan (a part of the cell wall of many different types of fungi) can also help diagnose PCP.

Treatment

PCP must be treated with prescription medicine. Without treatment, PCP can cause death. The most common form of treatment is trimethoprim/sulfamethoxazole (TMP/SMX), which is also known as co-trimoxazole and by several different brand names, including Bactrim, Septra, and Cotrim. This medicine is given by mouth or through a vein for 3 weeks.

TMP/SMX can cause side effects such as rash and fever. Other medicines are available for patients who cannot take TMP/SMX.

Chapter 44

HIV/AIDS and Co-Occurring Parasitic Infections

Chapter Contents

Section 44.1

Cryptosporidiosis

This section contains text excerpted from the following
sources: Text begins with excerpts from "Cryptosporidiosis,"
AIDSinfo, U.S. Department of Health and Human Services (HHS),
June 14, 2017; Text beginning with the heading "Who Might Be
Immunocompromised or Have a Weakened Immune System?"
is excerpted from "Parasites–*Cryptosporidium* (Also Known as
"Crypto")–General Information for Immunocompromised
Persons," Centers for Disease Control and
Prevention (CDC), March 20, 2015.

Cryptosporidiosis is caused by various species of the protozoan
parasite *Cryptosporidium*, which infect the small bowel mucosa and,
if symptomatic, typically cause diarrhea. *Cryptosporidium* can also
infect other gastrointestinal and extraintestinal sites, especially in
individuals whose immune systems are suppressed. Advanced immunosuppression—typically CD4 T lymphocyte cell (CD4) counts of <100
cells/μL1—is associated with the greatest risk for prolonged, severe,
or extraintestinal cryptosporidiosis. The three species that most commonly infect humans are *Cryptosporidium hominis*, *Cryptosporidium parvum*, and *Cryptosporidium meleagridis*. Infections are usually
caused by one species, but a mixed infection is possible.

Cryptosporidiosis remains a common cause of chronic diarrhea in
AIDS patients in developing countries, with up to 74% of diarrheal
stools demonstrating the organism. In developed countries with low
rates of environmental contamination and where potent antiretroviral
therapy (ART) is widely available, cryptosporidiosis has decreased and
occurs at an incidence of <1 case per 1000 person-years in patients with
AIDS. Infection occurs through ingestion of *Cryptosporidium* oocysts.
Viable oocysts in feces can be transmitted directly through contact with
infected humans or animals, particularly those with diarrhea. Oocysts
can contaminate recreational water sources such as swimming pools
and lakes, and public water supplies and may persist despite standard
chlorination. Person-to-person transmission is common, especially
among sexually active men who have sex with men.

Who Might Be Immunocompromised or Have a Weakened Immune System?

Examples of persons with weakened immune systems include
those with acquired immunodeficiency syndrome (AIDS); cancer

and transplant patients who are taking certain immunosuppressive drugs; and those with inherited diseases that affect the immune system (e.g., congenital agammaglobulinemia, congenital immunoglobulin A (IgA) deficiency). The risk of developing severe disease may differ depending on each person's degree of immune suppression.

What Is Cryptosporidiosis?

Cryptosporidiosis is a diarrheal disease caused by a microscopic parasite, *Cryptosporidium*, that can live in the intestine of humans and animals and is passed in the stool of an infected person or animal. Both the disease and the parasite are also known as "Crypto." The parasite is protected by an outer shell that allows it to survive outside the body for long periods of time and makes it very resistant to chlorine-based disinfectants. During the past 2 decades, Crypto has become recognized as one of the most common causes of waterborne disease (recreational water and drinking water) in humans in the United States. The parasite is found in every region of the United States and throughout the world.

What Are the Symptoms of Cryptosporidiosis?

The most common symptom of cryptosporidiosis is watery diarrhea. Other symptoms include:

- Stomach cramps or pain

- Dehydration

- Nausea

- Vomiting

- Fever

- Weight loss

Some people with Crypto will have no symptoms at all. While the small intestine is the site most commonly affected in immunocompromised persons, Crypto infections could possibly affect other areas of the digestive tract or the respiratory tract.

How Long after Infection Do Symptoms Appear?

Symptoms of cryptosporidiosis generally begin 2–10 days (average 7 days) after becoming infected with the parasite.

How Long Will Symptoms Last?

In persons with healthy immune systems, symptoms usually last about 1–2 weeks. The symptoms may go in cycles in which you may seem to get better for a few days, then feel worse before the illness ends. In persons with weakened immune systems, symptoms may last for much longer times.

How Does Cryptosporidiosis Affect You If Your Immune System Is Severely Weakened?

In persons with AIDS and in others whose immune system is weakened, Crypto can be serious, long-lasting, and sometimes fatal. If your CD4+ cell count is below 200/mm³, Crypto is more likely to cause severe symptoms and complications, including prolonged diarrhea, dehydration, and possibly death. If your CD4+ count is above 200/mm³, your illness may not last more than 1–3 weeks, or slightly longer. However, you could still carry the infection, which means that the Crypto parasites are living in your intestine but are not causing illness. As a carrier of Crypto, you could infect other people. If your CD4+ count later drops below 200/mm³, your symptoms may reappear. For persons taking immunosuppressive drugs, the Crypto infection usually resolves when the doses are reduced or the drugs are stopped. Persons taking immunosuppressive drugs need to consult their healthcare provider if they believe they have cryptosporidiosis.

Table 44.1. Immunosuppressed Persons

CD4+ cell count <200/mm³	• More likely to develop diarrhea and other symptoms that last for a long time
CD4+ cell count >200/mm³	• Symptoms may last 1–3 weeks, or slightly longer. • May carry Crypto parasites in their intestines but have no symptoms (these people could infect other people). • If their CD4+ counts drop below 200/mm³, their symptoms might reappear.

How Is Cryptosporidiosis Spread?

Cryptosporidium lives in the intestine of infected humans or animals. An infected person or animal sheds Crypto parasites in the stool. Millions of Crypto parasites can be released in a bowel movement from an infected human or animal. Shedding of Crypto in the stool begins when the symptoms begin and can last for weeks after the symptoms (e.g., diarrhea) stop. You can become infected after accidentally swallowing the parasite. Crypto may be found in soil, food, water, or surfaces that have been contaminated with the feces from infected humans or animals. Crypto is not spread by contact with blood. Crypto can be spread:

- By putting something in your mouth or accidentally swallowing something that has come in contact with the stool of a person or animal infected with Crypto

- By swallowing recreational water contaminated with Crypto. Recreational water is water in swimming pools, hot tubs, Jacuzzis, fountains, lakes, rivers, springs, ponds, or streams. Recreational water can be contaminated with sewage or feces from humans or animals.

- By swallowing water or beverages contaminated with stool from infected humans or animals.

- By eating uncooked food contaminated with Crypto. Thoroughly wash with uncontaminated water all vegetables and fruits you plan to eat raw.

- By touching your mouth with contaminated hands. Hands can become contaminated through a variety of activities, such as touching surfaces (e.g., toys, bathroom fixtures, changing tables, diaper pails) that have been contaminated by stool from an infected person, changing diapers, caring for an infected person, and handling an infected cow or calf.

- By contact with skin around an infected person's anus (especially important with sex partners)

What Should I Do If I Think I May Have Cryptosporidiosis?

See your healthcare provider.

How Is a Cryptosporidiosis Infection Diagnosed?

Your healthcare provider will ask you to submit stool samples to see if you are infected. Because testing for Crypto can be difficult, you may be asked to submit several stool specimens over several days. Tests for Crypto are not routinely done in most laboratories. Therefore, your healthcare provider should specifically request testing for the parasite.

What Is the Treatment for Cryptosporidiosis?

People who are in poor health or who have a weakened immune system are at higher risk for more severe and more prolonged illness. If you have diarrhea, drink plenty of fluids to prevent dehydration. Rapid loss of fluids because of diarrhea can be life-threatening in babies; parents should consult their healthcare provider about fluid replacement therapy options for babies. Antidiarrheal medicine may help slow down diarrhea, but consult with your healthcare provider before taking it.

Nitazoxanide has been the U.S. Food and Drug Administration (FDA)-approved for treatment of diarrhea caused by *Cryptosporidium* in people with healthy immune systems and is available by prescription. However, the effectiveness of nitazoxanide in immunosuppressed individuals is unclear. Some drugs, such as paromomycin, may reduce the symptoms of Crypto and new drugs are being tested. However, Crypto is usually not cured in people with immunosuppression and may come back if the immune status worsens.

For persons with acquired immunodeficiency syndrome (AIDS), antiretroviral therapy that improves immune status will also decrease or eliminate symptoms of Crypto infection. See your healthcare provider to discuss treatment and antiretroviral therapy used to improve immune status.

Section 44.2

Toxoplasmosis

This section includes text excerpted from "Parasites-
Toxoplasmosis (*Toxoplasma* Infection)—Toxoplasmosis Frequently
Asked Questions (FAQs)," Centers for Disease Control and
Prevention (CDC), August 25, 2017.

What Is Toxoplasmosis?

A single-celled parasite called *Toxoplasma gondii* causes a disease known as toxoplasmosis. While the parasite is found throughout the world, more than 60 million people in the United States may be infected with the *Toxoplasma* parasite. Of those who are infected, very few have symptoms because a healthy person's immune system usually keeps the parasite from causing illness. However, pregnant women and individuals who have compromised immune systems should be cautious; for them, a *Toxoplasma* infection could cause serious health problems.

How Do People Get Toxoplasmosis?

A *Toxoplasma* infection occurs by:

- Eating undercooked, contaminated meat (especially pork, lamb, and venison)

- Accidental ingestion of undercooked, contaminated meat after handling it and not washing hands thoroughly (*Toxoplasma* cannot be absorbed through intact skin)

- Eating food that was contaminated by knives, utensils, cutting boards, and other foods that have had contact with raw, contaminated meat

- Drinking water contaminated with *Toxoplasma gondii*

- Accidentally swallowing the parasite through contact with cat feces that contain *Toxoplasma*. This might happen by:

  - Cleaning a cat's litter box when the cat has shed *Toxoplasma* in its feces

  - Touching or ingesting anything that has come into contact with cat feces that contain *Toxoplasma*

- Accidentally ingesting contaminated soil (e.g., not washing hands after gardening or eating unwashed fruits or vegetables from a garden)

- Mother-to-child (congenital) transmission

- Receiving an infected organ transplant or infected blood via transfusion, though this is rare

What Are the Signs and Symptoms of Toxoplasmosis?

Symptoms of the infection vary.

- Most people who become infected with *Toxoplasma gondii* are not aware of it.

- Some people who have toxoplasmosis may feel as if they have the "flu" with swollen lymph glands or muscle aches and pains that last for a month or more.

- Severe toxoplasmosis, causing damage to the brain, eyes, or other organs, can develop from an acute *Toxoplasma* infection or one that had occurred earlier in life and is now reactivated. Severe cases are more likely in individuals who have weak immune systems, though occasionally, even persons with healthy immune systems may experience eye damage from toxoplasmosis.

- Signs and symptoms of ocular toxoplasmosis can include reduced vision, blurred vision, pain (often with bright light), redness of the eye, and sometimes tearing.

- Ophthalmologists sometimes prescribe medicine to treat active disease. Whether or not medication is recommended depends on the size of the eye lesion, the location, and the characteristics of the lesion (acute active, versus chronic not progressing). An ophthalmologist will provide the best care for ocular toxoplasmosis.

- Most infants who are infected while still in the womb have no symptoms at birth, but they may develop symptoms later in life. A small percentage of infected newborns have serious eye or brain damage at birth.

Who Is at Risk for Developing Severe Toxoplasmosis?

People who are most likely to develop severe toxoplasmosis include:

- Infants born to mothers who are newly infected with *Toxoplasma gondii* during or just before pregnancy

- Persons with severely weakened immune systems, such as individuals with acquired immunodeficiency syndrome (AIDS), those taking certain types of chemotherapy, and those who have recently received an organ transplant.

What Should I Do If I Think I Am at Risk for Severe Toxoplasmosis?

If you are planning to become pregnant, your healthcare provider may test you for *Toxoplasma gondii*. If the test is positive it means you have already been infected sometime in your life. There usually is little need to worry about passing the infection to your baby. If the test is negative, take necessary precautions to avoid infection.

If you are already pregnant, you and your healthcare provider should discuss your risk for toxoplasmosis. Your healthcare provider may order a blood sample for testing.

If you have a weakened immune system, ask your doctor about having your blood tested for *Toxoplasma*. If your test is positive, your doctor can tell you if and when you need to take medicine to prevent the infection from reactivating. If your test is negative, it means you need to take precautions to avoid infection.

What Should I Do If I Think I May Have Toxoplasmosis?

If you suspect that you may have toxoplasmosis, talk to your health-care provider. Your provider may order one or more varieties of blood tests specific for toxoplasmosis. The results from the different tests can help your provider determine if you have a *Toxoplasma gondii* infection and whether it is a recent (acute) infection.

What Is the Treatment for Toxoplasmosis?

Once a diagnosis of toxoplasmosis is confirmed, you and your healthcare provider can discuss whether treatment is necessary. In an otherwise healthy person who is not pregnant, treatment usually is not needed. If symptoms occur, they typically go away within a few weeks to months. For pregnant women or persons who have weakened immune systems, medications are available to treat toxoplasmosis.

How Can I Prevent Toxoplasmosis?

There are several general sanitation and food safety steps you can take to reduce your chances of becoming infected with *Toxoplasma gondii*.

Cook food to safe temperatures. A food thermometer should be used to measure the internal temperature of cooked meat. Do not sample meat until it is cooked. The U.S. Department of Agriculture (USDA) recommends the following for meat preparation.

For Whole Cuts of Meat (Excluding Poultry)

Cook to at least 145°F (63°C) as measured with a food thermometer placed in the thickest part of the meat, then allow the meat to rest* for three minutes before carving or consuming.

For Ground Meat (Excluding Poultry)

Cook to at least 160°F (71°C); ground meats do not require a rest* time.

For All Poultry (Whole Cuts and Ground)

Cook to at least 165°F (74°C), and for whole poultry allow the meat to rest* for three minutes before carving or consuming.

*According to USDA, "A 'rest time' is the amount of time the product remains at the final temperature, after it has been removed from a grill, oven, or other heat source. During the three minutes after meat is removed from the heat source, its temperature remains constant or continues to rise, which destroys pathogens."

Chapter 45

HIV/AIDS and Co-Occurring Viral Infections

Chapter Contents

Section 45.1

Cytomegalovirus

This section contains text excerpted from the following
sources: Text in this section begins with excerpts from
"Cytomegalovirus (CMV) and Congenital CMV Infection," Centers
for Disease Control and Prevention (CDC), June 17, 2016; Text
beginning with the heading "Transmission" is excerpted from "HIV/
AIDS—Cytomegalovirus (CMV)," U.S. Department of Veterans
Affairs (VA), February 8, 2018.

Cytomegalovirus, or CMV, is a common virus that infects people of all ages. In the United States, nearly one in three children are already infected with CMV by age 5 years. Over half of adults by age 40 have been infected with CMV. Once CMV is in a person's body, it stays there for life and can reactivate. A person can also be reinfected with a different strain (variety) of the virus.

Most people infected with CMV show no signs or symptoms. That's because a healthy person's immune system usually keeps the virus from causing illness. However, CMV infection can cause serious health problems for people with weakened immune systems, as well as babies infected with the virus before they are born (congenital CMV).

Transmission

Cytomegalovirus (or CMV) is passed by close contact through sex and through saliva, urine, and other body fluids. It can be passed from mother to child during pregnancy and by breastfeeding. If you are not infected, using condoms during sex may help prevent infection.

Signs and Symptoms

Many people are infected with this virus, though they have no symptoms. In people with HIV who have low CD4 counts, the infection can be extremely serious. Symptoms can include:

- Blind spots in vision, loss of peripheral vision

- Headache, difficulty concentrating, sleepiness

- Mouth ulcers

- Pain in the abdomen, bloody diarrhea

- Fever, fatigue, weight loss

- Shortness of breath

- Lower back pain

- Confusion, apathy, withdrawal, personality changes

Treatment

Drugs are available to keep symptoms of the infection under control. Anti-human immunodeficiency virus (HIV) drugs can improve the condition, too. If you have CMV and haven't started taking drugs for HIV, it may be best to wait until you have been on treatment for CMV for a few weeks.

Treatment can prevent further loss of vision but cannot reverse existing damage. If you experience any vision problems, tell your provider immediately.

Section 45.2

Genital Herpes

This section includes text excerpted from "Genital Herpes—Genital Herpes-CDC Fact Sheet (Detailed)," Centers for Disease Control and Prevention (CDC), January 31, 2017.

What Is Genital Herpes?

Genital herpes is a sexually transmitted disease (STD) caused by the herpes simplex virus type 1 (HSV-1) or type 2 (HSV-2).

How Common Is Genital Herpes?

Genital herpes infection is common in the United States. The Centers for Disease Control and Prevention (CDC) estimates that, annually, 776,000 people in the United States get new herpes infections. Nationwide, 15.7 percent of persons aged 14–49 years have HSV-2 infection, however, the prevalence of genital herpes infection is higher than that because an increasing number of genital herpes infections are caused by HSV-1. Oral HSV-1 infection is typically acquired in childhood; because the prevalence of oral HSV-1 infection has declined in recent decades, people may have become more susceptible to contracting a genital herpes infection from HSV-1.

HSV-2 infection is more common among women than among men (20.3% versus 10.6% in 14– 49-year-olds), possibly because genital infection is more easily transmitted from men to women than from women to men during penile-vaginal sex. HSV-2 infection is more common among non-Hispanic blacks (39.2%) than among non-Hispanic whites (12.3%). This disparity remains, even among persons with similar numbers of lifetime sexual partners. For example, among persons with 2– 4-lifetime sexual partners, HSV-2 is still more prevalent among non-Hispanic blacks (34.3%) than among non-Hispanic whites (9.1%) or Mexican Americans (13.0%). Most infected persons may be unaware of their infection; in the United States, an estimated 87.4 percent of 14– 49-year-olds infected with HSV-2 have never received a clinical diagnosis. The percentage of persons aged 14–49 in the United States who are infected with HSV-2 decreased from 21.0 percent in 1988–1994 to 15.7 percent in 2005–2010.

How Do People Get Genital Herpes?

Infections are transmitted through contact with HSV in herpes lesions, mucosal surfaces, genital secretions, or oral secretions. HSV-1 and HSV-2 can be shed from normal-appearing oral or genital mucosa or skin. Generally, a person can only get HSV-2 infection during genital contact with someone who has a genital HSV-2 infection. However, receiving oral sex from a person with an oral HSV-1 infection can result in getting a genital HSV-1 infection. Transmission commonly occurs from contact with an infected partner who does not have visible lesions and who may not know that he or she is infected. In persons with asymptomatic HSV-2 infections, genital HSV shedding occurs on 10.2 percent of days, compared to 20.1 percent of days among those with symptomatic infections.

What Are the Symptoms of Genital Herpes?

Most individuals infected with HSV are asymptomatic or have very mild symptoms that go unnoticed or are mistaken for another skin condition. When symptoms do occur, herpes lesions typically appear as one or more vesicles, or small blisters, on or around the genitals, rectum or mouth. The average incubation period for an initial herpes infection is 4 days (range, 2–12) after exposure. The vesicles break and leave painful ulcers that may take two to four weeks to heal after the initial herpes infection. Experiencing these symptoms is referred to as having first herpes "outbreak" or episode.

Clinical manifestations of genital herpes differ between the first and recurrent (i.e., subsequent) outbreaks. The first outbreak of herpes is often associated with a longer duration of herpetic lesions, increased viral shedding (making HSV transmission more likely) and systemic symptoms including fever, body aches, swollen lymph nodes, or headache. Recurrent outbreaks of genital herpes are common, and many patients who recognize recurrences have prodromal symptoms, either localized genital pain, or tingling or shooting pains in the legs, hips or buttocks, which occur hours to days before the eruption of herpetic lesions. Symptoms of recurrent outbreaks are typically shorter in duration and less severe than the first outbreak of genital herpes. Long-term studies have indicated that the number of symptomatic recurrent outbreaks may decrease over time. Recurrences and subclinical shedding are much less frequent for genital HSV-1 infection than for genital HSV-2 infection.

What Are the Complications of Genital Herpes?

Genital herpes may cause painful genital ulcers that can be severe and persistent in persons with suppressed immune systems, such as HIV-infected persons. Both HSV-1 and HSV-2 can also cause rare but serious complications such as aseptic meningitis (inflammation of the linings of the brain). Development of extragenital lesions (e.g., buttocks, groin, thigh, finger, or eye) may occur during the course of infection.

Some persons who contract genital herpes have concerns about how it will impact their overall health, sex life, and relationships. There can be can be considerable embarrassment, shame, and stigma associated with a herpes diagnosis that can substantially interfere with a patient's relationships. Clinicians can address these concerns by encouraging patients to recognize that while herpes is not curable, it is a manageable condition. Three important steps that providers can take for their newly-diagnosed patients are: giving information, providing support resources, and helping define treatment and prevention options. Patients can be counseled that risk of genital herpes transmission can be reduced, but not eliminated, by disclosure of infection to sexual partners, avoiding sex during a recurrent outbreak, use of suppressive antiviral therapy, and consistent condom use. Since a diagnosis of genital herpes may affect perceptions about existing or future sexual relationships, it is important for patients to understand how to talk to sexual partners about STDs.

There are also potential complications for a pregnant woman and her newborn child.

What Is the Link between Genital Herpes and Human Immunodeficiency Virus (HIV)?

Genital ulcerative disease caused by herpes makes it easier to transmit and acquire human immunodeficiency virus (HIV) infection sexually. There is an estimated 2- to 4-fold increased risk of acquiring HIV, if individuals with genital herpes infection are genitally exposed to HIV. Ulcers or breaks in the skin or mucous membranes (lining of the mouth, vagina, and rectum) from a herpes infection may compromise the protection normally provided by the skin and mucous membranes against infections, including HIV. In addition, having genital herpes increases the number of CD4 cells (the target cell for HIV entry) in the genital mucosa. In persons with both HIV and genital herpes, local activation of HIV replication at the site of genital herpes infection can increase the risk that HIV will be transmitted during contact with the mouth, vagina, or rectum of an HIV-uninfected sex partner.

How Does Genital Herpes Affect a Pregnant Woman and Her Baby?

Neonatal herpes is one of the most serious complications of genital herpes. Healthcare providers should ask all pregnant women if they have a history of genital herpes. Herpes infection can be passed from mother to child during pregnancy or childbirth, or babies may be infected shortly after birth, resulting in a potentially fatal neonatal herpes infection. Infants born to women who acquire genital herpes close to the time of delivery and are shedding virus at delivery are at a much higher risk for developing neonatal herpes, compared with women who have recurrent genital herpes. Thus, it is important that women avoid contracting herpes during pregnancy. Women should be counseled to abstain from intercourse during the third trimester with partners known to have or suspected of having genital herpes.

While women with genital herpes may be offered antiviral medication late in pregnancy through delivery to reduce the risk of a recurrent herpes outbreak, third-trimester antiviral prophylaxis has not been shown to decrease the risk of herpes transmission to the neonate. Routine serologic HSV screening of pregnant women is not recommended. However, at onset of labor, all women should undergo careful examination and questioning to evaluate for presence of prodromal symptoms or herpetic lesions. If herpes symptoms are present a cesarean delivery is recommended to prevent HSV transmission to the infant. There are detailed guidelines for how to manage asymptomatic infants born to women with active genital herpes lesions.

How Is Genital Herpes Diagnosed?

The preferred HSV tests for patients with active genital ulcers are detection of HSV deoxyribonucleic acid (DNA) by nucleic acid amplification tests such as polymerase chain reaction (PCR), or isolation by viral culture. HSV culture requires collection of a sample from the lesion and, once viral growth is seen, specific cell staining to differentiate between HSV-1 and HSV-2. However, culture sensitivity is low, especially for recurrent lesions, and declines as lesions heal. PCR is more sensitive, allows for more rapid and accurate results, and is increasingly being used. Because viral shedding is intermittent, failure to detect HSV by culture or PCR does not indicate an absence of HSV infection. Tzanck preparations are insensitive and nonspecific and should not be used.

Herpes serologic tests are blood tests that detect antibodies to the herpes virus. Providers should only request type-specific glycoprotein G (gG)-based serologic assays when serology is performed for their patients. Several enzyme-linked immunosorbent assay (ELISA)-based serologic tests are the U.S. Food and Administration (FDA) approved and available commercially. While the presence of HSV-2 antibody can be presumed to reflect genital infection, patients should be counseled that the presence of HSV-1 antibody may represent either oral or genital infection. The sensitivities of glycoprotein G type-specific serologic tests for HSV-2 vary from 80–98 percent; false-negative results might be more frequent at early stages of infection. The most commonly used test, HerpeSelect HSV-2 Elisa might be falsely positive at low index values (1.1–3.5).

Such low values should be confirmed with another test such as Biokit or the Western Blot (WB). Negative HSV-1 results should be interpreted with caution because some ELISA-based serologic tests are insensitive for detection of HSV-1 antibody. Immunoglobulin M (IgM) testing for HSV-1 or HSV-2 is not useful, because IgM tests are not type-specific and might be positive during recurrent genital or oral episodes of herpes.

For the symptomatic patient, testing with both virologic and serologic assays can determine whether it is a new infection or a newly-recognized old infection. A primary infection would be supported by a positive virologic test and a negative serologic test, while the diagnosis of recurrent disease would be supported by positive virologic and serologic test results.

CDC does not recommend screening for HSV-1 or HSV-2 in the general population. Several scenarios where type-specific serologic HSV tests may be useful include

- Patients with recurrent genital symptoms or atypical symptoms and negative HSV PCR or culture
- Patients with a clinical diagnosis of genital herpes but no laboratory confirmation
- Patients who report having a partner with genital herpes
- Patients presenting for an STD evaluation (especially those with multiple sex partners)
- Persons with HIV infection
- MSM at increased risk for HIV acquisition

Please note that while type-specific herpes testing can determine if a person is infected with HSV-1 or HSV-2 (or both), *there is no commercially available test to determine if a herpes infection in one individual was acquired from another specific person.* CDC encourages patients to discuss any herpes questions and concerns with their healthcare provider or seek counsel at an STD clinic.

Is There a Cure or Treatment for Herpes?

There is no cure for herpes. Antiviral medications can, however, prevent or shorten outbreaks during the period of time the person takes the medication. In addition, daily suppressive therapy (i.e., daily use of antiviral medication) for herpes can reduce the likelihood of transmission to partners.

There is currently no commercially available vaccine that is protective against genital herpes infection. Candidate vaccines are in clinical trials.

How Can Herpes Be Prevented?

Correct and consistent use of latex condoms can reduce, but not eliminate, the risk of transmitting or acquiring genital herpes because herpes virus shedding can occur in areas that are not covered by a condom.

The surest way to avoid transmission of STDs, including genital herpes, is to abstain from sexual contact, or to be in a long-term mutually monogamous relationship with a partner who has been tested for STDs and is known to be uninfected.

Persons with herpes should abstain from sexual activity with partners when herpes lesions or other symptoms of herpes are present. It is important to know that even if a person does not have any symptoms, he or she can still infect sex partners. Sex partners of infected persons should be advised that they may become infected and they should use condoms to reduce the risk. Sex partners can seek testing to determine if they are infected with HSV.

Daily treatment with valacyclovir decreases the rate of HSV-2 transmission in discordant, heterosexual couples in which the source partner has a history of genital HSV-2 infection. Such couples should be encouraged to consider suppressive antiviral therapy as part of a strategy to prevent transmission, in addition to consistent condom use and avoidance of sexual activity during recurrences.

Section 45.3

Herpes Zoster Virus

This section includes text excerpted from "Shingles (Herpes Zoster)—About Shingles (Herpes Zoster)," Centers for Disease Control and Prevention (CDC), October 17, 2017.

Almost 1 out of every 3 people in the United States will develop shingles, also known as herpes zoster, in their lifetime. There are an estimated 1 million cases of shingles each year in this country. Anyone who has recovered from chickenpox may develop shingles; even children can get shingles. However, the risk of shingles increases as you get older.

Some people have a greater risk of getting shingles. This includes people who:

- Have medical conditions that keep their immune systems from working properly, such as certain cancers like leukemia and lymphoma, and human immunodeficiency virus (HIV), and

- Receive immunosuppressive drugs, such as steroids and drugs that are given after organ transplantation.

Most people who develop shingles have only one episode during their lifetime. However, a person can have a second or even a third episode.

Cause

Shingles is caused by the varicella-zoster virus (VZV), the same virus that causes chickenpox. After a person recovers from chickenpox, the virus stays dormant (inactive) in the body. Scientists aren't sure why the virus can reactivate years later, causing shingles.

Signs and Symptoms

Shingles is a painful rash that develops on one side of the face or body. The rash consists of blisters that typically scab over in 7–10 days. The rash usually clears up within 2–4 weeks.

Before the rash develops, people often have pain, itching, or tingling in the area where the rash will develop. This may happen anywhere from 1–5 days before the rash appears.

Most commonly, the rash occurs in a single stripe around either the left or the right side of the body. In other cases, the rash occurs on one side of the face. In rare cases (usually among people with weakened immune systems), the rash may be more widespread and look similar to a chickenpox rash. Shingles can affect the eye and cause loss of vision.

Other symptoms of shingles can include

- Fever

- Headache

- Chills

- Upset stomach

Transmission

Shingles cannot be passed from one person to another. However, the virus that causes shingles, the varicella-zoster virus, can spread from a person with active shingles to cause chickenpox in someone who had never had chickenpox or received chickenpox vaccine. The virus is spread through direct contact with fluid from the rash blisters caused by shingles.

A person with active shingles can spread the virus when the rash is in the blister-phase. A person is not infectious before the blisters appear. Once the rash has developed crusts, the person is no longer infectious.

Shingles is less contagious than chickenpox and the risk of a person with shingles spreading the virus is low if the rash is covered.

If you have shingles, you should:

- Cover the rash

- Avoid touching or scratching the rash

- Wash your hands often to prevent the spread of varicella-zoster virus

- Avoid contact with the people below until your rash has developed crusts:

- pregnant women who have never had chickenpox or the chickenpox vaccine;

- premature or low birth weight infants; and

- people with weakened immune systems, such as people receiving immunosuppressive medications or undergoing chemotherapy, organ transplant recipients, and people with human immunodeficiency virus (HIV) infection.

Complications

The most common complication of shingles is a condition called postherpetic neuralgia (PHN). People with PHN have severe pain in the areas where they had the shingles rash, even after the rash clears up. The pain from PHN may be severe and debilitating, but it usually resolves in a few weeks or months. Some people can have pain from PHN for many years and it can interfere with daily life.

A person's risk of PHN also increases with age. Older adults are more likely to have PHN and to have longer lasting and more severe pain. About 10–13 percent of people who get shingles will experience PHN. PHN occurs rarely among people less than 40 years of age.

Shingles may lead to serious complications involving the eye such as vision loss. Very rarely, shingles can also lead to pneumonia, hearing problems, blindness, brain inflammation (encephalitis), or death.

Prevention

The only way to reduce the risk of developing shingles and the long-term pain from postherpetic neuralgia (PHN) is to get vaccinated. The Centers for Disease Control and Prevention (CDC) recommends that healthy adults 50 years and older get two doses of the shingles vaccine called Shingrix® to protect against shingles and the complications caused by the disease. Shingles vaccine is available in pharmacies and doctor's offices. Talk with your healthcare professional if you have questions about shingles vaccination.

Treatment

Several antiviral medicines—acyclovir, valacyclovir, and famciclovir—are available to treat shingles and shorten the length and severity of illness. People with shingles should start taking these medicines as soon as possible after the rash appears to be the most effective. People who have, or think they might have, shingles should call their healthcare provider as soon as possible to discuss treatment options.

Analgesics (pain medicine) may help relieve the pain caused by shingles. Wet compresses, calamine lotion, and colloidal oatmeal baths may help relieve some of the itching.

Section 45.4

Human Papillomavirus

This section includes text excerpted from "Human Papillomavirus (HPV)—Genital HPV Infection-Fact Sheet," Centers for Disease Control and Prevention (CDC), November 16, 2017.

What Is Human Papillomavirus (HPV)?

Human papillomavirus (HPV) is the most common sexually transmitted infection (STI). HPV is a different virus than human immunodeficiency virus (HIV) and herpes simplex virus (HSV) (herpes).

79 million Americans, most in their late teens and early 20s, are infected with HPV. There are many different types of HPV. Some types can cause health problems including genital warts and cancers. But there are vaccines that can stop these health problems from happening.

How Is HPV Spread?

You can get HPV by having vaginal, anal, or oral sex with someone who has the virus. It is most commonly spread during vaginal or anal sex. HPV can be passed even when an infected person has no signs or symptoms.

Anyone who is sexually active can get HPV, even if you have had sex with only one person. You also can develop symptoms years after you have sex with someone who is infected. This makes it hard to know when you first became infected.

Does HPV Cause Health Problems?

In most cases, HPV goes away on its own and does not cause any health problems. But when HPV does not go away, it can cause health problems like genital warts and cancer.

Genital warts usually appear as a small bump or group of bumps in the genital area. They can be small or large, raised or flat, or shaped like a cauliflower. A healthcare provider can usually diagnose warts by looking at the genital area.

Does HPV Cause Cancer?

HPV can cause cervical and other cancers including cancer of the vulva, vagina, penis, or anus. It can also cause cancer in the back of the throat, including the base of the tongue and tonsils (called oropharyngeal cancer).

Cancer often takes years, even decades, to develop after a person gets HPV. The types of HPV that can cause genital warts are not the same as the types of HPV that can cause cancers.

There is no way to know which people who have HPV will develop cancer or other health problems. People with weak immune systems (including those with human immunodeficiency virus (HIV) / acquired immunodeficiency syndrome (AIDS) may be less able to fight off HPV. They may also be more likely to develop health problems from HPV.

How Can I Avoid HPV and the Health Problems It Can Cause?

You can do several things to lower your chances of getting HPV.

Get vaccinated. The HPV vaccine is safe and effective. It can protect against diseases (including cancers) caused by HPV when given in the recommended age groups. The Centers for Disease Control and Prevention (CDC) recommends 11–12 year olds get two doses of HPV vaccine to protect against cancers caused by HPV.

Get screened for cervical cancer. Routine screening for women aged 21–65 years old can prevent cervical cancer.

If you are sexually active

- Use latex condoms the right way every time you have sex. This can lower your chances of getting HPV. But HPV can infect areas not covered by a condom—so condoms may not fully protect against getting HPV;

- Be in a mutually monogamous relationship—or have sex only with someone who only has sex with you.

Who Should Get Vaccinated?

All boys and girls ages 11 or 12 years should get vaccinated. Catch-up vaccines are recommended for boys and men through age 21 and for girls and women through age 26, if they did not get vaccinated when they were younger.

The vaccine is also recommended for gay and bisexual men (or any man who has sex with a man) through age 26. It is also recommended for men and women with compromised immune systems (including those living with HIV/AIDS) through age 26, if they did not get fully vaccinated when they were younger.

How Do I Know If I Have HPV?

There is no test to find out a person's "HPV status." Also, there is no approved HPV test to find HPV in the mouth or throat.

There are HPV tests that can be used to screen for cervical cancer. These tests are only recommended for screening in women aged 30 years and older. HPV tests are not recommended to screen men, adolescents, or women under the age of 30 years.

Most people with HPV do not know they are infected and never develop symptoms or health problems from it. Some people find out they have HPV when they get genital warts. Women may find out they have HPV when they get an abnormal Pap test result (during cervical cancer screening). Others may only find out once they've developed more serious problems from HPV, such as cancers.

How Common Is HPV and the Health Problems Caused by HPV?

HPV (the virus): About 79 million Americans are currently infected with HPV. About 14 million people become newly infected each year. HPV is so common that almost every person who is sexually-active will get HPV at some time in their life if they don't get the HPV vaccine.

Health problems related to HPV include genital warts and cervical cancer.

Genital warts: Before HPV vaccines were introduced, roughly 340,000–360,000 women and men were affected by genital warts caused by HPV every year.* Also, about one in 100 sexually active adults in the United States has genital warts at any given time.

Cervical cancer: Every year, nearly 12,000 women living in the United States will be diagnosed with cervical cancer, and more than 4,000 women die from cervical cancer—even with screening and treatment.

There are other conditions and cancers caused by HPV that occur in people living in the United States. Every year, approximately 19,400 women and 12,100 men are affected by cancers caused by HPV.

These figures only look at the number of people who sought care for genital warts. This could be an underestimate of the actual number of people who get genital warts.

I'm Pregnant. Will Having HPV Affect My Pregnancy?

If you are pregnant and have HPV, you can get genital warts or develop abnormal cell changes on your cervix. Abnormal cell changes can be found with routine cervical cancer screening. You should get routine cervical cancer screening even when you are pregnant.

Can I Be Treated for HPV or Health Problems Caused by HPV?

There is no treatment for the virus itself. However, there are treatments for the health problems that HPV can cause:

1. **Genital warts** can be treated by your healthcare provider or with prescription medication. If left untreated, genital warts may go away, stay the same, or grow in size or number.

2. **Cervical precancer** can be treated. Women who get routine Pap tests and follow up as needed can identify problems before cancer develops. Prevention is always better than treatment.

3. **Other HPV-related cancers** are also more treatable when diagnosed and treated early.

Section 45.5

Progressive Multifocal Leukoencephalopathy

This section includes text excerpted from "Progressive Multifocal Leukoencephalopathy Information Page," National Institute of Neurological Disorders and Stroke (NINDS), May 24, 2017.

Progressive multifocal leukoencephalopathy (PML) is a disease of the white matter of the brain, caused by a virus infection that targets cells that make myelin—the material that insulates nerve cells (neurons). Polyomavirus John Cunningham (JC) (often called JC virus) is carried by a majority of people and is harmless except among those with lowered immune defenses. The disease is rare and occurs in patients undergoing chronic corticosteroid or immunosuppressive therapy for organ transplant, or individuals with cancer (such as Hodgkin's disease or lymphoma). Individuals with autoimmune conditions such as multiple sclerosis, rheumatoid arthritis, and systemic lupus erythematosis—some of whom are treated with biological therapies that allow JC virus reactivation—are at risk for PML as well. PML is most common among individuals with HIV-1 infection / acquired immune deficiency syndrome (AIDS). Studies estimate that prior to effective antiretroviral therapy, as many as 5 percent of persons infected with HIV-1 eventually develop PML that is an AIDS-defining illness. However, current HIV therapy using antiretroviral drugs (ART), which effectively restores immune system function, allows as many as half of all HIV-PML patients to survive, although they may sometimes have an inflammatory reaction in the regions of the brain affected by PML. The symptoms of PML are diverse, since they are related to the location and amount of damage in the brain, and may evolve over the course of several weeks to months The most prominent symptoms are clumsiness; progressive weakness; and visual, speech, and sometimes personality changes. The progression of deficits leads to life-threatening disability and (frequently) death. A diagnosis of PML can be made following brain biopsy or by combining observations of a progressive course of the disease, consistent white matter lesions visible on a magnetic resonance imaging (MRI) scan, and the detection of the JC virus in spinal fluid.

Treatment

Currently, the best available therapy is reversal of the immune-deficient state, since there are no effective drugs that block virus infection without toxicity. Reversal may be achieved by using plasma exchange to accelerate the removal of the therapeutic agents that put patients at risk for PML. In the case of HIV-associated PML, immediately beginning antiretroviral therapy will benefit most individuals. Several new drugs that laboratory tests found effective against infection are being used in PML patients with special permission of the U.S. Food and Drug Administration (FDA). Hexadecyloxypropyl-Cidofovir (CMX001) is currently being studied as a treatment option for JVC because of its ability to suppress JVC by inhibiting viral deoxyribonucleic acid DNA replication.

Prognosis

In general, PML has a mortality rate of 30–50 percent in the first few months following diagnosis but depends on the severity of the underlying disease and treatment received. Those who survive PML can be left with severe neurological disabilities.

Section 45.6

Viral Hepatitis

This section contains text excerpted from the following
sources: Text beginning with the heading "What Is Viral
Hepatitis?" is excerpted from "Hepatitis (Viral)," National Institute
of Diabetes and Digestive and Kidney Diseases (NIDDK), May
2017; Text beginning with the heading What Is the Connection
between HIV and Hepatitis B Virus?" is excerpted from "HIV and
Hepatitis B," AIDSinfo, U.S. Department of Health and Human
Services (HHS), July 24, 2017; Text beginning with the heading
What Is the Connection between HIV and Hepatitis C Virus?" is
excerpted from "HIV and Hepatitis C," AIDSinfo, U.S. Department
of Health and Human Services (HHS), July 25, 2017.

What Is Viral Hepatitis?

Viral hepatitis is an infection that causes liver inflammation and
damage. Inflammation is swelling that occurs when tissues of the
body become injured or infected. Inflammation can damage organs.
Researchers have discovered several different viruses that cause hepatitis, including hepatitis A, B, C, D, and E.

Hepatitis A and hepatitis E typically spread through contact with
food or water that has been contaminated by an infected person's stool.
People may also get hepatitis E by eating undercooked pork, deer, or
shellfish.

Hepatitis B, hepatitis C, and hepatitis D spread through contact
with an infected person's blood. Hepatitis B and D may also spread
through contact with other body fluids. This contact can occur in many
ways, including sharing drug needles or having unprotected sex.

The hepatitis A and E viruses typically cause only acute, or short-
term, infections. In an acute infection, your body is able to fight off the
infection and the virus goes away.

The hepatitis B, C, and D viruses can cause acute and chronic,
or long-lasting, infections. Chronic hepatitis occurs when your body
isn't able to fight off the hepatitis virus and the virus does not go
away. Chronic hepatitis can lead to complications such as cirrhosis, liver failure, and liver cancer. Early diagnosis and treatment of
chronic hepatitis can prevent or lower your chances of developing
these complications.

When doctors can't find the cause of a person's hepatitis, they may
call this condition non-A–E hepatitis or hepatitis X. Experts think

that unknown viruses other than hepatitis A, B, C, D, and E may cause some cases of hepatitis. Researchers are working to identify these viruses.

Although non-A–E hepatitis is most often acute, it can become chronic.

What Is Hepatitis A?

Hepatitis A is a viral infection that causes liver inflammation and damage. Inflammation is swelling that occurs when tissues of the body become injured or infected. Inflammation can damage organs.

Viruses invade normal cells in your body. Many viruses cause infections that can be spread from person to person. The hepatitis A virus typically spreads through contact with food or water that has been contaminated by an infected person's stool.

Hepatitis A is an acute or short-term infection, which means people usually get better without treatment after a few weeks. Hepatitis A does not lead to long-term complications, such as cirrhosis, because the infection only lasts a short time.

You can take steps to protect yourself from hepatitis A, including getting the hepatitis A vaccine. If you have hepatitis A, you can take steps to prevent spreading hepatitis A to others.

What Is Hepatitis B?

Hepatitis B is a viral infection that causes liver inflammation and damage. Inflammation is swelling that occurs when tissues of the body become injured or infected. Inflammation can damage organs.

Viruses invade normal cells in your body. Many viruses cause infections that can be spread from person to person. The hepatitis B virus spreads through contact with an infected person's blood, semen, or other body fluids.

The hepatitis B virus can cause an acute or chronic infection. You can take steps to protect yourself from hepatitis B, including getting the hepatitis B vaccine. If you have hepatitis B, you can take steps to prevent spreading hepatitis B to others.

What Is Hepatitis C?

Hepatitis C is a viral infection that causes liver inflammation and damage. Inflammation is swelling that occurs when tissues of the body become injured or infected. Inflammation can damage organs.

Viruses invade normal cells in your body. Many viruses cause infections that can be spread from person to person. The hepatitis C virus spreads through contact with an infected person's blood.

Hepatitis C can cause an acute or chronic infection. Although no vaccine for hepatitis C is available, you can take steps to protect yourself from hepatitis C. If you have hepatitis C, talk with your doctor about treatment. Medicines can cure most cases of hepatitis C.

What Is Hepatitis D?

Hepatitis D is a viral infection that causes liver inflammation and damage. Inflammation is swelling that occurs when tissues of the body become injured or infected. Inflammation can damage organs.

Viruses invade normal cells in your body. Many viruses cause infections that can spread from person to person.

The hepatitis D virus is unusual because it can only infect you when you also have a hepatitis B virus infection. In this way, hepatitis D is a double infection. You can protect yourself from hepatitis D by protecting yourself from hepatitis B by getting the hepatitis B vaccine.

Hepatitis D spreads the same way that hepatitis B spreads, through contact with an infected person's blood or other body fluids. The hepatitis D virus can cause an acute or chronic infection, or both.

What Is Hepatitis E?

Hepatitis E is a viral infection that causes liver inflammation and damage. Inflammation is swelling that occurs when tissues of the body become injured or infected. Inflammation can damage organs.

Viruses invade normal cells in your body. The hepatitis E virus has different types that spread in different ways.

Some types are spread by drinking contaminated water. These types are more common in developing countries, including parts of Africa, Asia, Central America, and the Middle East.

Other types are spread by eating undercooked pork or wild game, such as deer. These types are more common in developed countries, such as the United States, Australia, Japan, and parts of Europe and East Asia. Hepatitis E typically causes short-term (acute) infection.

What Is the Connection between HIV and Hepatitis B Virus?

Both HIV and HBV spread in semen, blood, or other body fluids. Therefore, the main risk factors for HIV and HBV are the same: unprotected sex (sex without a condom) and injection drug use.

According to the Centers for Disease Control and Prevention (CDC), approximately 10% of people with HIV in the United States also have HBV. Infection with both HIV and HBV is called HIV/HBV coinfection.

Chronic HBV advances faster to cirrhosis, end-stage liver disease, and liver cancer in people with HIV/HBV coinfection than in people with only HBV infection. But chronic HBV doesn't appear to cause HIV to advance faster in people with HIV/HBV coinfection.

Should People with HIV Get Tested for Hepatitis B Virus?

Every person who has HIV should get tested for HBV. Testing can detect HBV infection even when a person has no symptoms of the disease.

There are several HBV blood tests. Results of different tests have different meanings. For example, a positive hepatitis B surface antigen (HBsAg) test result shows that a person has acute or chronic HBV and can spread the virus to others.

What Is the Connection between HIV and Hepatitis C Virus?

Because both HIV and HCV can spread in blood, a major risk factor for both HIV and HCV infection is injection drug use. Sharing needles or other drug injection equipment increases the risk of contact with HIV- or HCV-infected blood.

According to the Centers for Disease Control and Prevention (CDC), approximately 25% of people with HIV in the United States also have HCV. Among people with HIV who inject drugs, about 50% to 90% also have HCV. Infection with both HIV and HCV is called HIV/HCV coinfection.

In people with HIV/HCV coinfection, HIV may cause chronic HCV to advance faster. Whether HCV causes HIV to advance faster is unclear.

Should People with HIV Get Tested for Hepatitis C Virus?

Every person who has HIV should get tested for HCV. Usually, a person will first get an HCV antibody test. This test checks for HCV antibodies in the blood. (HCV antibodies are disease-fighting proteins that the body produces in response to HCV infection.) A positive result on an HCV antibody test means that the person has been exposed to HCV at some point in their life.

A positive result on an HCV antibody test must be confirmed by a second, follow-up test. The follow-up test checks to see if HCV is present in the person's blood. A positive result on this test confirms that a person has HCV.

Chapter 46

HIV/AIDS and Co-Occurring Cancers

Chapter Contents

Section 46.1

HIV Infection and Cancer Risk

This section includes text excerpted from "HIV Infection and
Cancer Risk," National Cancer Institute (NCI), September 14, 2017.

Do People Infected with Human Immunodeficiency Virus (HIV) Have an Increased Risk of Cancer?

Yes. People infected with human immunodeficiency virus (HIV)
have a substantially higher risk of some types of cancer compared
with uninfected people of the same age. The general term for these
cancers is "HIV-associated cancers." Three of these cancers are known
as "acquired immunodeficiency syndrome (AIDS)-defining cancers"
or "AIDS-defining malignancies": Kaposi sarcoma, aggressive B-cell
non-Hodgkin lymphoma, and cervical cancer. A diagnosis of any of these
cancers in someone infected with HIV confirms a diagnosis of AIDS.

Compared with the general population, people infected with HIV
are currently about 500 times more likely to be diagnosed with Kaposi
sarcoma, 12 times more likely to be diagnosed with non-Hodgkin lymphoma, and, among women, 3 times more likely to be diagnosed with
cervical cancer.

In addition, people infected with HIV are at higher risk of several
other types of cancer (collectively called "non–AIDS-defining cancers").
These other malignancies include cancers of the anus, liver, oral cavity/
pharynx, and lung, and Hodgkin lymphoma.

People infected with HIV are 19 times more likely to be diagnosed
with anal cancer, 3 times as likely to be diagnosed with liver cancer,
2 times as likely to be diagnosed with lung cancer, about 2 times as
likely to be diagnosed with oral cavity/pharynx cancer, and about 8
times more likely to be diagnosed with Hodgkin lymphoma compared
with the general population.

In addition to being linked to an increased risk of cancer, HIV
infection is associated with an increased risk of dying from cancer.
HIV-infected people with a range of cancer types are more likely to
die of their cancer than HIV-uninfected people with these cancers.

Why Might People Infected with HIV Have a Higher Risk of Some Types of Cancer?

Infection with HIV weakens the immune system and reduces
the body's ability to fight viral infections that may lead to cancer.

The viruses that are most likely to cause cancer in people with HIV are:

- Kaposi sarcoma-associated herpesvirus (KSHV), also known as human herpesvirus 8 (HHV-8), which causes Kaposi sarcoma and some subtypes of lymphoma

- Epstein-Barr virus (EBV), which causes some subtypes of non-Hodgkin and Hodgkin lymphoma

- Human papillomaviruses (HPV), high-risk types of which cause cervical cancer, most anal cancers, and oropharyngeal, penile, vaginal, and vulvar cancer

- Hepatitis B virus (HBV) and hepatitis C virus (HCV), which both cause liver cancer

- HIV-infected persons are more likely to be infected with these viruses than people in the general population.

In addition, the prevalence of some traditional risk factors for cancer, especially smoking (a known cause of lung and other cancers) and heavy alcohol use (which can increase the risk of liver cancer), is higher among people infected with HIV. Also, because people infected with HIV have compromised immune systems, both immunosuppression and inflammation may have direct or indirect roles in the development of some cancers that are elevated in people infected with HIV.

The poorer cancer survival of HIV-infected people may result, at least in part, from the weakened immune system in such individuals. The increased risk of death could also result from the cancer is more advanced at diagnosis, delays in cancer treatment, or poorer access to appropriate cancer treatment.

Has the Introduction of Antiretroviral Therapy Changed the Cancer Risk of People Infected with HIV?

The introduction of highly active antiretroviral therapy (HAART), also called combination antiretroviral therapy (cART), starting in the mid-1990s greatly reduced the incidence of certain cancers in HIV-infected patients, especially Kaposi sarcoma and non-Hodgkin lymphoma. The likely explanation for this reduced incidence is that cART lowers the amount of HIV circulating in the blood, thereby allowing partial restoration of immune system function to fight the viruses that cause many of these cancers.

Although the risk of these AIDS-defining cancers among people infected with HIV is lower than in the past, it is still much higher than among people in the general population. This persistently high risk may reflect the fact that cART does not completely restore immune system functioning. Also, many people infected with HIV are not aware they are infected, have had difficulty in accessing medical care, or for other reasons are not receiving adequate antiretroviral therapy.

The introduction of cART has not reduced the incidence of all HIV-related cancers, and in fact, there has been an increase in non–AIDS-defining cancers. For example, the incidence of liver and anal cancer may be increasing among HIV-infected individuals.

An important factor contributing to the increase in non–AIDS-defining cancers is that as cART has reduced the number of deaths from AIDS, the HIV-infected population has grown in size and become older. The fastest growing proportion of HIV-infected individuals is the over-40 age group. These individuals are now developing cancers common in older age and also have an increased cumulative risk of developing HIV-associated cancers.

What Can People Infected with HIV Do to Reduce Their Risk of Cancer or to Find Cancer Early?

Taking cART as indicated based on current HIV treatment guidelines lowers the risk of Kaposi sarcoma and non-Hodgkin lymphoma and increases overall survival.

The risk of lung, oral, and other cancers can be reduced by quitting smoking. Because HIV-infected people have a higher risk of lung cancer, it is especially important that they do not smoke. Help with quitting smoking is available through the National Cancer Institute's (NCI's) smoking quitline at 877-448-7848 (877-44U-QUIT) and other NCI resources.

The higher incidence of liver cancer among HIV-infected people appears to be related to more frequent infection with hepatitis virus (particularly HCV in the United States) than among HIV-uninfected people. Therefore, HIV-infected individuals should know their hepatitis status.

In addition, if HIV-infected people currently have viral hepatitis, they should discuss with their healthcare provider whether antiviral treatment is an option for them. Some drugs may be used for both HBV-suppressing therapy and cART.

Because HIV-infected women have a higher risk of cervical cancer, it is important that they be screened regularly for this disease. In addition, the Centers for Disease Control and Prevention (CDC) recommends vaccination against human papillomavirus (HPV) for women and men with HIV infection up to age 26 years. Cervical cancer screening guidelines that incorporate results of a Pap test and an human papillomavirus (HPV) deoxyribonucleic acid (DNA) test are evolving, and women should discuss screening options with their healthcare provider.

Some researchers recommend anal Pap test screening to detect and treat early lesions before they progress to anal cancer. However, it is not clear if this type of screening benefits all HIV-infected people or if treating such lesions prevents anal cancer. These questions are being addressed in an NCI-funded trial called the Anal Cancer/HSIL Outcomes Research (ANCHOR). This study is currently enrolling men and women with HIV to undergo anal Pap testing and then be randomly assigned to receive either treatment or observation (no treatment). The goal is to determine whether treatment of anal lesions prevents anal cancer in HIV-infected people with anal lesions.

Kaposi's sarcoma-associated herpesvirus (KSHV) is secreted in saliva, and transmission of this virus may occur through deep kissing, through the use of saliva as a lubricant in sex, or through oral-anal sex. Reducing contact through these routes may reduce the chance of being infected with KSHV.

Section 46.2

Kaposi Sarcoma

This section contains text excerpted from the following sources:
Text under the heading "Kaposi Sarcoma Is a Cancer That Causes
Lesions (Abnormal Tissue) to Grow in Different Parts of the Body"
is excerpted from "Kaposi Sarcoma Treatment (PDQ®)—Patient
Version," National Cancer Institute (NCI), February 14, 2018; Text
beginning with the heading "Kaposi Sarcoma among HIV Infected
People" is excerpted from "HIV/AIDS—Kaposi Sarcoma," U.S.
Department of Veterans Affairs (VA), February 8, 2018.

Kaposi Sarcoma Is a Cancer That Causes Lesions (Abnormal Tissue) to Grow in Different Parts of the Body

Kaposi sarcoma is cancer that causes lesions (abnormal tissue) to
grow in the skin; the mucous membranes lining the mouth, nose, and
throat; lymph nodes; or other organs. The lesions are usually purple
and are made of cancer cells, new blood vessels, red blood cells, and
white blood cells. Kaposi sarcoma is different from other cancers in
that lesions may begin in more than one place in the body at the same
time.

Human herpesvirus-8 (HHV-8) is found in the lesions of all patients
with Kaposi sarcoma. This virus is also called Kaposi sarcoma herpesvirus (KSHV). Most people infected with HHV-8 do not get Kaposi
sarcoma. Those infected with HHV-8 who are most likely to develop
Kaposi sarcoma have immune systems weakened by disease or by
drugs given after an organ transplant.

Human herpesvirus-8 (HHV-8) is found in the lesions of all patients
with Kaposi sarcoma. This virus is also called Kaposi sarcoma herpesvirus (KSHV). Most people infected with HHV-8 do not get Kaposi
sarcoma. Those infected with HHV-8 who are most likely to develop
Kaposi sarcoma have immune systems weakened by disease or by
drugs given after an organ transplant.

Kaposi Sarcoma among HIV-infected People

Kaposi sarcoma (KS) is the most common cancer seen in HIV. This
cancer is caused by the human herpesvirus 8 (HHV-8), also known
as Kaposi sarcoma-associated herpesvirus (KSHV). The virus can be
spread by deep kissing, unprotected sex, and sharing needles. It also

can be spread from mother to child. However, HIV-related KS usually develops only in people with relatively advanced HIV disease.

Symptoms

Symptoms include brown, purple, or pink lesions (or blotches) on the skin, usually on the arms and legs, neck or head, and sometimes in the mouth. KS can also affect the lungs and intestines and cause swelling in the legs. Sometimes there is tooth pain or tooth loss, weight loss, night sweats, or fever for longer than 2 weeks.

Treatment

HIV drugs can slow the growth of lesions, and even reverse the condition itself. KS has become less common and much more treatable since the development of effective HIV therapy. Other treatments for KS, such as laser therapy, are meant to relieve symptoms and improve the appearance of the lesions. There is also chemotherapy that helps control KS.

Section 46.3

AIDS-Related Lymphoma

This section includes text excerpted from "AIDS-Related Lymphoma Treatment (PDQ®)—Patient Version," National Cancer Institute (NCI), May 31, 2018.

Acquired immunodeficiency syndrome (AIDS)-related lymphoma is a disease in which malignant (Cancer) Cells form in the lymph system of patients who have AIDS.

Acquired immunodeficiency syndrome (AIDS) is caused by the human immunodeficiency virus (HIV), which attacks and weakens the body's immune system. The immune system is then unable to fight infection and disease. People with HIV disease have an increased risk of infection and lymphoma or other types of cancer. A person with HIV disease who develops certain types of infections or cancer is then diagnosed with AIDS. Sometimes, people are diagnosed with AIDS and AIDS-related lymphoma at the same time.

AIDS-related lymphoma is a type of cancer that affects the lymph system, which is part of the body's immune system. The immune system protects the body from foreign substances, infection, and diseases. The lymph system is made up of the following:

- **Lymph:** Colorless, watery fluid that carries white blood cells called lymphocytes through the lymph system. Lymphocytes protect the body against infections and the growth of tumors.

- **Lymph vessels:** A network of thin tubes that collect lymph from different parts of the body and return it to the bloodstream

- **Lymph nodes:** Small, bean-shaped structures that filter lymph and store white blood cells that help fight infection and disease. Lymph nodes are located along the network of lymph vessels found throughout the body. Clusters of lymph nodes are found in the neck, underarm, abdomen, pelvis, and groin.

- **Spleen:** An organ that makes lymphocytes, filters the blood, stores blood cells, and destroys old blood cells. The spleen is on the left side of the abdomen near the stomach.

- **Thymus:** An organ in which lymphocytes grow and multiply. The thymus is in the chest behind the breastbone

- **Tonsils:** Two small masses of lymph tissue at the back of the throat. The tonsils make lymphocytes.

- **Bone marrow:** The soft, spongy tissue in the center of large bones. Bone marrow makes white blood cells, red blood cells, and platelets.

Lymph tissue is also found in other parts of the body such as the brain, stomach, thyroid gland, and skin.

Sometimes AIDS-related lymphoma occurs outside the lymph nodes in the bone marrow, liver, meninges (thin membranes that cover the brain) and gastrointestinal tract. Less often, it may occur in the anus, heart, bile duct, gingiva, and muscles.

Types of Lymphoma

Lymphomas are divided into two general types:

- Hodgkin lymphoma

- Non-Hodgkin lymphoma

Both Hodgkin lymphoma and non-Hodgkin lymphoma may occur in patients with AIDS, but non-Hodgkin lymphoma is more common. When a person with AIDS has non-Hodgkin lymphoma, it is called AIDS-related lymphoma. When AIDS-related lymphoma occurs in the central nervous system (CNS), it is called AIDS-related primary CNS lymphoma.

Non-Hodgkin lymphomas are grouped by the way their cells look under a microscope. They may be indolent (slow-growing) or aggressive (fast-growing). AIDS-related lymphomas are aggressive. There are two main types of AIDS-related non-Hodgkin lymphoma:

- Diffuse large B-cell lymphoma (including B-cell immunoblastic lymphoma)

- Burkitt or Burkitt-like lymphoma

Signs of AIDS-related lymphoma include weight loss, fever, and night sweats.

These and other signs and symptoms may be caused by AIDS-related lymphoma or by other conditions. Check with your doctor if you have any of the following:

- Weight loss or fever for no known reason

- Night Sweats

- Painless, swollen lymph nodes in the neck, chest, underarm, or groin

- A feeling of fullness below the ribs

Tests that examine the lymph system and other parts of the body are used to help detect (find) and diagnose AIDS-related lymphoma. The following tests and procedures may be used:

- **Physical exam and history:** An exam of the body to check general signs of health, including checking for signs of disease, such as lumps or anything else that seems unusual. A history of the patient's health habits and past illnesses and treatments will also be taken.

- **Complete blood count (CBC):** A procedure in which a sample of blood is drawn and checked for the following:

  - The number of red blood cells, white blood cells, and platelets

- The amount of hemoglobin (the protein that carries oxygen) in the red blood cells

- The portion of the sample made up of red blood cells

- **HIV test:** A test to measure the level of HIV antibodies in a sample of blood. Antibodies are made by the body when it is invaded by a foreign substance. A high level of HIV antibodies may mean the body has been infected with HIV.

- **Lymph node biopsy:** The removal of all or part of a lymph node. A pathologist views the tissue under a microscope to look for cancer cells. One of the following types of biopsies may be done:

  - Excisional biopsy: The removal of an entire lymph node

  - Incisional biopsy: The removal of part of a lymph node

  - Core biopsy: The removal of tissue from a lymph node using a wide needle

- **Fine-needle aspiration (FNA) biopsy:** The removal of tissue from a lymph node using a thin needle

- **Bone marrow aspiration and biopsy:** The removal of bone marrow and a small piece of bone by inserting a hollow needle into the hipbone or breastbone. A pathologist views the bone marrow and bone under a microscope to look for signs of cancer.

- **Chest X-ray:** An X-ray of the organs and bones inside the chest. An X-ray is a type of energy beam that can go through the body and onto film, making a picture of areas inside the body.

Factors Affecting Prognosis, Recovery and Treatment Options

The prognosis (chance of recovery) and treatment options depend on the following:

- The stage of the cancer

- The age of the patient

- The number of CD4 lymphocytes (a type of white blood cell) in the blood

- The number of places in the body lymphoma is found outside the lymph system

- Whether the patient has a history of intravenous (IV) drug use

- The patient's ability to carry out regular daily activities

Stages of AIDS-Related Lymphoma

After AIDS-related lymphoma has been diagnosed, tests are done to find out if cancer cells have spread within the lymph system or to other parts of the body.

The process used to find out if cancer cells have spread within the lymph system or to other parts of the body is called staging. The information gathered from the staging process determines the stage of the disease. It is important to know the stage in order to plan treatment, but AIDS-related lymphoma is usually advanced when it is diagnosed.

The following tests and procedures may be used in the staging process:

- **Blood chemistry studies:** A procedure in which a blood sample is checked to measure the amounts of certain substances released into the blood by organs and tissues in the body. An unusual (higher or lower than normal) amount of a substance can be a sign of disease. The blood sample will be checked for the level of LDH (lactate dehydrogenase).

- **Computed tomography (CT) scan/Computed axial tomography (CAT) scan:** A procedure that makes a series of detailed pictures of areas inside the body, such as the lung, lymph nodes, and liver, taken from different angles. The pictures are made by a computer linked to an X-ray machine. A dye may be injected into a vein or swallowed to help the organs or tissues show up more clearly.

- **Positron emission tomography (PET) scan:** A procedure to find malignant tumor cells in the body. A small amount of radioactive glucose (sugar) is injected into a vein. The PET scanner rotates around the body and makes a picture of where glucose is being used in the body. Malignant tumor cells show up brighter in the picture because they are more active and take up more glucose than normal cells do.

- **Magnetic resonance imaging (MRI) with gadolinium:** A procedure that uses a magnet, radio waves, and a computer to make a series of detailed pictures of areas inside the body. A substance called gadolinium is injected into the patient through a vein. The gadolinium collects around the cancer cells so they show up brighter in the picture. This procedure is also called nuclear magnetic resonance imaging (NMRI).

- **Lumbar puncture:** A procedure used to collect cerebrospinal fluid (CSF) from the spinal column. This is done by placing a needle between two bones in the spine and into the CSF around the spinal cord and removing a sample of the fluid. The sample of CSF is checked under a microscope for signs that cancer has spread to the brain and spinal cord. The sample may also be checked for Epstein-Barr virus. This procedure is also called an LP or spinal tap.

There are three ways that cancer spreads in the body.

Cancer can spread through tissue, the lymph system, and the blood:

- **Tissue.** Cancer spreads from where it began by growing into nearby areas

- **Lymph system.** Cancer spreads from where it began by getting into the lymph system. Cancer travels through the lymph vessels to other parts of the body.

- **Blood.** Cancer spreads from where it began by getting into the blood. Cancer travels through the blood vessels to other parts of the body.

Stages of AIDS-related lymphoma may include E and S.

AIDS-related lymphoma may be described as follows:

- E: "E" stands for extranodal and means the cancer is found in an area or organ other than the lymph nodes or has spread to tissues beyond, but near, the major lymphatic areas.

- S: "S" stands for spleen and means the cancer is found in the spleen

The following stages are used for AIDS-related lymphoma:

Stage I

Stage I AIDS-related lymphoma is divided into stage I and stage IE.

- Stage I: Cancer is found in one lymphatic area (lymph node group, tonsils and nearby tissue, thymus, or spleen)

- Stage IE: Cancer is found in one organ or area outside the lymph nodes

Stage II

Stage II AIDS-related lymphoma is divided into stage II and stage IIE.

- Stage II: Cancer is found in two or more lymph node groups either above or below the diaphragm (the thin muscle below the lungs that helps breathing and separates the chest from the abdomen).
- Stage IIE: Cancer is found in one or more lymph node groups either above or below the diaphragm. Cancer is also found outside the lymph nodes in one organ or area on the same side of the diaphragm as the affected lymph nodes.

Stage III

Stage III AIDS-related lymphoma is divided into stage III, stage IIIE, stage IIIS, and stage IIIE+S.

- Stage III: Cancer is found in lymph node groups above and below the diaphragm (the thin muscle below the lungs that helps breathing and separates the chest from the abdomen).
- Stage IIIE: Cancer is found in lymph node groups above and below the diaphragm and outside the lymph nodes in a nearby organ or area
- Stage IIIS: Cancer is found in lymph node groups above and below the diaphragm, and in the spleen
- Stage IIIE+S: Cancer is found in lymph node groups above and below the diaphragm, outside the lymph nodes in a nearby organ or area, and in the spleen

Stage IV

In stage IV AIDS-related lymphoma, cancer:

- is found throughout one or more organs that are not part of a lymphatic area (lymph node group, tonsils and nearby tissue, thymus, or spleen) and may be in lymph nodes near those organs; or
- is found in one organ that is not part of a lymphatic area and has spread to organs or lymph nodes far away from that organ; or
- is found in the liver, bone marrow, cerebrospinal fluid (CSF), or lungs (other than cancer that has spread to the lungs from nearby areas).

Patients who are infected with the Epstein-Barr virus (EPV) or whose AIDS-related lymphoma affects the bone marrow have an increased risk of cancer spreading to the central nervous system (CNS).

For treatment, AIDS-related lymphomas are grouped based on where they started in the body, as follows:

Peripheral/Systemic Lymphoma

Lymphoma that starts in the lymph system or elsewhere in the body, other than the brain, is called peripheral/systemic lymphoma. It may spread throughout the body, including to the brain or bone marrow. It is often diagnosed in an advanced stage.

Primary CNS Lymphoma

Primary CNS lymphoma starts in the central nervous system (brain and spinal cord). It is linked to the Epstein-Barr virus. Lymphoma that starts somewhere else in the body and spreads to the central nervous system is not primary CNS lymphoma.

Treatment Option Overview

There are different types of treatment for patients with AIDS-related lymphoma.

Different types of treatment are available for patients with AIDS-related lymphoma. Some treatments are standard (the currently used treatment), and some are being tested in clinical trials. A treatment clinical trial is a research study meant to help improve current treatments or obtain information on new treatments for patients with cancer. When clinical trials show that a new treatment is better than the standard treatment, the new treatment may become the standard treatment. Patients may want to think about taking part in a clinical trial. Some clinical trials are open only to patients who have not started treatment.

Treatment of AIDS-related lymphoma combines treatment of the lymphoma with treatment for AIDS.

Patients with AIDS have weakened immune systems and treatment can cause the immune system to become even weaker. For this reason, treating patients who have AIDS-related lymphoma is difficult and some patients may be treated with lower doses of drugs than lymphoma patients who do not have AIDS.

Combined antiretroviral therapy (cART) is used to lessen the damage to the immune system caused by HIV. Treatment with combined antiretroviral therapy may allow some patients with AIDS-related lymphoma to safely receive anticancer drugs in standard or higher doses. In these patients, treatment may work as well as it does in lymphoma patients who do not have AIDS. Medicine to prevent and treat infections, which can be serious, is also used.

Four types of standard treatment are used:

Chemotherapy

Chemotherapy is a cancer treatment that uses drugs to stop the growth of cancer cells, either by killing the cells or by stopping them from dividing. When chemotherapy is taken by mouth or injected into a vein or muscle, the drugs enter the bloodstream and can reach cancer cells throughout the body (systemic chemotherapy). When chemotherapy is placed directly into the cerebrospinal fluid (intrathecal chemotherapy), an organ, or a body cavity such as the abdomen, the drugs mainly affect cancer cells in those areas (regional chemotherapy). Combination chemotherapy is treatment using more than one anticancer drug.

The way the chemotherapy is given depends on where cancer has formed. Intrathecal chemotherapy may be used in patients who are more likely to have lymphoma in the central nervous system (CNS).

Chemotherapy is used in the treatment of AIDS-related peripheral/systemic lymphoma. It is not yet known whether it is best to give combined antiretroviral therapy at the same time as chemotherapy or after chemotherapy ends.

Colony-stimulating factors are sometimes given together with chemotherapy. This helps lessen the side effects chemotherapy may have on the bone marrow.

Radiation Therapy

Radiation therapy is a cancer treatment that uses high-energy X-rays or other types of radiation to kill cancer cells or keep them from growing. There are two types of radiation therapy:

- External radiation therapy uses a machine outside the body to send radiation toward the cancer

- Internal radiation therapy uses a radioactive substance sealed in needles, seeds, wires, or catheters that are placed directly into or near the cancer

The way the radiation therapy is given depends on where cancer has formed. External radiation therapy is used to treat AIDS-related primary CNS lymphoma.

High-Dose Chemotherapy with Stem Cell Transplant

High-dose chemotherapy with stem cell transplant is a way of giving high doses of chemotherapy and replacing blood-forming cells destroyed by the cancer treatment. Stem cells (immature blood cells) are removed from the blood or bone marrow of the patient or a donor and are frozen and stored. After the chemotherapy is completed, the stored stem cells are thawed and given back to the patient through an infusion. These reinfused stem cells grow into (and restore) the body's blood cells.

Targeted Therapy

Targeted therapy is a type of treatment that uses drugs or other substances to identify and attack specific cancer cells without harming normal cells. Monoclonal antibody therapy is a type of targeted therapy.

Monoclonal antibody therapy is a cancer treatment that uses antibodies made in the laboratory from a single type of immune system cell. These antibodies can identify substances on cancer cells or normal substances that may help cancer cells grow. The antibodies attach to the substances and kill the cancer cells, block their growth, or keep them from spreading. Monoclonal antibodies are given by infusion. These may be used alone or to carry drugs, toxins, or radioactive material directly to cancer cells. Rituximab is used in the treatment of AIDS-related peripheral/systemic lymphoma.

Patients May Want to Think about Taking Part in a Clinical Trial

For some patients, taking part in a clinical trial may be the best treatment choice. Clinical trials are part of the cancer research process. Clinical trials are done to find out if new cancer treatments are safe and effective or better than the standard treatment.

Many of today's standard treatments for cancer are based on earlier clinical trials. Patients who take part in a clinical trial may receive the standard treatment or be among the first to receive a new treatment.

Patients who take part in clinical trials also help improve the way cancer will be treated in the future. Even when clinical trials do not lead to effective new treatments, they often answer important questions and help move research forward.

Patients Can Enter Clinical Trials before, during, or after Starting Their Cancer Treatment

Some clinical trials only include patients who have not yet received treatment. Other trials test treatments for patients whose cancer has not gotten better. There are also clinical trials that test new ways to stop cancer from recurring (coming back) or reduce the side effects of cancer treatment.

Follow-Up Tests May Be Needed

Some of the tests that were done to diagnose cancer or to find out the stage of cancer may be repeated. Some tests will be repeated in order to see how well the treatment is working. Decisions about whether to continue, change or stop treatment may be based on the results of these tests.

Some of the tests will continue to be done from time to time after treatment has ended. The results of these tests can show if your condition has changed or if cancer has recurred (come back). These tests are sometimes called follow-up tests or check-ups.

Chapter 47

Other AIDS-Related Health Concerns

Chapter Contents

Section 47.1

HIV-Associated Neurocognitive Disorders

This section includes text excerpted from "HIV-Associated
Neurocognitive Disorders in the Combination Antiretroviral Therapy
Era," HIV/AIDS Bureau (HAB), Health Resources and Services
Administration (HRSA), July 2014. Reviewed June 2018.

Since the beginning of the epidemic, human immunodeficiency virus
(HIV) infection has been associated with neurologic and neurocognitive complications. HIV-associated neurocognitive disorders (HAND),
the term used to describe these manifestations, describes a spectrum
ranging from mild, asymptomatic neurologic impairment to severe,
HIV-associated dementia (HAD).

Symptoms of HIV-Associated Neurocognitive Disorders (HAND)

Symptoms of HAND include:

- Behavioral changes
- Difficulties with decision-making
- Problem-solving
- Concentration
- Learning
- Language memory
- Loss of coordination
- Weakness
- Tremors

Combination antiretroviral therapy (cART) use has changed the
pattern—but not the overall prevalence—of neurocognitive impairment among people living with HIV (PLWH). In the pre-cART era,
moderate-to-severe impairment was more common among people with
acquired immunodeficiency syndrome (AIDS) than those with less
advanced HIV disease (ranging from 4% in asymptomatic persons
to 17% in people with AIDS). "We are simply not seeing new cases of
AIDS dementia in treated patients, but mild cognitive impairment

remains a challenge," says Dr. David B. Clifford, Professor of Clinical Neuropharmacology in Neurology and Professor of Medicine at Washington University School of Medicine.

In the cART era, both the rate and severity of cognitive impairment have doubled among people with asymptomatic HIV, possibly due to prolonged immunosuppression and lower cluster of differentiation 4 (CD4) count prior to commencement of cART. According to Dr. Victor Valcour, Associate Professor of Geriatric Medicine and Neurology at the University of California, San Francisco, "Cognitive impairment is quite frequent in HIV. If you test 100 people, about 50 percent of them will test below what we expect, yet only a quarter or a third of them will have symptoms."

In the pre-cART era, patients with the more serious form of HAND—HIV-associated dementia or HAD—progressed rapidly and their prognosis was poor. Fortunately, cART use has decreased the incidence of HAD (from 15–2%), and dramatically extended median survival among people with this condition, from five months to four years. Impairment in motor skills, verbal fluency, and cognitive speed were common in the pre-cART era; nowadays, HAND appears more similar to Alzheimer disease (AD). In the cART era, PLWH are still vulnerable to neurological complications, even when HIV is undetectable. Researchers have reported that the presence of inflammatory markers—rather than the HIV RNA (ribonucleic acid) or CD4 cell count—are associated with HAND in people on cART. In fact, immunologic recovery and virologic suppression have been associated with increased abnormalities in white and gray matter, which supports the role of neuroinflammation as a cause of HAND.

Prevalence of HAND

It is estimated that at least 50 percent of HIV-positive people have some degree of neurocognitive impairment. An estimated 33 percent of HIV-positive people experience mild neurocognitive impairment.

The most common presentations of HAND are impaired memory and executive function (the ability to remember details, make plans, organize, focus, manage time, and control behavior). But even in mild cases, HAND may cause real-life consequences, such as poor adherence to HIV treatment and difficulty with everyday functioning (e.g., shopping, cooking, driving, multitasking, and financial management).

Fortunately, progression from the milder forms of HAND to severe impairment is rare; in fact, most people with mild HAND remain stable or improve after starting cART. Neurocognitive impairment and white matter abnormalities are common among HIV-infected children, regardless of cART use, although neurocognitive benefits of cART have been demonstrated in perinatally infected children.

What Causes HAND?

Many factors can cause or worsen HAND, including HIV itself. Shortly after infection, HIV enters the brain and the central nervous system (CNS); this is called neuroinvasion.

Certain types of white blood cells (WBCs)—macrophages and monocytes—carry the virus throughout the body, including into the CNS and the brain, causing inflammation and persistent infection. Infected macrophages and monocytes pass HIV into microglia (immune cells found only in the brain) and astrocytes (star-shaped cells found in the brain and spinal cord); when these cells are activated in response to HIV, they release neurotoxins that are harmful to brain tissue.

Although HAND is seen more frequently in people with AIDS, it also occurs in people with asymptomatic HIV and has been reported in people with recent HIV infection. But the risk of neurologic complication is higher among people with a low CD4 cell nadir (<200 cells/ mm^3), even after initiation of and response to cART.

HIV is not the only cause of cognitive impairment. Opportunistic infections (OIs), inflammatory immune reconstitution syndrome (IRIS), and other comorbidities that are more prevalent among PLWH than their HIV-negative counterparts (hepatitis C virus (HCV) coinfection, cardiovascular disease, type 2 diabetes, certain cancers, and syphilis) have been implicated in HAND. In addition, aging, antiretroviral drug toxicity, and long-term, heavy illicit drug and alcohol use are potential contributing factors in HAND.

HIV and Aging: HAND in HAND?

The risk for neurodegenerative diseases increases with age. By 2020, 50 percent of PLWH in the United States will be over 50 years old. Older HIV-positive people may be long-term survivors or newly infected; in 2010, the Centers for Disease Control and Prevention (CDC) reported that 5 percent of all new HIV infections occurred in people aged 55 and over. Older adults are often diagnosed later, since they are often not perceived to be at high risk; delayed initiation of cART, lower CD4 nadir, and blunted immune response increase the risk for HAND.

The risk factors for AD in elderly people—immune dysfunction, inflammation, and hyperlipidemia—are also associated with HIV. Comorbidities that become more common as people age—metabolic disorders, and cardiovascular and cerebrovascular disease—are also associated with neurocognitive impairment.

Cumulative toxicity from certain antiretroviral agents may contribute to or increase the risk of HAND among long-term survivors as they age. In fact, HAND is almost twice as prevalent among HIV-positive people over 50 years of age than their younger counterparts, and they are three times more likely to experience HIV-associated dementia.

Although age-related comorbidities may complicate adherence to cART, older patients are usually more adherent than those under 50 years of age—unless they are experiencing neurocognitive impairment. HAND associated poor adherence could result in a vicious cycle that may limit the benefits of cART among older people by worsening neurocognitive impairment.

The complexity of cART regimens varies, according to the number of medications, actual pill count, dosing schedule, and special instructions (such as food requirements). Treatment simplification may improve cART adherence, especially for older people who are likely to be taking other medications.

Use of five or more drugs for various comorbid conditions—known as polypharmacy—is common among HIV-positive people as they age; 55 percent of people over 50 years of age are on at least five medications. Polypharmacy can have a negative impact on adherence and increases the risk of drug-drug interactions that may lower the effectiveness of cART or worsen drug toxicity.

Late diagnosis and untreated HIV increase the risk for opportunistic infections, particularly in people with advanced immunosuppression. Fortunately, cART has decreased the incidence of and mortality from several of the opportunistic infections known to cause HAND: progressive multifocal leukoencephalopathy, HIV encephalopathy, cytomegalovirus, and primary CNS lymphoma.

Delaying cART initiation also increases the risk for IRIS. Usually, this syndrome occurs in people with advanced immunosuppression (CD4 cell count of <50 cells/mm^3), most frequently within months of starting, restarting, or switching cART. After the immune system begins to recover, it may mount a fierce response to pathogens.

Sometimes, IRIS manifests in the nervous system. Although this can occur in the absence of any pathogen, it is usually a response to tuberculosis (TB); progressive multifocal leukoencephalopathy;

toxoplasmic encephalitis; cryptococcal meningitis; or cytomegalovirus. IRIS is usually manageable, but it can be life threatening, depending on cause and severity.

Diagnosing HAND

At present, only clinical criteria and neuropsychiatric testing are used to diagnose HAND; no single laboratory test or biomarker has been established. Experts in the field have practical ideas about screening for HAND.

A combination of simple, paper-based tests has been used to screen for mild neurocognitive impairment, although the tests are not always reliable. In clinical settings, simple tests are used for screening and to diagnose mild-to-moderate neurologic impairment and severe neurologic impairment.

Who, When, and How Often to Screen

Although screening for HAND is an important part of HIV care, it is not always clear who should be screened and how often to perform screening. The Mind Exchange Working Group has developed guidance for assessing, diagnosing, and treating HAND; screening for HAND is recommended every 6–12 months in higher risk patients, and every 12–24 months in lower risk patients; immediate screening is recommended at initiation of cART, upon diagnosis with a psychiatric disorder, or if a patient's health has deteriorated.

What to Do about HAND

Combination Antiretroviral Therapy (cART)

Although several approaches are being studied, initiation of and adherence to cART are the most successful interventions to prevent, delay, or improve HAND. The brain is known to be a reservoir for HIV, even in the context of effective cART. Researchers have found HIV deoxyribonucleic acid (DNA) in peripheral blood (despite undetectable HIV RNA after more than a year of cART) and linked it with decreases in brain gray matter. Antiretroviral agents with activity against HIV-infected macrophages may prevent or improve HAND, since these cells deliver HIV to the brain.

Sometimes, high levels of HIV RNA can be detected in the CNS even when cART has suppressed HIV to very low or undetectable levels in the blood stream; this is known as CNS escape. Researchers are studying the relationship between the degree of CNS penetration in cART and improvement of neurocognitive function. They devised a CNS penetration-effectiveness (CPE) index to classify antiretroviral agents according to their ability to cross the blood-brain barrier. The scoring is based on the properties of individual drugs, their concentration in cerebrospinal fluid, and/or their effectiveness in clinical studies. Regimens with higher CPE scores are more likely to fully suppress HIV in the CNS.

Although regimens with a high CPE score may improve neurocognitive function, this remains controversial; the usual selection criteria for cART is often related to more practical concerns, such as pill burden, dosing schedule, and side effect profile. Antiretroviral agents themselves can have side effects, despite their lifesaving benefits: Efavirenz, for example, is associated with CNS side effect

Healthy Living

Healthy weight. The risk for multiple morbidities increases with higher body mass index (BMI). In the United States, obesity has become more common than wasting among PLWH. A study of 681 HIV-positive treatment-naïve adults in Alabama found an obesity rate of 20 percent, signaling that clinicians have an opportunity to discuss healthy lifestyles with HIV patients. Obesity, HIV, and the use of certain antiretroviral agents are risk factors for type 2 diabetes and cardiovascular disease, which are also associated with HAND.

Diet. Clearly, diet has an important role in the overall health of PLWH. In particular, diet can promote cognitive function. Antioxidant-laden foods (e.g., dark chocolate, dark berries, and many other fruits, as well as vegetables and legumes) and beverages (e.g., coffee, green and black tea) reduce inflammation and may preserve or improve cognitive functioning in older HIV-negative adults.

Physical exercise is known to improve neurological impairment in HIV-negative adults and is likely to offer the same benefit for HIV-positive adults; a recent study reported lower rates of impairment among HIV-positive people who exercise than those who are sedentary.

Section 47.2

Oral Health Issues

This section includes text excerpted from "HIV/AIDS,"
National Institute of Dental and Craniofacial
Research (NIDCR), February 2018.

People with human immunodeficiency virus (HIV), the virus that
causes acquired immunodeficiency syndrome (AIDS), are at special
risk for oral health problems. Some of the most common oral problems
for people with HIV/AIDS are:

- Chronic dry mouth

- Gingivitis

- Bone loss around the teeth (periodontitis)

- Canker sores

- Oral warts

- Fever blisters

- Oral candidiasis (thrush)

- Hairy leukoplakia (which causes a rough, white patch on the
  tongue)

- Dental caries

Combination antiretroviral therapy (cART), which is used to treat
the HIV condition and restore immune system function, has made
some oral problems less common. Oral conditions can be painful,
annoying, and can lead to other problems.

Causes

People with HIV/AIDS have an increased risk for oral health problems because HIV/AIDS weakens the immune system and makes it
harder to fight off infection.

Symptoms

Oral health problems may include:

Table 46.1. Oral Health Problems

Description	It Could Be	What and Where?	Painful?	Contagious?	Treatment
Red sores ulcers	Aphthous ulcers. Also known as canker sores	Red sores that might also have a yellow-gray film on top. They are usually on the moveable parts of the mouth such as the tongue or inside of the cheeks and lips.	Yes	No	Mild cases—Over-the-counter (OTC) cream or prescription mouthwash that contains corticosteroids; More severe cases—corticosteroids in a pill form
Red sores ulcers	Herpes: A viral infection	Red sores usually on the roof of the mouth. They are sometimes on the outside of the lips, where they are called fever blisters.	Sometimes	Yes	Prescription pill can reduce healing time and frequency of outbreaks.
White hairlike growth	Hairy leukoplakia caused by the Epstein-Barr virus	White patches that do not wipe away; sometimes very thick and "hairlike." Usually appear on the side of the tongue or sometimes inside the cheeks and lower lip.	Not usually	No	Mild cases—not usually required; More severe cases—a prescription pill that may reduce severity of symptoms. In some severe cases, a pain reliever might also be required.

Table 46.1. Continued

Description	It Could Be	What and Where?	Painful?	Contagious?	Treatment
White creamy or bumpy patches like cottage cheese	Candidiasis, a fungal (yeast) infection—Also known as thrush	White or yellowish patches (or can sometimes be red). If wiped away, there will be redness or bleeding underneath. They can appear anywhere in the mouth.	Sometimes, a burning feeling	No	Mild cases— prescription antifungal lozenge or mouthwash; More severe cases— prescription antifungal pills.
Warts		Small, white, gray, or pinkish rough bumps that look like cauliflower. They can appear inside the lips and on other parts of the mouth.	Not usually	Possibly	Inside the mouth—a doctor can remove them surgically or use "cryosurgery"—a way of freezing them off; On the lips—a prescription cream that will wear away the wart. Warts can return after treatment.

Treatment

The most common oral problems linked with HIV can be treated. So, talk with your doctor or dentist about what treatment might work for you.

Helpful Tips

In addition to the problems listed in the table above, you may experience dry mouth. Dry mouth happens when you don't have enough saliva, or spit, to keep your mouth wet. Saliva helps you chew and digest food, protects teeth from decay, and prevents infections by controlling bacteria and fungi in the mouth. Without enough saliva, you could develop tooth decay or other infections and might have trouble chewing and swallowing. Your mouth might also feel sticky or dry and have a burning feeling, and you may have cracked, chapped lips.

To help with a dry mouth, try these things:

- Sip water or sugarless drinks often
- Chew sugarless gum or suck on sugarless hard candy
- Avoid tobacco
- Avoid alcohol
- Avoid salty foods
- Use a humidifier at night

Talk to your doctor or dentist about prescribing artificial saliva, which may help keep your mouth moist.

Section 47.3

Kidney Disease

This section includes text excerpted from "HIV and Kidney
Disease," AIDS*info*, U.S. Department of Health and
Human Services (HHS), November 13, 2017.

The kidneys are two fist-sized organs in the body. They are located
near the middle of the back on either side of the spine. The main job of
the kidneys is to filter harmful waste and extra water from the blood.
The waste and water become urine, which is flushed from the body.
The kidneys also release hormones that help control blood pressure,
make red blood cells, and keep bones strong.

Kidney function declines as people age. Injury or disease, including
human immunodeficiency virus (HIV) infection, can also damage the
kidneys. Damage to the kidneys can lead to kidney disease (also called
renal disease). Kidney disease can advance to kidney failure.

Causes of Kidney Disease

Diabetes and high blood pressure are the leading causes of kidney
disease. Other factors that increase the risk of kidney disease include
heart disease and a family history of kidney disease or kidney failure.

A person's risk of kidney disease increases as they get older. The
longer a person has diabetes, high blood pressure, or heart disease,
the greater their risk of kidney disease.

Anyone can get kidney disease but the risk is greatest for African
Americans, Hispanics, and American Indians, mainly because of the
high rates of high blood pressure and diabetes among these population
groups.

People with Human Immunodeficiency Virus (HIV) and Risk of Kidney Disease

The risk factors for kidney disease in people with HIV include all
those listed above. In addition, poorly controlled HIV infection and
coinfection with the hepatitis C virus (HCV) increase the risk of kidney
disease in people with HIV.

Antiretroviral therapy (ART) is the use of HIV medicines to treat
HIV infection. People on ART take a combination of HIV medicines
(called an HIV regimen) every day. ART is recommended for everyone

infected with HIV. Some HIV medicines can affect the kidneys. Health-care providers carefully consider the risk of kidney damage when recommending specific HIV medicines to include in an HIV regimen. If a person on ART shows signs of kidney disease, the type or dose of HIV medicine in their HIV regimen may change.

Symptoms of Kidney Disease

Kidney disease can advance very slowly. Slowly worsening kidney disease is called chronic kidney disease. Chronic kidney disease may not cause symptoms for many years.

Sudden damage to the kidneys, often because of an illness or injury, is called acute kidney injury.

Symptoms of worsening kidney disease can include:

- Swelling of the legs, feet, or ankles (called edema)

- Increased or decreased urination

- Feeling tired or having trouble sleeping

- Nausea and vomiting

- Itching or numbness

Blood and urine tests are often the only way to detect kidney disease. Care for people with HIV includes testing for kidney disease.

Treatment for Kidney Disease

People with kidney disease often take medicines to slow down the disease and delay kidney failure. They may also change what they eat and drink to manage their kidney disease. For example, they may need to reduce the amount of salt and protein in their diet.

The treatments for kidney failure are dialysis and a kidney transplant. Both treatments take over the job of the failed kidneys.

- Dialysis is a process that uses a machine (called hemodialysis) or the lining of the abdomen (called peritoneal dialysis) to filter harmful waste and extra water from the blood.

- A kidney transplant is surgery to place a healthy kidney from a donor into the body of a person with kidney disease. The donated kidney can be from a person who just died or a living person.

Both dialysis and a kidney transplant are used to treat kidney failure in people with HIV.

Living with HIV—Reducing Risk of Kidney Disease

Take the following steps to reduce your risk of kidney disease:

- Take your HIV medicines every day to keep your HIV under control.

- Eat a healthy diet that includes fresh fruits, fresh or frozen vegetables, whole grains, and low-fat dairy foods. Avoid processed foods high in salt, such as deli meats, soups, and chips.

- Make physical activity a part of every day.

- Keep all of your medical appointments. During your visits, talk to your healthcare provider about your risk for kidney disease.

Section 47.4

Wasting Syndrome

This section includes text excerpted from "HIV Wasting Syndrome," U.S. Department of Veterans Affairs (VA), February 8, 2018.

Wasting syndrome refers to unwanted weight loss of more than 10 percent of a person's body weight, with either diarrhea or weakness and fever that have lasted at least 30 days. For a 150-pound man, this means a weight loss of 15 pounds or more. Weight loss can result in loss of both fat and muscle. Once lost, the weight is difficult to regain.

Causes of Wasting Syndrome

The condition may occur in people with advanced human immunodeficiency virus (HIV) disease, and can be caused by many things:

- HIV

- Inflammation

- Opportunistic infections (OIs)

The person may get full easily or have no appetite at all.

Treatment and Ways to Control Wasting Syndrome

The most important treatment for wasting syndrome is effective treatment of HIV with antiretroviral medications. In addition, the condition may be controlled, to some degree, by eating a good diet. A "good diet" for an HIV-positive person may not be the low-fat, low-calorie diet recommended for healthy people. Compared with other people, you may need to take in more calories and protein to keep from losing muscle mass. To do this, you can add to your meals:

- Peanut butter
- Legumes (dried beans and peas)
- Cheeses
- Eggs
- Instant breakfast drinks
- Milkshakes
- Sauces

You can also maintain or increase muscle mass through exercise, especially with progressive strength-building exercises. These include resistance and weight-lifting exercise.

Part Six

Living with HIV Infection

Chapter 48

Coping with an HIV/AIDS Diagnosis

Finding out that you have human immunodeficiency virus (HIV) can be scary and overwhelming. If you feel overwhelmed, try to remember that you can get help and that these feelings will get better with time.

Testing positive for HIV is a serious matter but one that you can deal with. Starting HIV medications early is one of the best ways to take care of your health. This chapter will take you through the steps you need to take to protect your health:

- Understand your diagnosis

- Find support

- Work with your doctor

- Monitor your health

- Be aware of possible complications

- Protect others

- Start treatment

- Move forward with your life

This chapter includes text excerpted from "HIV/AIDS—Your Next Steps: Entire Lesson," U.S. Department of Veterans Affairs (VA), February 8, 2018.

There are some things that you should know about HIV that may ease some of the stress or confusion you are feeling. Remember:

- **You are not alone.** Many people are living with HIV, even if you don't know that they are.

- **HIV does not equal death.** Having HIV does not mean that you are going to die of it. Most people with HIV live long and healthy lives if they get medical treatment and take care of themselves.

- **HIV does not means acquired immunodeficiency syndrome (AIDS).** A diagnosis of HIV does not automatically mean that you have AIDS.

- **Don't freeze.** Learning how to live with HIV and getting into care and onto medications will help you to feel better and get on with your life. Your VA care provider can help you connect with a healthcare team that knows how to manage HIV.

Understand Your Diagnosis

When your medical provider tells you that you are HIV positive, it means that you have been infected with the HIV. However, the HIV test does not tell you if you have AIDS or how long you have been infected or how sick you might be. Soon after your diagnosis, your provider will run other tests to determine your overall health, and the condition of your immune system.

Learn about Human Immunodeficiency Virus (HIV) and Acquired Immunodeficiency Syndrome (AIDS)

The more you know about HIV and how to treat it, the less confused and anxious you will be about your diagnosis. The more you learn, the better you will be at making decisions about your health. You don't have to learn it all at once, however, it is important to go at a pace you are comfortable with. This may be fast, slow, or in-between. You may want to go over the same information several times.

There are many ways to learn about HIV and AIDS:

- **Read information online.** Remember that there is a lot of Internet information that can be inaccurate or misleading—be sure to look for reputable sites whose content can be trusted. Check out government or nonprofit educational organizations that deal with HIV and AIDS issues.

- **Use your local library.** The most updated information will be in the library's collection of newspapers and magazines (books about HIV and AIDS may be out of date by the time they are published).

- **Check for on-site library in local medical center.** Check with your local medical center to see if there's an on-site library where you can find patient materials on HIV and AIDS.

Find Support

Talk with others who have been diagnosed with HIV and AIDS. Ask your healthcare provider if they know of any support groups. Or you can go online, where you can find message boards and chat rooms. Always discuss what you learn from these sources with your provider. The information may not be accurate; and even if it is, it may not be right for your particular situation.

Finding support means finding people who are willing to help you through the emotional and physical issues you are facing. If you let the right people in your life know that you are HIV positive, they can:

- offer you support and understanding

- provide you with assistance, such as helping with child care, doctor visits, and work

- learn from you how HIV is spread and work with you to prevent the virus from spreading

Telling Others

Deciding to tell others that you are HIV positive is an important personal choice. It can make a big difference in how you cope with the disease. It can also affect your relationships with people.

If you decide to share information about your diagnosis, it is best to tell people you trust or people who are directly affected. These include:

- family members

- people you spend a lot of time with, such as good friends

- all your healthcare providers, such as doctors, nurses, and dentists

- sex partner(s)

You don't have to tell everyone about your HIV status right away. You might want to talk with a counselor or social worker first.

Join a Support Group

Some medical centers have support groups for veterans with HIV, so you may want to ask your provider if your center has one that you can join for support and for more information about living with HIV. Joining a group of people who are facing the same challenges you are facing can have important benefits. These include:

- feeling better about yourself
- finding or strengthening your life focus
- making new friendships
- improving your mood
- better understanding your needs and those of your family

People in support groups often help each other deal with common experiences associated with being HIV positive. Support groups are especially helpful if you live alone or don't have family and friends nearby. There are different types of support groups, from hotlines to face-to-face encounter groups. Here are descriptions of some of the most popular types, and suggestions about how to find them.

Hotlines

Hotlines can provide information, support, or link you with local services. Find a hotline in your area by talking to a social worker in your hospital. Or look in the telephone book, in the yellow pages under "Social Service Organizations."

Professional Help

You can get referrals to mental health professionals, such as psychologists, nurse therapists, clinical social workers, or psychiatrists. You also will likely have a social worker who is part of the HIV clinic team where you will receive care. You can also get help for substance use.

Self-Help Organizations

Self-help groups enable people to share experiences and pool their knowledge to help each other and themselves. They are run by members, not by professionals (though professionals are involved). You may, for example, be able to find groups specifically for women, African

Americans, gay men, transgender individuals, or other specific groups of people. Because members face similar challenges, they may feel an instant sense of community. These groups are volunteer, nonprofit organizations, with no fees (though sometimes there are small dues).

Work with Your Provider

HIV is the virus that causes AIDS. If ignored, it can lead to illness and death. This is why it is so important to get medical care and start treatment if you find out you have HIV. Please see a doctor or nurse practitioner with experience in treating people with HIV—he or she can help you to stay well. Most VA clinicians who treat HIV are specialists in infectious disease. They work with a team of other health professionals who focus on HIV as a chronic, or lifelong, disease.

Treatments for HIV are not perfect (no medicine is), but are very tolerable and extremely effective for most people. They also work very well to minimize the chance that you may transmit HIV to sex partners (for pregnant women they also decrease the risk of infecting the baby). A doctor or other healthcare provider can explain the best options for you. If you work with your healthcare provider in planning your care, you can deal with the disease in a way that is best for you.

Before Appointments

Start with a list or notebook. Prepare for your appointment with your doctor by writing down:

1. any questions that you have (print out questions to ask your doctor and take it to your appointment)

2. any symptoms or problems you want to tell the doctor about (include symptoms such as poor sleep, trouble concentrating, feeling tired)

3. a list of the medications that you are taking (include herbs and vitamins), including a list of any HIV medications you have taken in the past and any HIV-related problems you have had when taking them

4. upcoming tests or new information you've heard about

5. changes in your living situation, such as a job change

That way you won't forget anything during the appointment. You may want to ask a friend or family member to come with you and take notes. It can be difficult for you to take notes and pay attention to what your doctor is saying at the same time.

During Appointments

Go over your lab results, and keep track of them. If your health-care provider wants you to have some medical tests, make sure you understand what the test is for and what your provider will do with the results. If you don't understand what your medical provider is saying, ask him/her to explain it in everyday terms. If you feel your provider has forgotten something during the appointment, it is better to ask about it than to leave wondering whether something was supposed to happen that didn't. It's your right to ask questions of your provider. You also have a legal right to see your medical records. After all, it's your body. Be honest. Your provider isn't there to judge you, but to make decisions based on your particular circumstances. Tell your doctor about your sexual or drug use history. These behaviors can put you at risk of getting other sexually transmitted diseases as well as hepatitis. If your body is fighting off these other diseases, it will not be able to fight off HIV as effectively. You may get sicker, faster. If you have sex with someone of the same sex or someone other than your spouse, it's OK to tell your medical provider.

Monitor Your Health

Once you have been diagnosed with HIV, you need to pay closer attention to your health than you did before. You can keep track of your immune system in two ways:

1. Have regular lab tests done. Lab tests often can show signs of illness before you have any noticeable symptoms.

2. Listen to what your body is telling you, and be on the alert for signs that something isn't right. Note any change in your health—good or bad. And don't be afraid to call a doctor.

Have Regular Lab Tests

Your medical provider will use laboratory tests to check your health. Some of these tests will be done soon after you learn you are HIV positive.

The lab tests look at several things:

*   how well your immune system is functioning

- how well your medications are controlling the HIV (or, if you are not taking HIV medications, how rapidly HIV is progressing)

- certain basic body functions (tests look at your kidneys, liver, cholesterol, and blood cells)

- whether you have other diseases that are associated with HIV

For your first few doctor visits, be prepared to have a lot of blood drawn. Don't worry. You are not going to have so much blood drawn at every appointment.

Be Aware of Possible Complications

By weakening your immune system, HIV can leave you vulnerable to certain cancers and infections. These infections are called "opportunistic" because they take the opportunity to attack you when your immune system is weak. HIV also is an inflammatory disease that affects many parts of the body, not just the immune system. That means that HIV can affect organs like the brain, kidneys, liver, and heart and may increase the risk of some cancers. HIV medicines can sometimes have side effects. Sometimes these can raise the risk of heart disease or kidney disease. It is important that you let your medical providers know if you notice any concerning symptoms.

Know When to Call a Medical Provider

You don't need to panic every time you have a headache or get a runny nose. But if a symptom is concerning you or is not going away, it is always best to have a provider check it out even if it doesn't feel like a big deal. The earlier you see a provider when you have unusual symptoms, the better off you are likely to be.

The following symptoms may or may not be serious, but don't wait until your next appointment before calling a doctor if you are experiencing them.

Breathing problems:

- persistent cough

- wheezing or noisy breathing

- sharp pain when breathing

- difficulty catching your breath

Skin problems:

- Appearance of brownish, purple or pink blotches on the skin
- New or worsening rash—especially important if you are taking medication

Eye or vision problems:

- blurring, wavy lines, sudden blind spots
- eye pain
- sensitivity to light

Aches and pains:

- numbness, tingling, or pain in hands and feet
- headache, especially when accompanied by a fever
- stiffness in neck
- severe or persistent cough
- persistent cramps
- pain in lower abdomen, often during sex (women in particular)

Other symptoms:

- mental changes—confusion, disorientation, loss of memory or balance
- appearance of swollen lymph nodes (glands), especially when larger on one side of the body
- diarrhea—when severe, accompanied by fever, or lasting more than 3 days
- weight loss
- high or persistent fever
- fatigue
- frequent urination

Protect Others

Once you have HIV, it is important that you take measures so you don't pass the virus to sex partners, to injecting drug partners, or (for women who wish to become pregnant) to a baby during pregnancy or delivery, or by breast-feeding. Starting and staying on HIV medications (antiretroviral therapy, or ART) is a hugely effective way to minimize the risk of transmitting the HIV virus. Using condoms and clean injection equipment also can prevent HIV from passing to other people and condoms can also protect you from getting other sexually transmitted diseases. Partners who do not have HIV also can use PrEP (preexposure prophylaxis), a daily pill that can prevent HIV infection.

Sometimes it can be difficult to explain that you have HIV to people you have had sex with or shared syringes with in the past. However, it is important that they know so they can get tested. If you need help telling people that you may have exposed them to HIV, many city or county health departments will tell them for you, without using your name. Ask your provider about this service.

Before telling your partner that you have HIV, take some time alone to think about how you want to bring up the subject.

- Decide when and where would be the best time and place to have a conversation. Choose a time when you expect that you will both be comfortable, rested, and as relaxed as possible.

- Think about how your partner may react to stressful situations. If there is a history of violence in your relationship, consider your safety first and plan the situation with a case manager or counselor.

Consider Treatment

When or whether to start treatment for HIV is a decision that each person must make with his or her providers. In general, experts recommend starting HIV treatment very soon after your diagnosis; this can help prevent some of the damage that HIV causes in many parts of the body. HIV treatment (ART) is strongly recommended for all HIV-infected people, and more urgently for anyone who has evidence of immune suppression (a cluster of differentiation 4+ (CD4+) cell count that is below normal) or an AIDS diagnosis (an infection or cancer associated with HIV). It also is more urgently recommended for anyone who has a sex partner who is not infected with HIV, and for women who may become pregnant.

Move Forward with Your Life

Life does not end with a diagnosis of HIV. In fact, with proper treatment, people with HIV usually live long healthy lives. HIV can be a manageable chronic disease, like diabetes or heart disease. Taking care of your overall health can help you deal with HIV:

- Take your medicines every day
- Get regular medical and dental checkups
- Eat a healthy diet
- Exercise regularly
- Avoid smoking and recreational drug use
- Go easy on alcohol
- Use condoms during sex (it can protect others from getting HIV, prevent unintended pregnancy, and protect you from other sexually transmitted diseases)

Chapter 49

Staying Healthy When You Have HIV/AIDS

Chapter Contents

Section 49.1

HIV and Nutrition

This section includes text excerpted from "HIV/AIDS—
Diet and Nutrition and HIV: Entire Lesson,"
U.S. Department of Veterans Affairs (VA), February 8, 2018.

Nutrition and Its Importance

Nutrition is important for everyone because food gives our bodies the nutrients they need to stay healthy, grow, and work properly. Foods are made up of six classes of nutrients, each with its own special role in the body:

- Protein builds muscles and a strong immune system

- Carbohydrates (including vegetables, fruits, grains) give you energy

- Fat gives you extra energy

- Vitamins regulate body processes

- Minerals regulate body processes and also makeup body tissues

- Water gives cells shape and acts as a medium where body processes can occur

Having good nutrition means eating the right types of foods in the right amounts so you get these important nutrients.

Do I Need a Special Diet?

There are no special diets, or particular foods, that will directly boost your immune system. But there are things you can do to keep your immunity up.

When you are infected with human immunodeficiency virus (HIV), your immune system has to work very hard to fight off infections—and this takes energy (measured in calories). For some people, this may mean you need to eat more food than you used to.

If you are underweight—or you have advanced HIV disease, high viral loads, or opportunistic infections—you should include more protein as well as extra calories (in the form of carbohydrates and fats).

Keep in mind, you may need to eat more nutritious foods to meet your body's needs.

Preventing Weight Loss

Weight loss can be a common problem for people with relatively advanced stages of HIV infection, and it should be taken very seriously. It usually improves with effective antiretroviral therapy (ART). Losing weight can be dangerous because it makes it harder for your body to fight infections and to get well after you're sick.

People with advanced HIV often do not eat enough because:

- HIV may reduce your appetite, make food taste bad, and prevent the body from absorbing food in the right way. Some HIV medicines may also cause these symptoms (if this is so, tell your HIV specialist—you may be able to change to medications that do not have these side effects).

- Symptoms like a sore mouth, nausea, and vomiting make it difficult to eat

- Fatigue from HIV or medicines may make it hard to prepare food and eat regularly

- To keep your weight up, you will need to take in more protein and calories. What follows are ways to do that.

To Add Protein to Your Diet

Protein-rich foods include meats, fish, beans, dairy products, and nuts. To boost the protein in your meals:

- Spread nut butter on toast, crackers, fruit, or vegetables

- Add cottage cheese to fruit and tomatoes

- Add canned tuna to casseroles and salads.

- Add shredded cheese to sauces, soups, omelets, baked potatoes, and steamed vegetables

- Eat yogurt on your cereal or fruit

- Eat hard-boiled (hard-cooked) eggs. Use them in egg-salad sandwiches or slice and dice them for tossed salads.

- Eat beans and legumes (pinto and other beans, lentils, etc.), nuts, and seeds

- Add diced or chopped meats to soups, salads, and sauces

- Add dried milk powder or egg white powder to foods (like scrambled eggs, casseroles, and milkshakes)

To Add Calories to Your Diet

The best way to increase calories is to add extra fat and carbohydrates to your meals. Fats are more concentrated sources of calories. Add moderate amounts of the following to your meals:

- Butter, margarine, sour cream, cream cheese, peanut butter
- Gravy, sour cream, cream cheese, grated cheese
- Avocados, olives, salad dressing

  Carbohydrates include both starches and simple sugars. Starches are in:

- Bread, muffins, biscuits, crackers
- Oatmeal and cold cereals
- Pasta
- Potatoes
- Rice

  Simple sugars are in:

- Fresh or dried fruit (raisins, dates, apricots, etc.)
- Jelly, honey, and maple syrup added to cereal, pancakes, and waffles

Maintaining Appetite

When you become ill, you often lose your appetite. This can lead to weight loss, which can make it harder for your body to fight infection. Here are some tips for increasing your appetite:

- Try a little exercise, like walking or doing yoga. This can often stimulate your appetite and make you feel like eating more.

- Eat smaller meals more often. For instance, try to snack between meals.

- Eat whenever your appetite is good.

- Avoid drinking too much right before or during meals. This can make you feel full.

- Avoid carbonated (fizzy) drinks and foods such as cabbage, broccoli, and beans. These foods and drinks can create gas in your stomach and make you feel full and bloated.

- Eat with your family or friends.

- Choose your favorite foods, and make meals as attractive to you as possible. Try to eat in a pleasant location.

Water Intake

Drinking enough liquids is very important when you have HIV. Fluids transport the nutrients you need through your body. Extra water can:

- Reduce the side effects of medications

- Help flush out the medicines that have already been used by your body

- Help you avoid dehydration (fluid loss), dry mouth, and constipation

- Make you feel less tired

Many of us don't drink enough water every day. You should be getting at least 8–10 glasses of water (or other fluids, such as juices or soups) a day.

Here are some tips on getting the extra fluids you need:

- Drink more water than usual. Try other fluids, too, like noncaffeinated teas, flavored waters, or fruit juice mixed with water.

- Avoid colas, coffee, tea, and cocoa. These may contain caffeine and can actually dehydrate you. Read the labels on drinks to see if they have caffeine in them.

- Avoid alcohol

- Begin and end each day by drinking a glass of water

- Suck on ice cubes and popsicles

Note: If you have diarrhea or are vomiting, you will lose a lot of fluids and will need to drink more than usual.

Do I Need Supplements?

Our bodies need vitamins and minerals, in small amounts, to keep our cells working properly. They are essential to our staying healthy. People with HIV may need extra vitamins and minerals to help repair and heal cells that have been damaged.

Even though vitamins and minerals are present in many foods, your healthcare provider may recommend a vitamin and mineral supplement (a pill or other form of concentrated vitamins and minerals). While vitamin and mineral supplements can be useful, they can't replace eating a healthy diet.

If you are taking a supplement, here are some things to remember:

- Do not take vitamin pills on an empty stomach. Take them regularly.

- Some vitamins and minerals, if taken in high doses, can be harmful

- Some minerals (like calcium, magnesium, and iron) may interfere with certain HIV medicines—talk with your healthcare provider about whether or when to take these minerals.

What You Should Know about Food Safety

Paying attention to food and water safety is important when you have HIV, because your immune system is already weakened and working hard to fight off infections. If food is not handled or prepared in a safe way, germs from the food can be passed on to you. These germs can make you sick.

You need to handle and cook food properly to keep those germs from getting to you. Here are some food safety guidelines:

- Keep everything clean. Clean your counters and utensils often.

- Wash your hands with soap and warm water before and after preparing and eating food.

- Check expiration dates on food packaging. Do not eat foods that are past the expiration date.

- Rinse all fresh fruits and vegetables with clean water.

- Thaw frozen meats and other frozen foods in the refrigerator or in a microwave. Never thaw foods at room temperature. Germs that grow at room temperature can make you very sick.

- Clean all cutting boards and knives (especially those that touch chicken and meat) with soap and hot water before using them again.

- Make sure you cook all meat, fish, and poultry "well-done." You might want to buy a meat thermometer to help you know for sure that it is done. Put the thermometer in the thickest part of the meat and not touching a bone. Cook the meat until it reaches 165–212 degrees Fahrenheit on your thermometer.

- Do not eat raw, soft-boiled, or "over easy" eggs, or Caesar salads with raw egg in the dressing.

- Do not eat sushi, raw seafood, or raw meats, or unpasteurized milk or dairy products.

- Keep your refrigerator cold, set no higher than 40 degrees. Your freezer should be at 0 degrees.

- Refrigerate leftovers at temperatures below 40°F. Do not eat leftovers that have been sitting in the refrigerator for more than 3 days.

- Keep hot items heated to over 140°F, and completely reheat leftovers before eating.

- Throw away any foods (like fruit, vegetables, and cheese) that you think might be old. If food has a moldy or rotten spot, throw it out. When in doubt, throw it out.

- Some germs are spread through tap water. If your public water supply isn't totally pure, drink bottled water.

Diet Helps in Easing Side Effects and Symptoms

Many symptoms of HIV, as well as the side effects caused by HIV medicines, can be helped by using (or avoiding) certain types of foods and drinks.

Below are some tips for dealing with common problems people with HIV face.

Nausea

- Try the BRAT diet (Bananas, Rice, Applesauce, and Toast)

- Try some ginger—in tea, ginger ale, or ginger snaps (these need to be made with real ginger root)

- Don't drink liquids at the same time you eat your meals

- Eat something small, like crackers, before getting out of bed

- Keep something in your stomach; eat a small snack every 1–2 hours

- Avoid foods like:
  - Fatty, greasy, or fried foods
  - Very sweet foods (candy, cookies, or cake)
  - Spicy foods
  - Foods with strong odors

Mouth and Swallowing Problem

- Avoid hard or crunchy foods such as raw vegetables
- Try eating cooked vegetables and soft fruits (like bananas and pears)
- Avoid very hot foods and beverages. Cold and room temperature foods will be more comfortable to your mouth.
- Do not eat spicy foods. They can sting your mouth.
- Try soft foods like mashed potatoes, yogurt, and oatmeal
- Also try scrambled eggs, cottage cheese, macaroni and cheese, and canned fruits
- Rinse your mouth with water. This can moisten your mouth, remove bits of food, and make food taste better to you.
- Stay away from oranges, grapefruit, and tomatoes. They have a lot of acids and can sting your mouth.

Diarrhea

- Try the BRAT diet (Bananas, Rice, Applesauce, and Toast)
- Keep your body's fluids up (hydrated) with water or other fluids (those that don't have caffeine)
- Limit sodas and other sugary drinks
- Avoid greasy and spicy foods
- Avoid milk and other dairy products
- Eat small meals and snacks every hour or two

Remember, there is no one "right" way to eat. Eating well means getting the right amount of nutrients for your particular needs. Your healthcare provider can refer you to a dietitian or nutritionist who can help design a good diet for you.

Section 49.2

HIV and Exercise

This section includes text excerpted from "HIV/AIDS—
Exercise and HIV: Entire Lesson," U.S. Department of
Veterans Affairs (VA), February 8, 2018.

Being human immunodeficiency virus (HIV)-positive is no different
from being human immunodeficiency virus (HIV)-negative when it
comes to exercise. Regular exercise is part of a healthy lifestyle.

Benefits of Exercise

Following are some of the benefits of exercise:

• Maintains or builds muscle mass

• Reduces cholesterol and triglyceride levels (less risk of heart
disease)

• Increases energy

• Regulates bowel function

• Strengthens bones (less risk of osteoporosis)

• Improves blood circulation

• Increases lung capacity

• Helps with sound, restful sleep

• Lowers stress

• Improves appetite

Before Starting

Before starting an exercise program, talk to your healthcare provider about what you have done in the past for exercise; mention
any problems that you had. Consider your current health status
and other medical conditions that may affect the type of exercise
you can do.

Make sure you can set aside time for your exercise program. Experts
recommend about 150 minutes (2–1/2 hours) of moderately vigorous
exercise per week. That means about 30 minutes of brisk walking,
bicycling, or working around the house, 5 days a week. This amount

of exercise can reduce risks of developing coronary heart disease, high blood pressure, colon cancer, and diabetes.

If this amount of time seems too much, consider starting with 3 times a week. The important thing is consistency. This is an ongoing program and you will not benefit without consistency.

Types of Exercise

Two types of exercise are resistance training and aerobic exercise. Resistance training—sometimes called strength training—helps to build muscle strength and mass. Aerobic exercise is important because it strengthens your lungs and your heart.

Resistance Training

Resistance or strength training is important for people with HIV because it can help offset the loss of muscle sometimes caused by the disease. This form of exercise involves exertion of force by moving (pushing or pulling) objects of weight. They can be barbells, dumbbells, or machines in gyms. You can also use safe, common household objects such as plastic milk containers filled with water or sand, or you can use your own body weight in exercises such as push-ups or pull-ups. The purpose of resistance training is to build muscle mass.

Use the correct amount of weight for the exercise you are performing. You should not feel pain during the exercise. When starting a resistance training program, you should feel a little sore for a day or two, but not enough to limit your regular activities. If you do feel very sore, you have used too much weight or have done too many repetitions. Rest an extra day and start again using less weight.

Aerobic Exercise

Aerobic exercise strengthens your lungs and heart. Walking, jogging, running, swimming, hiking, and cycling are forms of this exercise.

This movement increases your heart rate and the rate and depth of your breathing, which in turn increases how much blood and oxygen your heart pumps to your muscles. To achieve the maximum benefit of this kind of exercise, most experts recommend that your heart rate should reach the target rate for at least 20 minutes. It may take you weeks to reach this level if you haven't been exercising much.

Designing a Program

When beginning an exercise program, start slow and build. Start any exercise session with a warmup. This can be as short as a few stretches, if you are working out later in the day when your muscles and joints are already loose, or a short 10-minute stretch session if you are working out first thing in the morning, when your muscles and joints are still tight. Your warm-up should not tire you out but invigorate you and decrease the risk of joint or muscle injury.

If you join a gym, ask about what comes with the membership. Many gyms offer a free evaluation that includes weighing and measuring you and asking what your goals are. Some gym memberships come with a free workout with a personal trainer and advice to help you achieve your goals.

Finding a workout partner can be helpful for support and encouragement, and your workout partner can help motivate you with the last repetitions of an exercise, which can help improve your strength.

A balanced exercise program is best. Starting with anaerobic exercise is a good warmup to a resistance training session. Remember that learning the correct form in a weight training program will lessen the chance of injury. Go at your own pace. You are not competing with anyone. Listen to your body. If it hurts, stop.

Exercise Cautions

After an exercise session, you should feel a little tired. A little while later, however, you should have some energy.

Water. Drink it before, during, and after you exercise. When you feel thirsty you have already lost important fluids and electrolytes and may be dehydrated.

Eat well. Exercising tears down muscle in order to build it up stronger. You need nutrition to provide the raw materials to rebuild your muscles.

Sleep. While you sleep, your body is rebuilding.

Listen to your body. It will tell you to slow down or speed up.

If you are sick or have a cold, take a break. Your body will thank you.

Section 49.3

Mental Health

This section contains text excerpted from the following sources:
Text under the heading "What Is Mental Health?" is excerpted from
"Living with HIV," AIDS*info*, U.S. Department of Health and Human
Services (HHS), June 7, 2018; Text under the heading "People with
Human Immunodeficiency Virus (HIV) / Acquired Immunodeficiency
Syndrome (AIDS) Are at a Higher Risk for Mental Health Disorders"
is excerpted from "HIV/AIDS and Mental Health," National Institute
of Mental Health (NIMH), November 2016; Text beginning with the
heading "What Are Common Types of Mental Health Conditions
and Symptoms?" is excerpted from "Act against AIDS," Centers for
Disease Control and Prevention (CDC), February 12, 2018.

What Is Mental Health?

Mental health is defined as a state of overall well-being in which
every individual realizes his or her own potential, can cope with the
normal stresses of life, can work productively and fruitfully, and is
able to make a contribution to his or her community.

Mental health has three main areas:

1. Emotional well-being (life satisfaction, happiness,
   cheerfulness, peacefulness)

2. Psychological well-being (self-acceptance, optimism,
   hopefulness, purpose in life, spirituality, self-direction, positive
   relationships)

3. Social well-being (social acceptance, believing in the potential
   of people and society as a whole, personal self-worth and
   usefulness to society, sense of community)

If you are living with human immunodeficiency virus (HIV), it is
important to take care of not only your physical health but also your
mental health.

People with HIV/AIDS Are at a Higher Risk for Mental Health Disorders

If you are living with human immunodeficiency virus (HIV), it is
important for you to be aware that you have an increased risk for
developing mood, anxiety, and cognitive disorders. For example, people

living with HIV are twice as likely to have depression compared to those who are not infected with HIV. These conditions may be treatable. Many people with mental health conditions recover completely.

Some forms of stress can contribute to mental health problems for people living with HIV, including:

- Having trouble getting the services you need

- Experiencing a loss of social support, resulting in isolation

- Experiencing a loss of employment or worries about whether you will be able to perform your work as you did before

- Having to tell others you are HIV-positive

- Managing your HIV medicines

- Going through changes in your physical appearance or abilities due to HIV/AIDS

- Dealing with loss, including the loss of relationships or even death

- Facing the stigma and discrimination associated with HIV/AIDS

The HIV virus itself also can contribute to mental health problems because it enters and resides in your brain. Some other opportunistic infections can also affect your nervous system and lead to changes in your behavior and functioning. Similarly, neuropsychological disorders, such as mild cognitive changes or more severe cognitive conditions, such as dementia, are associated with HIV disease.

You can better manage your overall health and well-being if you know how having HIV can affect your mental health and what resources are available to help you if you need them.

Common Types of Mental Health Conditions and Symptoms

One of the most common mental health conditions that people living with HIV face is depression. Depression can range from mild to severe, and the symptoms of depression can affect your day-to-day life. Symptoms can include:

- Persistent sadness

- Anxiety

- Feeling "empty"

- Helplessness

- Negativity

- Loss of appetite

- Disinterest in engaging with others

The good news is that depression is treatable.

Finding Treatment and Support for Mental Health

Because mental health conditions are common, many outlets can help you maintain good mental health. If you are having symptoms of depression or another mental health condition, talk to your healthcare provider, social worker, or case manager. These people can refer you to a mental health provider who can give you the care you need.

Types of mental health providers include:

- **Psychiatrists.** Medically trained physicians who treat mental health problems with various therapies, like talk therapy, and by prescribing medicine.

- **Psychologists.** Trained professionals who help people cope with life challenges and mental health problems with therapies, like talk therapy, but usually cannot prescribe medicines.

- **Therapists.** Mental health or marriage and family counselors who help people cope with life issues and mental health problems.

You may also choose to join a support group. Support groups include:

- **Mental health support groups.** An organized group of peers who meet in a safe and supportive environment to provide mental health support to members of the group.

- **HIV support groups.** An organized group of peers living with HIV who meet in a safe and supportive environment to provide support to other people living with HIV.

Work with a trained mental health professional to learn about treatment options such as therapy and/or medicine. You and your provider can develop a plan that will help you regain and maintain good mental health.

Other ways to help improve mental health and well-being include:

- **Exercise.** Regular exercise may help improve symptoms of depression and decrease stress. When you exercise, your brain releases chemicals called endorphins. These chemicals help improve your mood.

- **Meditation.** Studies suggest that mindfulness meditation can help ease depression, anxiety, and stress.

Resources for Finding Mental Health Treatment and Support

Many organizations have websites and telephone hotlines that can help you find treatment for mental health conditions.

- Substance Abuse and Mental Health Services Administration (SAMHSA)'s Find Help website provides a list of organizations and contact numbers that can help you find mental health treatment and support in your local area.

- The Womenshealth.gov mental health and HIV resource provides useful information for all people living with HIV.

Steps to Take before Starting Treatment for a Mental Health Condition

Talk to your HIV healthcare provider before starting any mental health treatment. If you are taking antiretroviral therapy (ART) or plan to take ART, consider the following:

- Your HIV treatment may contribute to mental health conditions. Talk to your healthcare provider to better understand how your HIV treatment might affect your mental health and if anything can be done to address the side effects.

- Some medicines for mental health conditions or mood disorders can interact with ART.

Communicate openly and honestly with your healthcare provider about your mental health so that he or she can help you find the support you need.

Section 49.4

HIV, Alcohol, and Drugs

This section includes text excerpted from "HIV/AIDS—
Drugs, Alcohol and HIV," U.S. Department of Veterans
Affairs (VA), February 8, 2018.

If you've just found out that you are human immunodeficiency virus (HIV) positive, you might be wondering what alcohol and other "recreational" drugs will do to your body. (Recreational drugs are drugs that aren't being used for medical purposes, such as beer, cocaine, amphetamines, and pot; this also includes prescription medicines that are being used for pleasure.)

You may be wondering whether these drugs are bad for your immune system. And what about your HIV medications—can recreational drugs affect those?

Is using alcohol or other drugs is bad for you? Each person is different, and a lot depends on which drugs you use, how much you use, and how often you use them.

However, most experts would agree that, in large amounts, drugs and alcohol are bad for your immune system and your overall health. Remember, if you have HIV, your immune system is already weakened.

Here, in this section, you can read about what alcohol and drugs can do to your overall health.

Your Immune System

Drinking too much alcohol can weaken your immune system. A weaker immune system will have a harder time fighting off common infections (such as a cold), as well as HIV-related infections. A weaker immune system also increases the chance that you will experience more side effects from your HIV medications.

Smoking marijuana (pot) or any other drug irritates the lungs. You may be more likely to get serious lung infections, such as pneumonia.

Other common recreational drugs, such as cocaine or crystal methamphetamine ("meth," "speed"), can leave your body dehydrated and exhausted, as well as lead to skin irritation. All of these things can make it easier for you to get infections.

The organ in your body that alcohol and other drugs affect most is your liver. The liver rounds up waste from chemicals that you put in your body. Those chemicals include recreational drugs as well as prescription drugs, such as your HIV medications. A weaker liver means less efficient "housekeeping" and, probably, a weaker you.

If you also have hepatitis C (or any other kind of hepatitis), your liver is already working very hard to fight the disease itself and deal with the strong drugs that you may be taking for your hepatitis treatment.

Interactions with Meds

HIV medications can be hard on your body, so when you are taking these medications, it is important that your liver works as well as possible. The liver is responsible for getting rid of waste products from the medications.

Once you are HIV positive, your body may react differently to alcohol and drugs. Many people find that it takes longer to recover from using pot, alcohol, or other recreational drugs than it did before they had HIV.

Remember that having HIV means a major change has taken place in your body. You may choose to use alcohol and drugs in moderation, but be sure to respect your body. Pay attention to what and how much you eat, drink, smoke, and take into your body.

Certain HIV medications can boost the level of recreational drugs in your system in unexpected and potentially dangerous ways. For example, amphetamines (such as crystal meth) can be present at 3–22 times their normal levels in the bloodstream when mixed with an HIV drug called ritonavir (Norvir). That's because ritonavir hampers the body's ability to break down these other drugs.

If you are going to take a recreational drug while you are on HIV medication, it is better to start with a very low amount of the recreational drug (as low as 1/4 the normal amount) and allow time to see how it affects you before increasing the amount. Keep in mind that recreational drugs aren't regulated, so you never know exactly how much you are getting.

Although you may feel uncomfortable at first, you should tell your doctor what recreational drugs you are using. That way, your doctor will know how the substances you are using affect your HIV drugs and your overall health. Most likely, your doctor will then be able to explain some things going on in your body.

Safer Sex

Many drugs, including alcohol and methamphetamine, may affect your ability to make decisions.

Even though you take your HIV medications regularly and practice safer sex when you're not high, when you're under the influence of methamphetamine or other drugs you may be willing to take more risks and, for example, not use a condom or not take your HIV medications.

Alcohol also can affect the decisions you make about safer sex. For example, if you have too much to drink, you may not be able to remember where you put the condoms, and decide simply not to use them. These are decisions you probably would not make if you were sober.

These actions put your partner at risk for HIV and put you at risk for other sexually transmitted diseases or for pregnancy.

Remember to take your HIV medications every day, and to keep condoms handy in places where you might have sex. Also, try to limit the amount of drugs you use or alcohol you drink if you know you are going to have sex.

Injection Drug Use

Sharing a needle or any equipment when injecting drugs is dangerous for you and for the people you are sharing with. They could get HIV from you, and you could get another disease, such as hepatitis, from them.

The safest option is not to share. Use clean needles and syringes each time, and keep your own equipment to yourself. Because of the dangers of injection drug use, the best way to lower your risk is to stop injecting drugs and to enter and complete a substance abuse treatment plan. You can talk to your healthcare provider about this.

If you do inject drugs, follow these reminders:

- Never reuse or "share" syringes, water, or drug preparation equipment.

- Use only syringes obtained from a reliable source (such as pharmacies and needle or syringe exchange programs).

- Use a new, sterile syringe each time to prepare and inject drugs. If this is not possible, sterilize your syringe or disinfect your syringe and other equipment with bleach.

- If possible, use sterile water to prepare drugs; otherwise, use clean water from a reliable source (such as fresh tap water).

- Use a new or disinfected container ("cooker") and a new filter ("cotton") to prepare drugs.

- Clean the injection site with a new alcohol swab prior to injection.

- Safely dispose of syringes after one use.

Section 49.5

HIV and Smoking

This section includes text excerpted from "HIV/AIDS—
Kicking the Habit: HIV and Smoking," U.S. Department of
Veterans Affairs (VA), February 8, 2018.

Smoking cigarettes is the leading cause of preventable death in the United States. And smoking is even worse for people with human immunodeficiency virus (HIV) than it is for people without HIV. Among persons living with HIV/AIDS (acquired immunodeficiency syndrome), smoking is closely linked with heart disease and serious lung diseases such as chronic obstructive pulmonary disease (COPD), emphysema, chronic bronchitis, and asthma. It also is associated with a number of types of cancer.

By-the-Numbers

People with HIV are more than twice as likely to smoke as people in the general population. In the United States, 40–75 percent of HIV-positive people smoke, while only 18 percent of the general population smokes. Many HIV-positive people who smoke are highly dependent on nicotine (55–65%). Quitting smoking is a powerful way you can improve your health.

Nicotine Replacement Therapies

The most common way people try to quit smoking is by gradually decreasing the body's dependence on and cravings for nicotine. Nicotine replacement therapies can help. These therapies are meant to replace cigarettes. They work by delivering a specific dose of nicotine to your body. When it is time, you switch to a lower dose of nicotine. Over time, the dose of nicotine gets lower and lower. Nicotine replacement therapies come in many different forms, including patches, gum, lozenges, nasal inhalers, and false cigarettes.

Nicotine patches are the most commonly used. Patches typically come in 3 different strengths, sometimes referred to as "steps." Choosing the right step at which to start depends on how much you smoke. How much you smoke also influences how long you'll need to wear the patches. It usually takes about 3 months to quit smoking by using patches. The patches may cause side effects that are similar to those of cigarettes, including insomnia, headaches, and nausea. Some people are allergic to the tape used in patches and may get a skin reaction such as swelling or redness around the patch area.

E-cigarettes may help some smokers quit smoking regular cigarettes, but their role in stop-smoking programs, and their overall safety, have not been studied thoroughly.

A Pill to Stop Smoking

If you would rather take a daily medicine to help you stop smoking, there are two options. Both require a prescription from your doctor.

Bupropion is an antidepressant that also helps people stop smoking when it is taken at higher doses. It's not known exactly how bupropion reduces nicotine cravings, but it's known that it works on many chemicals in the brain. You begin taking bupropion 1 week before you want to quit smoking and continue taking it for at least 12 weeks. Some people take it for up to 6 months to make sure they do not begin smoking again. Possible side effects of bupropion include headache, insomnia, dizziness, rapid heartbeat, weight loss, and nausea. Some antiretroviral therapies (HIV medicines) may lower the levels of bupropion in the body. Check with your doctor or pharmacist to see if your medications interact with bupropion. If they interact, that does not mean you can't use bupropion; it may just mean that you will need close monitoring, extra support, or combination therapy with nicotine replacement to reach your goal of quitting.

Varenicline is another prescription medicine used to help people quit smoking. It reduces cravings and lessens the good feelings people get from smoking. You begin taking varenicline at least 1 week before you want to quit smoking and continue taking it for at least 12 weeks, maybe longer if you're worried about relapse. It does not interact with HIV medicines. However, people who have depression or heart disease should use varenicline very carefully. Some people have experienced changes in mood such as feeling agitated, hostile, or depressed; in rare cases, people have experienced psychosis or the desire to commit suicide. A study found that patients who used varenicline were slightly more likely to have heart attacks or strokes, although these heart attacks and strokes did not occur very often.

These severe side effects are rare, but it is important to talk with your doctor about which medicine might be best for you.

These medicines can be used with nicotine replacement therapies.

Beyond Medications

Although there are several good medicines to support your goals of quitting smoking, the other "nonmedicine" parts of your plan are equally important. These include having a supportive team around you. Friends, family members, and healthcare providers can help keep you on track. Your plan should include talking about reasons why you want to quit smoking, so you can remain inspired. Your plan should also include understanding when you typically smoke, how much you smoke, and why you smoke. Knowing these things can help you identify situations that tempt you to reach for a cigarette, so that you can avoid or work around them. You also can take advantage of many great telephone resources such as 800-QUIT-NOW (800-784-8669) for free counseling, advice, and services. It is not easy to quit smoking, but it is important for your health over the long run. If you've been thinking about quitting, start the conversation with your healthcare provider.

Chapter 50

Avoiding Infections When You Have HIV/AIDS

Chapter Contents

Section 50.1

Preventing Exposure

This section includes text excerpted from "Guidelines for Prevention and Treatment of Opportunistic Infections in HIV-Infected Adults and Adolescents," AIDS*info*, U.S. Department of Health and Human Services (HHS), May 29, 2018.

Sexual Exposures

Male latex condoms, when used consistently and correctly during every act of sexual intercourse, are highly effective in preventing the sexual transmission of human immunodeficiency virus (HIV) and can reduce the risk for acquiring other sexually transmitted diseases (STDs), including chlamydia, gonorrhea, and trichomoniasis. Correct and consistent use of male latex condoms not only reduces the risk of HIV transmission but might reduce the risk for transmission of herpes simplex virus, syphilis, and chancroid when the infected area or potential site of exposure is covered, although data for this effect are more limited. Male condoms also appear to reduce the risk for human papillomavirus (HPV) associated diseases (i.e., genital warts, cervical cancer) and thereby mitigate the adverse consequences of infection with HPV. Although data for female condoms are limited, women should consider using them to prevent the acquisition of STDs and reduce their risk of transmitting HIV. Spermicides containing nonoxynol-9 are not effective for HIV/STD prevention and may increase risk of transmission to uninfected partners; nonoxynol-9 should not be used as a microbicide or lubricant during vaginal or anal intercourse.

As with many nonsexually transmitted opportunistic infections, intercurrent infections with sexually transmitted pathogens (especially pathogens that cause genital ulcers such as herpes simplex, syphilis, and chancroid) can, if untreated, stimulate increases in HIV viral load and consequent declines in cluster of differentiation 4 (CD4) T lymphocyte count. Furthermore, acquisition of STDs by HIV infected patients indicates participation in high-risk sexual behavior that is capable of transmitting HIV to others, the risk for which is substantially increased in the presence of genital tract inflammation (e.g., from gonorrhea or chlamydia) and genital ulcer disease (e.g., herpes simplex virus-2 infection, syphilis). All HIV-infected persons, including those who are asymptomatic, should be tested at initial evaluation for trichomoniasis in women; syphilis, urogenital gonorrhea, and chlamydia in men and women; and oral gonorrhea, rectal gonorrhea, and rectal chlamydia for male patients reporting receptive sex at these anatomic sites. Nucleic acid amplification testing methods are the most sensitive and specific method for the diagnosis of anogenital, oral, and rectal chlamydia and gonorrhea infection. For all sexually active patients, screening should be repeated at least annually and more frequently depending on individual risk or symptoms. In addition to identifying and treating STDs, providers should communicate prevention messages, discuss sexual and drug-use behaviors, positively reinforce safer behaviors, refer patients for services such as substance abuse treatment, and facilitate partner notification, counseling, and testing.

Specific sex practices should be avoided that might result in oral exposure to feces (e.g., oral-anal contact) to reduce the risk for intestinal infections (e.g., cryptosporidiosis, shigellosis, campylobacteriosis, amebiasis, giardiasis, lymphogranuloma venereum (LGV) serovars of chlamydia, hepatitis A (HAV)). Persons who wish to reduce their risk for exposure might consider using dental dams or similar barrier methods for oral-anal and oral-genital contact, changing condoms after anal intercourse, and wearing latex gloves during digital-anal contact. Frequent washing of hands and genitals with warm soapy water during and after activities that might bring these body parts in contact with feces might further reduce risk for illness.

Sexual transmission of hepatitis C virus (HCV) and infection can occur, especially among HIV-infected men who have sex with men (MSM). HIV-infected MSM not known to be infected with HCV, and who present with new and unexplained increases in alanine aminotransferase, should be tested for HCV virus infection. Routine (e.g., annual) HCV testing should be considered for MSM with high-risk sexual behaviors or with a diagnosis of an ulcerative STD.

HAV can be transmitted sexually, therefore, vaccination is recommended for all susceptible MSM, as well as others with indications for HAV vaccination (e.g., injection-drug users, persons with chronic liver disease or who are infected with hepatitis B [HBV]). HAV vaccination is also recommended for other HIV-infected persons (e.g., injection-drug users, persons with chronic liver disease or who are infected with HBV or HCV). HBV vaccination is recommended for all susceptible HIV-infected patients. HBV infection can occur when mucous membranes are exposed to blood or body fluids that contain blood, which might occur during some types of sexual contact. HIV infected patients coinfected with HBV or HCV should be reminded that use of latex condoms not only reduces their risk of transmitting HIV to sexual partners but reduces their risk of transmitting these viral hepatitis infections as well.

Injection-Drug-Use Exposures

Injection-drug use is a complex behavior that puts HIV-infected persons at risk for HBV and HCV infection, additional possibly drug-resistant strains of HIV, and other bloodborne pathogens. Providers should assess a person's readiness to change this practice and encourage activities to provide education and support directed at recovery. Patients should be counseled to stop using injection drugs and to enter and complete substance abuse treatment, including relapse prevention programs. For patients who continue to inject drugs, healthcare providers should advise them to adhere to the following practices:

- Never reuse or share syringes, needles, water, or drug-preparation equipment; if injection equipment that has been used by other persons is shared, the implements should first be cleaned with bleach and water before use.

- Use only sterile syringes and needles obtained from a reliable source (e.g., pharmacies or syringe-exchange programs).

- Use sterile (e.g., boiled) water to prepare drugs, and if this is not feasible, use clean water from a reliable source (e.g., fresh tap water); use a new or disinfected container (i.e., cooker) and a new filter (i.e., cotton) to prepare drugs.

- Clean the injection site with a new alcohol swab before injection.

- Safely dispose of syringes and needles after one use.

All susceptible injection-drug-users should be vaccinated against HBV and HAV infection. HIV-infected injection drug users not known to be HCV infected who present with new and unexplained increases in alanine aminotransferase should be tested for HCV infection. Routine (e.g., annual) HCV testing should be considered for injection drug users who continue to inject drugs.

Environmental and Occupational Exposures

Certain activities or types of employment might increase the risk for exposure to tuberculosis (TB). These include residency or occupation in correctional institutions and shelters for the homeless, other settings identified as high risk by local health authorities, as well as volunteer work or employment in healthcare facilities where patients with TB are treated. Decisions regarding the risk of occupational exposure to TB should be made in conjunction with a healthcare provider and should be based on such factors as the patient's specific duties in the workplace, the prevalence of TB in the community, and the degree to which precautions designed to prevent the transmission of TB are taken in the workplace. These decisions will affect the frequency with which the patient should be screened for TB.

Day care providers and parents of children in child care are at increased risk for acquiring cytomegalovirus infection, cryptosporidiosis, and other infections (e.g., HAV, giardiasis) from children. The risk for acquiring infection can be diminished by practicing optimal hygienic practices (e.g., washing hands with soap and water, or alcohol-based hand sanitizers if soap and water are unavailable) after fecal contact (e.g., during diaper changing) and after contact with urine or saliva.

Occupations involving contact with animals (e.g., veterinary work and employment in pet stores, farms, or slaughterhouses) might pose a risk for toxoplasmosis, cryptosporidiosis, salmonellosis, campylobacteriosis, Bartonella infection, *E. coli* infection, and other infections of concern to any immunocompromised host (e.g., leptospirosis, brucellosis, Capnocytophaga spp.). However, available data are insufficient to justify a recommendation against HIV-infected persons working in such settings. Wearing gloves and good hand hygiene can reduce the risk of infection.

Contact with young farm animals, specifically animals with diarrhea, should be avoided to reduce the risk for cryptosporidiosis. Since soils and sands can be contaminated with *Toxoplasma gondii* and *Cryptosporidium parvum*, persons who have extended contact with these materials (e.g., gardening; playing in or cleaning sandboxes) should wash their hands thoroughly with soap and water following exposure. In areas where histoplasmosis is endemic, patients should avoid activities known to be associated with increased risk (e.g., creating dust when working with surface soil; cleaning chicken coops that are heavily contaminated with compost droppings; disturbing soil beneath bird-roosting sites; cleaning, remodeling or demolishing old buildings; and cave exploring). In areas where coccidioidomycosis is endemic, when possible, patients should avoid activities associated with increased risk, including extensive exposure to disturbed native soil (e.g., building excavation sites, during dust storms).

Pet-Related Exposures

Healthcare providers should advise HIV-infected persons of the potential risk posed by pet ownership. However, they should be sensitive to the psychological benefits of pet ownership and should not routinely advise HIV-infected persons to part with their pets. Specifically, providers should advise HIV-infected patients of the following precautions.

General

HIV-infected persons should avoid direct contact with stool from pets or stray animals. Veterinary care should be sought when a pet develops diarrheal illness. If possible, HIV-infected persons should avoid contact with animals that have diarrhea.

When obtaining a new pet, HIV-infected patients should avoid animals that are younger than 6 months (or younger than 1 year for cats) and specifically animals with diarrhea. Because the hygienic and sanitary conditions in pet-breeding facilities, pet stores, and animal shelters vary, patients should be cautious when obtaining pets from these sources. Stray animals should also be avoided, and specifically those with diarrhea.

Gloves should always be worn when handling feces or cleaning areas that might have been contaminated by feces from pets. Patients should wash their hands after handling pets and also before eating. Patients, especially those with CD4 cell counts below 200 cells/μL should avoid direct contact with all animal feces to reduce the risk for toxoplasmosis, cryptosporidiosis, salmonellosis, campylobacteriosis, *E. coli* infection, and other infectious illnesses. HIV-infected persons should limit or avoid direct exposure to calves and lambs (e.g., farms, petting zoos). Paying attention to hand hygiene (i.e., washing hands with soap and water, or alcohol-based hand sanitizers if soap and water are unavailable) and avoiding direct contact with stool are important when visiting premises where these animals are housed or exhibited.

Patients should not allow pets, particularly cats, to lick patients' open cuts or wounds and should take care to avoid any animal bites. Patients should wash all animal bites, animal scratches, or wounds licked by animals promptly with soap and water and seek medical attention. A course of antimicrobial therapy might be recommended if the wounds are moderate or severe, demonstrate crush injury and edema, involve the bones of a joint, involve a puncture of the skin near a joint, or involve a puncture of a joint directly.

Cats

Patients should be aware that cat ownership may under some circumstances increase their risk for toxoplasmosis and Bartonella infection, and enteric infections. Patients who elect to obtain a cat should adopt or purchase an animal at least a year old and in good health to reduce the risk for cryptosporidiosis, Bartonella infection, salmonellosis, campylobacteriosis, and *E. coli* infection.

Litter boxes should be cleaned daily, preferably by an HIV-negative, nonpregnant person; if HIV-infected patients perform this task, they should wear gloves and wash their hands thoroughly afterward to reduce the risk for toxoplasmosis. To further reduce the risk for toxoplasmosis, HIV-infected patients should keep cats indoors, not allow them to hunt, and not feed them raw or undercooked meat. Although declawing is not usually advised, patients should avoid activities that might result in cat scratches or bites to reduce the risk for Bartonella infection. Patients should also wash sites of cat scratches or bites promptly and should not allow cats to lick patients' open cuts or wounds. Care of cats should include flea control to reduce the risk for Bartonella infection. Testing cats for toxoplasmosis or Bartonella infection is not recommended, as such tests cannot accurately identify animals that pose a current risk for human infection.

Birds

Screening healthy birds for Cryptococcus neoformans, Mycobacterium avium, or Histoplasma capsulatum is not recommended.

Other

HIV-infected persons should avoid or limit contact with reptiles (e.g., snakes, lizards, iguanas, and turtles) and chicks and ducklings because of the high risk for exposure to Salmonella spp. Gloves should be used during aquarium cleaning to reduce the risk for infection with Mycobacterium marinum. Contact with exotic pets (e.g., nonhuman primates) should be avoided.

Food- and Water-Related Exposures

Food

Contaminated food is a common source of enteric infections. Transmission most often occurs by ingestion of undercooked foods or by cross-contamination of foods in the kitchen.

Healthcare providers should advise HIV-infected persons, particularly those with a CD4 count below 200 cells/μL, not to eat raw or undercooked eggs, including specific foods that might contain raw eggs (e.g., certain preparation of Hollandaise sauce, Caesar salad dressings, homemade mayonnaises, uncooked cookie and cake batter, eggnog); raw or undercooked poultry, meat, and seafood (raw shellfish in particular); unpasteurized dairy products (including milk and cheese); unpasteurized fruit juices; and raw seed sprouts (e.g., alfalfa sprouts or mung bean sprouts).

Meat and poultry are safest when adequate cooking is confirmed by thermometer. The U.S. Department of Agriculture (USDA) guidance is that the internal temperature be at least 145°F (63°C) for whole cuts of meat, 160°F (71°C) for ground meat excluding poultry, and 165°F (74°C) for poultry; whole cuts of meat and poultry should rest at least three minutes before carving and consuming. Immunocompromised persons who wish to maximally ensure their cooked meats are safe to eat may choose to use the following recommendations: the internal temperature should be at least 165°F (74°C) for all types of red meats and 180°F (82°C) for poultry. If a thermometer is not used when cooking meats, the risk for illness is decreased by eating poultry and meat that have no trace of pink color. However, color change of the meat (e.g., absence of pink) does not always correlate with internal temperature. Irradiated meats, if available, are predicted to eliminate the risk of foodborne enteric infection. Use of microwaves as a primary means of cooking of potentially contaminated foods (e.g., meats, hot dogs) should be avoided because microwave cooking is not uniform.

Produce items should be washed thoroughly; providers may wish to advise patients that produce is safest when cooked.

Healthcare providers should advise HIV-infected persons to avoid cross-contamination of foods. Salad preparation prior to handling of raw meats or other uncooked, potentially contaminated foods decreases risk. Uncooked meats, including hot dogs, and their juices should not come into contact with other foods. Hands, cutting boards, counters, knives, and other utensils should be washed thoroughly (preferably in a dishwasher on hot cycle) after contact with uncooked foods.

Soft cheeses (e.g., feta, Brie, Camembert, blue-veined, and Mexican-style cheese such as queso fresco) and prepared deli foods (including cold cuts, salads, hummus, hot dogs, pâtés) are potential sources of *Listeria monocytogenes* infection, which can lead to serious, even fatal, systemic infection in HIV-infected patients with low CD4 cell counts; consumption of these foods should be avoided.

Hard cheeses, processed cheeses, cream cheese, including slices and spreads; cottage cheese or yogurt; and canned or shelf-stable pâté and meat spreads need not be avoided. Avoid raw or unpasteurized milk, including goat's milk, or foods that contain unpasteurized milk or milk products.

Water

Patients should not drink water directly from lakes or rivers because of the risk for cryptosporidiosis, giardiasis, and toxoplasmosis. Waterborne infection can also result from swallowing water during recreational activities. All HIV-infected patients should avoid swimming in water that is probably contaminated with human or animal waste and should avoid swallowing water during swimming. Patients, especially those with CD4 cell counts below 200 cells/ μ L, should also be made aware that swimming or playing in lakes, rivers, and oceans, as well as some swimming pools, recreational water parks, and ornamental water fountains, can expose them to enteric pathogens (e.g., *Cryptosporidium*, *Giardia*, norovirus, Shiga toxin-producing *E. coli*) that cause diarrheal illness and to which their HIV infection makes them more susceptible.

Outbreaks of diarrheal illness have been linked to drinking water from municipal water supplies. During outbreaks or in other situations in which a community boil-water advisory is issued, boiling water for >1 minute will eliminate the risk for most viral, bacterial, and parasitic causes of diarrhea, including cryptosporidiosis. Using submicron, personal-use water filters (home/office types) or drinking bottled water might also reduce the risk from municipal and from well water.

Available data are inadequate to support a recommendation that all HIV-infected persons boil or otherwise avoid drinking tap water in non-outbreak settings. However, persons who wish to take independent action to reduce their risk for waterborne cryptosporidiosis might take precautions similar to those recommended during outbreaks. Such decisions are best made in conjunction with a healthcare provider. Persons who choose to use a personal-use filter or bottled water should be aware of the complexities involved in selecting the appropriate products, the lack of enforceable standards for destruction or removal of oocysts, product cost, and the difficulty of using these products consistently.

Patients taking precautions to avoid acquiring pathogens from drinking water should be advised that ice made from contaminated tap water also can be a source of infection. Patients should also be made aware that fountain beverages served in restaurants, bars, theaters, and other public places also might pose a risk, because these beverages, and the ice they might contain, are usually made from tap water. Nationally distributed brands of bottled or canned water and carbonated soft drinks are safe to drink. Commercially packaged (i.e., sealed at the factory and unopened), noncarbonated soft drinks and fruit juices that do not require refrigeration until after they are opened (i.e., those that can be stored unrefrigerated on grocery shelves) also are safe. Nationally distributed brands of frozen fruit juice concentrate are safe if they are reconstituted by users with water from a safe source. Fruit juices that must be kept refrigerated from the time they are processed to the time they are consumed might be either fresh (i.e., unpasteurized) or heat treated (i.e., pasteurized); only juices labeled as pasteurized should be considered safe to consume. Other pasteurized beverages and beers also are considered safe.

Travel-Related Exposures

HIV-infected travelers to developing countries, especially travelers who are severely immunosuppressed, risk exposure to both opportunistic and nonopportunistic pathogens not prevalent in the United States. Healthcare providers or specialists in travel medicine should be consulted 4–6 weeks in advance of travel to fully review and implement all measures necessary to prevent illness abroad. The Centers for Disease Control and Prevention (CDC) maintain a website accessible to travelers and their care providers at www.cdc.gov/travel and regularly publishes recommendations for prevention of disease while traveling in the CDC's Yellow Book (Health Information for International Travel). The CDC's travel website allows users to locate prevention recommendations according to geographic destination and to find updates on international disease outbreaks that might pose a health threat to travelers.

The following advice should be considered for all HIV-infected travelers but does substitute for destination-specific consultation with a travel medicine specialist.

The risk for foodborne and waterborne infections among HIV-infected persons is magnified during travel to economically developing countries. Specifically, persons who travel to economically developing areas should avoid foods and beverages that might be contaminated, as well as tap water, ice made with tap water, and items sold by street vendors. Raw fruits or vegetables that might have been washed in tap water should be avoided. Foods and beverages that are usually safe include steaming hot foods, fruits that are peeled by the traveler, unopened and properly bottled (including carbonated) beverages, hot coffee and tea, beer, wine, and water that is brought to a rolling boil for 1 minute. Treating water with iodine or chlorine can be as effective as boiling for preventing infections with most pathogens. Iodine and chlorine treatments may not prevent infection with *Cryptosporidium*; however, these treatments can be used when boiling is not practical.

Waterborne infections might result from swallowing water during recreational activities. To reduce the risk for parasitic (e.g., cryptosporidiosis, giardiasis, toxoplasmosis) and bacterial infections, patients should avoid swallowing water during swimming and should not swim in water that might be contaminated (e.g., with sewage or animal waste). HIV-infected persons traveling to developing countries should also be advised to not use tap water to brush their teeth.

Scrupulous attention to safe food and water consumption and good hygiene (i.e., regularly washing hands with soap and water, or alcohol-based hand sanitizers if soap and water are unavailable) are the most effective methods for reducing risk of traveler's diarrhea. Antimicrobial prophylaxis for travelers' diarrhea is not recommended routinely for HIV-infected persons traveling to developing countries. Such preventive therapy can have adverse effects, can promote the emergence of drug-resistant organisms, and can increase the risk of C. difficile-associated diarrhea. Nonetheless, studies (none involving an HIV-infected population) have reported that prophylaxis can reduce the risk for diarrhea among travelers. Under selected circumstances (e.g., those in which the risk for infection is high and the period of travel brief), the healthcare provider and patient might weigh the potential risks and benefits and decide that antibiotic prophylaxis is warranted.

HIV-infected travelers to developing countries should consider carrying a sufficient supply of an antimicrobial agent to be taken empirically if diarrhea occurs. Antimicrobial resistance among enteric bacterial pathogens outside the United States is a growing public health problem; therefore, the choice of antibiotic should be made in consultation with a clinician based on the traveler's destination. Travelers should consult a physician if they develop severe diarrhea that does not respond to empirical therapy, if their stools contain blood, they develop fever with shaking chills, or dehydration occurs. Antiperistaltic agents (e.g., diphenoxylate and loperamide) are used for treating diarrhea; however, they should not be used by patients with high fever or with blood in the stool, and their use should be discontinued if symptoms persist for more than 48 hours.

Live-virus vaccines should, in general, not be used. An exception is measles vaccine, which is recommended for nonimmune persons. However, measles vaccine is not recommended for persons who are severely immunosuppressed. Severely immunosuppressed persons who must travel to measles-endemic countries should consult a travel medicine specialist regarding possible utility of prophylaxis with immune globulin. Another exception is varicella vaccine, which can be administered to asymptomatic susceptible persons with a CD4 cell count ≥200 cells/μL. For adults and adolescents with CD4 cell counts <200 cells/μL, varicella-zoster immunoglobulin (VariZIG™) is indicated after close contact with a person who has active varicella or zoster and anti-herpetic antiviral therapy (e.g., acyclovir, famciclovir, valacyclovir) is recommended in the event vaccination or exposure results in clinical disease. Persons at risk for and nonimmune to polio and typhoid fever or who require influenza vaccination should be administered only inactivated formulations of these vaccines, not live-attenuated preparations.

Yellow fever vaccine is a live-virus vaccine with uncertain safety and efficacy among HIV-infected persons. Travelers with asymptomatic HIV infection who cannot avoid potential exposure to yellow fever should be offered vaccination. If travel to a zone with yellow fever is necessary and vaccination is not administered, patients should be advised of the risk, instructed in methods for avoiding the bites of vector mosquitoes, and provided a vaccination waiver letter. Preparation for travel should include a review and updating of routine vaccinations, including diphtheria, tetanus, acellular pertussis, and influenza.

Killed and recombinant vaccines (e.g., influenza, diphtheria, tetanus, rabies, HAV, HBV, Japanese encephalitis, meningococcal vaccines) should usually be used for HIV-infected persons just as they would be used for non-HIV-infected persons anticipating travel.

Section 50.2

Safe Food and Water

This section includes text excerpted from "Food Safety for
People with HIV/AIDS," U.S. Food and Drug
Administration (FDA), November 8, 2017.

Food safety is important for everyone—but it's especially important
for you. This section will provide practical guidance on how to reduce
your risk of foodborne illness. In addition to content in this section, you
are encouraged to check with your physician or healthcare provider to
identify foods and other products that you should avoid.

Foodborne Illness in the United States

When certain disease-causing bacteria, viruses or parasites contaminate food, they can cause foodborne illness. Another word for such
a bacteria, virus, or parasite is "pathogen." Foodborne illness, often
called food poisoning, is an illness that comes from a food you eat.

- The food supply in the United States is among the safest in the
  world—but it can still be a source of infection for all persons.

- According to the Centers for Disease Control and Prevention
  (CDC), 48 million persons get sick, 128,000 are hospitalized,
  and 3,000 die from foodborne infection and illness in the United
  States each year. Many of these people are children, older
  adults, or have weakened immune systems and may not be able
  to fight infection normally.

Since foodborne illness can be serious—or even fatal—it is important for you to know and practice safe food-handling behaviors to help
reduce your risk of getting sick from contaminated food.

Importance of Food Safety

As a person with the human immunodeficiency virus (HIV) / acquired
immunodeficiency syndrome (AIDS), you are susceptible to many types
of infection, like those that can be brought on by disease-causing bacteria and other pathogens that cause foodborne illness.

- A properly functioning immune system works to clear the
  infection and other foreign agents from your body. When the

HIV virus that causes AIDS damages or destroys the body's immune system, you become more vulnerable to developing and opportunistic infection, such as *Pneumocystis carinii* pneumonia, or contracting an infection, such as foodborne illness.

- As with many types of infection, because you have HIV/AIDS, you are more likely to have a lengthier illness, undergo hospitalization, or even die, should you contract a foodborne illness.

- Because your immune system is weakened, you must be especially vigilant when handling, preparing and consuming foods.

- To avoid contracting a foodborne illness, you must be vigilant when handling, preparing and consuming foods.

Make safe handling a lifelong commitment to minimize your risk of foodborne illness. Be aware that as you age, your immunity to infection naturally is weakened.

Major Pathogens That Cause Foodborne Illness

Table 50.1. Pathogens Causing Foodborne Illness

Campylobacter	
Associated Foods • Untreated or contaminated water • Unpasteurized ("raw") milk • Raw or undercooked meat, poultry, or shellfish	Symptoms and Potential Impact • Fever, headache, and muscle pain followed by diarrhea (sometimes bloody), abdominal pain, and nausea. Symptoms appear 2–5 days after eating and may last 2–10 days. May spread to bloodstream and cause life-threatening infection.
Cryptosporidium	
Associated Foods/Sources • Swallowing contaminated water, including that from recreational sources (e.g., swimming pool or lake) • Eating uncooked or contaminated food • Placing a contaminated object in the mouth • Soil, food, water, contaminated surfaces	Symptoms and Potential Impact • Watery diarrhea, dehydration, weight loss, stomach cramps or pain, fever, nausea, and vomiting; respiratory symptoms may also be present. • Symptoms begin 7–10 days after becoming infected and may last 2–14 days. In those with a weakened immune system, including people with HIV/AIDS, symptoms may subside and return over weeks to months.

Table 50.1. Continued

Clostridium perfringens	
Associated Foods/Sources	Symptoms and Potential Impact
• Many outbreaks result from food left for long periods in steam tables or at room temperature and time and/or temperature abused foods. • Meats, meat products, poultry, poultry products, and gravy	• Onset of watery diarrhea and abdominal cramps within about 16 hours. The illness usually begins suddenly and lasts for 12–24 hours. In elderly, symptoms may last 1–2 weeks. • Complications and/or death occur only very rarely.

Listeria monocytogenes Can grow slowly at refrigerator temperatures	
Associated Foods	Symptoms and Potential Impact
• Improperly reheated hot dogs, luncheon meats, cold cuts, fermented or dry sausage, and other deli-style meat and poultry • Unpasteurized (raw) milk and soft cheeses made with unpasteurized (raw) milk • Smoked seafood and salads made in the store such as ham salad, chicken salad, or seafood salads • Raw vegetable	• Fever, chills, headache, backache, sometimes upset stomach, abdominal pain, and diarrhea. May take up to 2 months to become ill. • Gastrointestinal symptoms may appear within a few hours to 2–3 days and disease may appear 2–6 weeks after ingestion. The duration is variable. • Those at-risk (including people with HIV/AIDS and others with weakened immune systems) may later develop more serious illness; death can result from this bacteria. • Can cause problems with pregnancy, including miscarriage, fetal death, or severe illness or death in newborns.

Escherichia coli O157: H7 One of several strains of E. coli that can cause human illness	
Associated Foods	Symptoms and Potential Impact
• Undercooked beef, especially ground beef • Unpasteurized milk and juices, like "fresh" apple cider • Contaminated raw fruits and vegetables, and water • Person-to-person contact	• Severe diarrhea that is often bloody, abdominal cramps, and vomiting. Usually little or no fever. • Can begin 1 to 9 days after contaminated food is eaten and lasts about 2 to 9 days. • Some, especially the very young, may develop hemolytic-uremic syndrome (HUS), which cause acute kidney failure, and can lead to permanent kidney damage or even death.

Table 50.1. Continued

Noroviruses (and other caliciviruses)	
Associated Foods	Symptoms and Potential Impact
• Shellfish and fecally-contaminated foods or water • Ready-to-eat foods touched by infected food workers; for example, salads, sandwiches, ice, cookies, fruit	• Nausea, vomiting, stomach pain usually start between 24 and 48 hours, but cases can occur within 12 hours of exposure. Symptoms usually last 12–60 hours. • Diarrhea is more prevalent in adults and vomiting is more prevalent in children.
Salmonella (over 2,300 types)	
Associated Foods	Symptoms and Potential Impact
• Raw or undercooked eggs, poultry, and meat • Unpasteurized (raw) milk or juice • Cheese and seafood • Fresh fruits and vegetable	• Stomach pain, diarrhea (can be bloody), nausea, chills, fever, and/or headache usually appear 6–72 hours after eating; may last 4–7 days. • In people with a weakened immune system, such as people with HIV/AIDS, the infection may be more severe and lead to serious complications including death.
Toxoplasma gondii	
Associated Foods/Sources	Symptoms and Potential Impact
• Accidental contact of cat feces through touching hands to mouth after gardening, handling cats, cleaning cat's litter box, or touching anything that has come in contact with cat feces. • Raw or undercooked meat.	• Flu-like illness that usually appears 10–13 days after eating, may last months. Those with a weakened immune system, including people with HIV/AIDS, may develop more serious illness. • Can cause problems with pregnancy, including miscarriage and birth defects.
Vibrio vulnificus	

Eating at Home—Making Wise Food Choices

Some foods are more risky for you than others. In general, the foods that are most likely to contain harmful bacteria or viruses fall in two categories:

1. Uncooked fresh fruits and vegetables

2. Some animal products, such as unpasteurized (raw) milk; soft cheeses made with raw milk; and raw or undercooked eggs, raw meat, raw poultry, raw fish, raw shellfish and their juices; luncheon meats and deli-type salads (without added preservatives) prepared on site in a deli-type establishment.

Interestingly, the risk these foods may actually pose depends on the origin or source of the food and how the food is processed, stored, and prepared. Follow these guidelines for safe selection and preparation of your favorite foods.

- If you have questions about wise food choices, be sure to consult with your doctor or healthcare provider. He or she can answer any specific questions or help you in your choices.

- If you are not sure about the safety of a food in your refrigerator, don't take the risk.

- When in doubt, throw it out!

Wise choices in your food selections are important.

Common Foods—Select the Lower Risk Options

Table 50.2. Foods and Risk Levels

Type of Food	Higher Risk	Lower Risk
Meat and Poultry	• Raw or undercooked meat or poultry	• Meat or poultry cooked to a safe minimum internal temperature
Tip: Use a food thermometer to check the internal temperature on the "Is It Done Yet?" chart for specific safe minimum internal temperature.		
Seafood	• Any raw or undercooked fish, or shellfish, or food containing raw or undercooked seafood e.g., sashimi, found in some sushi or ceviche. Refrigerated smoked fish • Partially cooked seafood, such as shrimp and crab	• Previously cooked seafood heated to 165°F • Canned fish and seafood • Seafood cooked to 145°F
Milk	• Unpasteurized (raw) milk	• Pasteurized milk
Eggs	Foods that contain raw/undercooked eggs, such as: • Homemade Caesar salad dressings* • Homemade raw cookie dough* • Homemade eggnog*	At home: • Use pasteurized eggs/egg products when preparing recipes that call for raw or undercooked eggs • When eating out: • Ask if pasteurized eggs were used
*Tip: Most premade foods from grocery stores, such as Caesar dressing, premade cookie dough, or packaged eggnog are made with pasteurized eggs.		

Table 50.2. Continued

Type of Food	Higher Risk	Lower Risk
Sprouts	• Raw sprouts (alfalfa, bean, or any other sprout)	• Cooked sprouts
Vegetables	• Unwashed fresh vegetables, including lettuce/salads	• Washed fresh vegetables, including salads • Cooked vegetables

Cheese	• Soft cheeses made from unpasteurized (raw) milk, such as:
	  • Feta
	  • Brie
	  • Camembert
	  • Blue-veined
	  • Queso fresco
		• Hard cheeses
		• Processed cheeses
		• Cream cheese
		• Mozzarella
		• Soft cheeses that are clearly labeled "made from pasteurized milk"

Hot Dogs and Deli Meats	• Hot dogs, deli and luncheon meats that have not been reheated	• Hot dogs, luncheon meats, and deli meats reheated to steaming hot or 165°F
Tip: You need to reheat hot dogs, deli meats and luncheon meats before eating them because the bacteria, *Listeria monocytogenes* grows at refrigerated temperatures (40°F or below). This bacteria may cause severe illness, hospitalization, or even death. Reheating these foods until they are steaming hot destroys these dangerous bacteria and makes these foods safe for you to eat.		
Pâtés	• Unpasteurized, refrigerated pâtés or meat spreads	• Canned or shelf-stable pâtés or meat spreads

Taking Care—Handling and Preparing Food Safely

Foodborne pathogens are sneaky. Food that appears completely fine can contain pathogens—disease-causing bacteria, viruses, or parasites—that can make you sick. You should never taste a food to determine if it is safe to eat.

As a person with HIV/AIDS, it is especially important that you—or those preparing your food—are always careful with food handling and preparation.

Four Basic Steps to Food Safety

1. Clean—Wash Hand Surfaces Often

Bacteria can spread throughout the kitchen and get onto cutting boards, utensils, counter tops, and food.

To ensure that your hands and surfaces are clean, be sure to:

- Wash hands in warm soapy water for at least 20 seconds before and after handling food and using the bathroom, changing diapers, or handling pets.

- Wash cutting boards, dishes, utensils, and counter tops with hot soapy water between the preparation of raw meat, poultry, and seafood products and preparation of any other food that will not be cooked. As an added precaution, sanitize cutting boards and countertops by rinsing them in a solution made of one tablespoon of unscented liquid chlorine bleach per gallon of water, or, as an alternative, you may run the plastic board through the wash cycle in your automatic dishwasher.

- Use paper towels to clean up kitchen surfaces. If using cloth towels, you should wash them often in the hot cycle of the washing machine.

- Wash produce. Rinse fruits and vegetables, and rub firm-skin fruits and vegetables under running tap water, including those with skins and rinds that are not eaten.

- With canned goods: remember to clean lids before opening.

2. Separate—Don't Cross-Contaminate

Cross-contamination occurs when bacteria are spread from one food product to another. This is especially common when handling raw meat, poultry, seafood, and eggs. The key is to keep these foods—and their juices—away from ready-to-eat foods.

To prevent cross-contamination, remember to:

- Separate raw meat, poultry, seafood, and eggs from other foods in your grocery shopping cart, grocery bags, and in your refrigerator.

- Never place cooked food on a plate that previously held raw meat, poultry, seafood, or eggs without first washing the plate with hot soapy water.

- Don't reuse marinades used on raw foods unless you bring them to a boil first.

- Consider using one cutting board only for raw foods and another only for ready-to-eat foods, such as bread, fresh fruits and vegetables, and cooked meat.

3. Cook to Safe Temperatures

Foods are safely cooked when they are heated to the USDA-FDA recommended safe minimum internal temperatures, as shown on the "Is it Done Yet" table.

To ensure that your foods are cooked safely, always:

- Use a food thermometer to measure the internal temperature of cooked foods. Check the internal temperature in several places to make sure that the meat, poultry, seafood, or egg product is cooked to safe minimum internal temperatures.

- Cook ground beef to at least 160°F and ground poultry to a safe minimum internal temperature of 165°F. Color of food is not a reliable indicator of safety or doneness.

- Reheat fully cooked hams packaged at a USDA-inspected plant to 140°F. For fully cooked ham that has been repackaged in any other location or for leftover fully cooked ham, heat to 165°F.

- Cook seafood to 145°F. Cook shrimp, lobster, and crab until they turn red and the flesh is pearly opaque. Cook clams, mussels, and oysters until the shells open. If the shells do not open, do not eat the seafood inside.

- Cook eggs until the yolks and whites are firm. Use only recipes in which the eggs are cooked or heated to 160°F.

- Cook all raw beef, lamb, pork, and veal steaks, roasts, and chops to 145°F with a 3-minute rest time after removal from the heat source.

- Bring sauces, soups, and gravy to a boil when reheating. Heat other leftovers to 165°F.

- Reheat hot dogs, luncheon meats, bologna, and other deli meats until steaming hot or 165°F.

- When cooking in a microwave oven, cover food, stir, and rotate for even cooking. If there is no turntable, rotate the dish by hand once or twice during cooking. Always allow standing time, which completes the cooking, before checking the internal temperature with a food thermometer. Food is done when it reaches the USDA-FDA recommended safe minimum internal temperature.

Is it done yet?

Use a food thermometer to be most accurate. You can't always tell by looking.

4. Chill—Refrigerate Promptly

Cold temperatures slow the growth of harmful bacteria. Keeping a constant refrigerator temperature of 40°F or below is one of the most effective ways to reduce risk of foodborne illness. Use an appliance thermometer to be sure the refrigerator temperature is consistently 40°F or below and the freezer temperature is 0°F or below.

To chill foods properly:

- Refrigerate or freeze meat, poultry, eggs, seafood, and other perishables within 2 hours of cooking or purchasing. Refrigerate within 1 hour if the temperature outside is above 90°F.

- Never thaw food at room temperature, such as on the countertop. It is safe to thaw food in the refrigerator, in cold water, or in the microwave. If you thaw food in cold water or in the microwave, you should cook it immediately.

- Divide large amounts of food into shallow containers for quicker cooling in the refrigerator.

- Follow the recommendations in the abridged USDA-FDA Cold Storage Chart (Table 50.3). These time limit guidelines will help keep refrigerated food safe to eat. Because freezing keeps food safe indefinitely, recommended storage times for frozen foods are for quality only.

Table 50.3. USDA-FDA Cold Storage Chart

Product	Refrigerator (40°F)	Freezer (0°F)
Eggs		
Fresh, in shell	3–5 weeks	Don't freeze
Hard-cooked	1 week	Don't freeze well
Liquid Pasteurized Eggs, Egg Substitutes		
Opened	3 days	Don't freeze well
Unopened	10 days	1 year
Deli and Vacuum-Packed Products		
Egg, chicken, ham, tuna, and macaroni salads	3–5 days	Don't freeze well
Hot Dogs		
Opened package	1 week	1–2 months
Unopened package	2 weeks	1–2 months

Table 50.3. Continued

Product	Refrigerator (40°F)	Freezer (0°F)
Luncheon Meat		
Opened package	3–5 days	1–2 months
Unopened package	2 weeks	1–2 months
Bacon and Sausage		
Bacon	7 days	1 month
Sausage, raw—from chicken, turkey, pork, beef	1–2 days	1–2 months
Hamburger and Other Ground Meats		
Hamburger, ground beef, turkey, veal, pork, lamb, and mixtures of them	1–2 days	3–4 months
Fresh Beef, Veal, Lamb, Pork		
Steaks	3–5 days	6–12 months
Chops	3–5 days	4–6 months
Roast	3–5 days	4–12 months
Fresh Poultry		
Chicken or turkey, whole	1–2 days	1 year
Chicken or turkey, pieces	1 to 2 days	9 months
Seafood		
Lean fish (flounder, haddock, halibut, etc.)	1 to 2 days	6 to 8 months
Fatty fish (salmon, tuna, etc.)	1 to 2 days	2 to 3 months
Leftovers		
Cooked meat or poultry	3 to 4 days	2 to 6 months
Chicken nuggets, patties	3 to 4 days	1 to 3 months
Pizza	3 to 4 days	1 to 2 months

Become a Better Shopper

Follow these safe food-handling practices while you shop.

- Carefully read food labels while in the store to make sure food is not past its "sell by" date

- Put raw packaged meat, poultry, or seafood into a plastic bag before placing it in the shopping cart so that its juices will not drip on—and contaminate—other foods. If the meat counter does not offer plastic bags, pick some up from the produce section before you select your meat, poultry, and seafood.

- Buy only pasteurized milk, cheese, and other dairy products from the refrigerated section. When buying fruit juice from the refrigerated section of the store, be sure that the juice label says it is pasteurized.

- Purchase eggs in the shell from the refrigerated section of the store. (Note: store the eggs in their original carton in the main part of your refrigerator once you are home.) For recipes that call for eggs that are raw or undercooked when the dish is served—homemade Caesar salad dressing and homemade ice cream are two examples—use either shell eggs that have been treated to destroy *Salmonella* by pasteurization or pasteurized egg products. When consuming raw eggs, using pasteurized eggs is the safer choice.

- Never buy food that is displayed in unsafe or unclean conditions.

- When purchasing canned goods, make sure that they are free of dents, cracks, or bulging lids. (Once you are home, remember to clean each lid before opening the can.)

- Purchase produce that is not bruised or damaged.

- Check Your Steps:

  - Check "Sell-By" date

  - Put raw meat, poultry, or seafood in plastic bags.

  - Buy only pasteurized milk, soft cheeses made with pasteurized milk, and pasteurized or juices that have been otherwise treated to control harmful bacteria.

  - When buying eggs, purchase refrigerated shell eggs. If your recipe calls for raw eggs, purchase pasteurized, refrigerated liquid eggs.

  - Don't buy food displayed in unsafe or unclean conditions.

  - Food Product Dating

Open dating is found primarily on perishable foods such as meat, poultry, eggs, and dairy products.

- A"Sell-By" date tells the store how long to display the product for sale. You should buy the product before the date expires.

- A "Best if Used By (or Before)" date is recommended for best flavor or quality. It is not a purchase or safety date.

- A "Use-By" date is the last date recommended for the use of the product while at peak quality. The date has been determined by the manufacturer of the product.

"Closed or coded dates" are packing numbers for use by the manufacturer. "Closed" or "coded" dating might appear on shelf-stable products such as cans and boxes of food.

Transporting Your Groceries

Follow these tips for safe transporting of your groceries:

- Pick up perishable foods last, and plan to go directly home from the grocery store

- Always refrigerate perishable foods within 2 hours of cooking or purchasing

- Refrigerate within 1 hour if the temperature outside is above 90°F

- In hot weather, take a cooler with ice or another cold source to transport foods safely

Being Smart When Eating Out

Eating out can be lots of fun—so make it an enjoyable experience by following some simple guidelines to avoid foodborne illness. Remember to observe your food when it is served, and don't ever hesitate to ask questions before you order. Waiters and waitresses can be quite helpful if you ask how a food is prepared. Also, let them know you don't want any food item containing raw meat, poultry, seafood, sprouts, or eggs.

Basic Rules for Ordering

- Ask whether the food contains uncooked ingredients such as eggs, sprouts, meat, poultry, or seafood. If so, choose something else.

- Ask how these foods have been cooked. If the server does not know the answer, ask to speak to the chef to be sure your food has been cooked to a safe minimum internal temperature.

- If you plan to get a "doggy bag" or save leftovers to eat at a later time, refrigerate perishable foods as soon as possible—and always within 2 hours after purchase or delivery. If the leftover is in air temperatures above 90°F, refrigerate within 1 hour.

If in doubt, make another selection.

Table 50.4. Smart Menu Choices

Higher Risk	Lower Risk
Soft cheese made from unpasteurized (raw) milk.	Hard or processed cheeses. Soft cheeses only if they are made from pasteurized milk.
Refrigerated smoked seafood and raw or undercooked seafood.	Fully cooked fish or seafood.
Cold or improperly heated hot dogs.	Hot dogs reheated to steaming hot. If the hot dogs are served cold or lukewarm, ask to have them reheated until steaming, or choose something else.
Sandwiches with cold deli or luncheon meat.	Grilled sandwiches in which the meat or poultry is heated until steaming.
Raw or undercooked fish, such as sashimi, nonvegetarian sushi or ceviche.	Fully cooked fish that is firm and flaky.
Soft-boiled or "over-easy" eggs, as the yolks are not fully cooked.	Fully cooked eggs with firm yolk and whites.
Salads, wraps, or sandwiches containing raw (uncooked) or lightly cooked sprouts	Salads, wraps, or sandwiches containing cooked sprouts.

Tips for Transporting Food

The following tips will be useful for you for transporting food.

- Keep cold food cold, at 40°F or below. To be safest, place cold food in cooler with ice or frozen gel packs. Use plenty of ice or frozen gel packs. Cold food should be at 40°F or below the entire time you are transporting it.

- Hot food should be kept at 140°F or above. Wrap the food well and place in an insulated container.

Stay "Food Safe" When Traveling Internationally

Discuss your travel plans with your physician before traveling to other countries. Your physician may have specific recommendations for the places you are visiting, and may suggest extra precautions or medications to take on your travels.

Foodborne Illness: Know the Symptoms

Despite your best efforts, you may find yourself in a situation where you suspect you have a foodborne illness. Foodborne illness often presents itself with flu-like symptoms.

These symptoms include:

- Nausea

- Vomiting

- Diarrhea

- Fever

If you suspect that you could have a foodborne illness, there are four key steps that you should take. Follow the guidelines in the Foodborne Illness Action Plan provided below, which begins with contacting your physician or healthcare provider right away.

When in doubt—contact your physician or healthcare provider.

Foodborne Illness Action Plan

If you suspect you have a foodborne illness, follow these general guidelines:

1. Consult your physician or healthcare provider, or seek medical treatment as appropriate. As a person with HIV/AIDS, you are at increased risk for severe infection.

   - Contact your physician immediately if you develop symptoms or think you may be at risk.

   - If you develop signs of infection as discussed with your physician, seek out medical advice and/or treatment immediately.

2. Preserve the food.

   - If a portion of the suspect food is available, wrap it securely, label it to say "DANGER," and freeze it.

   - The remaining food may be used in diagnosing your illness and in preventing others from becoming ill.

3. Save all the packaging materials, such as cans or cartons.

- Write down the food type, the date and time consumed, and when the onset of symptoms occurred. Write down as many foods and beverages you can recall consuming in the past week (or longer), since the onset time for various foodborne illnesses differ.

- Save any identical unopened products.

- If the suspect food is a USDA-inspected meat, poultry, or egg product, call the USDA Meat and Poultry Hotline, 888-MPHotline (888-674-6854). For all other foods, call the FDA Office of Emergency Operations at 866-300-4374 or 301-796-8240.

4. Call your local health department if you believe you became ill from food you ate in a restaurant or other food establishment.

- The health department staff will be able to assist you in determining whether any further investigation is warranted.

- To locate your local health department, visit Health Guide USA (www.healthguideusa.org/local_health_departments.htm).

Section 50.3

Staying Healthy while Traveling

This section includes text excerpted from "HIV/AIDS—
Travelling with HIV," Centers for Disease Control and
Prevention (CDC), May 21, 2018.

Each year, millions of Americans travel abroad. Even though travel outside the United States can be risky for anyone, it may require special precautions for individuals living with HIV infection. For example, travel to some developing countries can increase the risk of getting an opportunistic infection. For some destinations, certain vaccines that contain live viruses may be required, and your healthcare provider needs to review your medical record to ensure they are safe for you.

The most important things you can do is see your healthcare provider before you travel, know the medical risks you might face, and learn how to protect yourself.

Before You Travel

- Talk to your healthcare provider or an expert in travel medicine about health risks in the places you plan to visit. Ideally, this conversation should take place at least 4–6 weeks before your scheduled departure. Your healthcare provider can advise you on preventive medicines you may need, specific measures you need to take to stay healthy, and what to watch out for. He or she may also be able to provide you with the name(s) of healthcare providers or clinics that treat people with HIV infection in the region you plan to visit. Your healthcare provider may also:

- recommend you pack a supply of medicine, such as antibiotics to treat travelers' diarrhea;

- recommend certain vaccinations.

- Consult CDC Health Information for International Travel (commonly called the Yellow Book).

- If you are traveling to an area where insect-borne diseases (such as dengue fever, yellow fever, or malaria) are common, minimize the risk of getting bitten by mosquitoes or ticks. Remember to:

  - Pack a good supply of insect repellant that contains at least 30 percent DEET;

  - Wear lightweight long pants and shirts with long sleeves;

  - Wear a hat and inspect your scalp and body daily for ticks.

  - Your doctor may also recommend:

    - Sleeping under a mosquito net to prevent mosquito bites;

    - Taking medicine to prevent getting malaria.

- Educate and prepare yourself

  - About your destination:

    - Make sure you know if the countries you plan to visit have special health rules for visitors, especially visitors with human immunodeficiency virus (HIV) infection.

- About your insurance policies:
  - Review your medical insurance to see what coverage it provides when you are away from home. You may purchase supplemental traveler's insurance to cover the cost of emergency medical evacuation by air and the cost of in-country care, if these costs may are not covered by your regular insurance.
  - Take proof of insurance, such as a photocopy or scan your policy and send the image to an e-mail address you can access both in the United States and abroad. Leave a copy at home and tell your friends or family where it is located.

When You Travel Abroad

- Food and water in developing countries may contain germs that could make you sick.
- Do not:
  - eat raw fruit or vegetables that you do not peel yourself
  - eat raw or undercooked seafood or meat
  - eat unpasteurized dairy products
  - eat anything from a street vendor
  - drink tap water (in developing countries some hotels may purify their own water but it is safer to avoid it), drinks made with tap water, or ice made from tap water
- Do eat and drink:
  - hot foods
  - hot coffee or tea
  - bottled water and drinks (make sure the seals are original and have not been tampered with)
  - water that you bring to a rolling boil for one full minute then cool in a covered and clean vessel
  - fruits that you peel
  - wine, beer, and other alcoholic beverages are also safe
- Tuberculosis (TB) is very common worldwide, and can be severe in people with HIV. Avoid hospitals and clinics where coughing

TB patients are treated. See your doctor upon your return to discuss whether you should be tested for TB.

- Animal wastes, such as fecal droppings in soil or on sidewalks, can pose hazards to individuals with weakened immune systems. Physical barriers, such as shoes, can protect you from direct contact. Likewise, towels can protect you from direct contact when lying on a beach or in parks. If you are in physical contact with animals, wash your hands thoroughly afterward with soap and water.

- Take all your medications on schedule, as usual

- Stick to your special diet, if you are on one

- Take the same precautions that you take at home to prevent transmitting HIV to others

Section 50.4

Vaccinations

This section includes text excerpted from "Immunizations Recommended for People Living with HIV," HIV.gov, U.S. Department of Health and Human Services (HHS), May 15, 2017.

Immunizations (also called "vaccines") protect people from diseases such as chicken pox, flu, and polio. Vaccines are given by needle injection (a shot), by mouth, or sprayed into the nose.

Most vaccines are designed to prevent a person from ever having a disease or so that a person will only have a mild case of the disease. When a person gets a vaccine, his or her body responds by mounting an immune system response to defend the body against the infection.

Since human immunodeficiency virus (HIV) can make it difficult for your immune system to fight infections, people living with HIV could benefit greatly from vaccines against preventable infections.

Also, vaccines don't just protect individuals from disease. They also protect communities. When most people in a community get immunized against a disease, there is little chance of a disease outbreak.

Vaccines Recommended for People Living with HIV?

The following vaccines are recommended for people living with HIV:

- Hepatitis B

- Influenza (flu)

- Pneumococcal (pneumonia)

- Tetanus, diphtheria, and pertussis (whooping cough). A single vaccine called Tdap protects adolescents and adults against the three diseases. Every 10 years, a repeat vaccine against tetanus and diphtheria (called Td) is recommended.

- Human papillomavirus (HPV) (for those up to age 26)

Additional vaccines may be recommended based on an HIV-infected person's age, previous vaccinations, risk factors for a particular disease, or certain HIV-related factors. Talk to your healthcare provider about which vaccines are recommended for you.

Vaccines Safety for People Living with HIV?

There are two basic types of vaccines:

1. Live, attenuated vaccines are vaccines that contain a weakened but live form of a disease-causing microbe. Although the weakened microbe cannot cause the disease (or can cause only mild disease), the vaccine can still trigger an immune response.

2. Inactivated vaccines are vaccines that are made from dead microbes. There is no chance that an inactivated vaccine can cause the disease it was designed to prevent.

In general, to be safe, people with HIV should get inactivated vaccines to avoid even the remote chance of getting a disease from a live, attenuated vaccine. However, for some diseases, only live, attenuated vaccines are available. In this case, the protection offered by the live vaccine may outweigh the risks. Vaccines against chickenpox and shingles are examples of live, attenuated vaccines that, in certain situations, may be recommended for people with HIV. Talk to your healthcare provider about what is recommended for you.

HIV and Its Impact on How a Vaccine Works

HIV can weaken your body's immune response to a vaccine, making the vaccine less effective. In general, vaccines work best when your CD4 count is above 200 copies/mm^3. Also, by stimulating your immune system, vaccines may cause your HIV viral load to increase temporarily.

Because HIV medicines strengthen the immune system and reduce HIV viral load, people living with HIV may want to start antiretroviral therapy (ART) before getting vaccinated whenever possible. In some situations, however, immunizations should be given even if ART has not been started. For example, it's important for people with HIV to get vaccinated against the flu at the time of year when the risk of flu is greatest. Talk to your healthcare provider about what is recommended for you.

Vaccines and Their Side Effects

Any vaccine can cause side effects. Side effects from vaccines are generally minor (for example, soreness at the location of an injection or a low-grade fever) and go away within a few days. Severe reactions to vaccines are rare. Before getting a vaccine, talk to your healthcare provider about the benefits and risks of the vaccine and possible side effects.

Travel and Vaccines

You should be up to date on routine vaccinations, no matter where you are going. If you are planning a trip outside the United States, you may need immunizations against diseases that are present in other parts of the world, such as cholera or yellow fever.

If you have HIV, talk to your healthcare provider about any vaccines you may need before you travel. He or she will know which vaccines are safe for you. Keep in mind:

If a required immunization is available only as a live, attenuated vaccine, ask your healthcare provider if the potential benefits are greater than the potential risks. If so, your provider may be willing to give you a letter excusing you from getting the vaccine (although not all countries accept waiver letters.)

If your CD4 count is less than 200 copies/mm^3, your healthcare provider may recommend that you delay travel to give your HIV medicines time to strengthen your immune system.

Vaccine against HIV

There is currently no vaccine that has been approved by the FDA to prevent HIV infection or treat those who have it. However, scientists are working to develop one.

Chapter 51

Life Issues When You Have HIV/AIDS

Chapter Contents

Section 51.1

Standing Up to HIV-Related Stigma

This section contains text excerpted from the following sources: Text under the heading "How Can I Stand up to Human Immunodeficiency Virus (HIV)-Related Stigma?" is excerpted from "Standing up to Stigma," HIV.gov, U.S. Department of Health and Human Services (HHS), March 12, 2018; Text under the heading "Internalized HIV-Related Stigma" is excerpted from "Internalized HIV-Related Stigma," Centers for Disease Control and Prevention (CDC), February 2018.

How Can I Stand up to Human Immunodeficiency Virus (HIV)-Related Stigma?

HIV-related stigma and discrimination still persist in the United States and negatively affect the health and well-being of people living with human immunodeficiency virus (HIV). You can play an important role in reducing stigma and discrimination by offering your support to people living with HIV and speaking out to correct myths and stereotypes that you hear from others in your community.

Almost 8 in 10 HIV patients in the United States report feeling internalized HIV-related stigma, according to a Centers for Disease Control and Prevention (CDC) study. Internalized stigma is when a person living with HIV experiences negative feelings or thoughts about their HIV status.

Internalized HIV-Related Stigma

It is when a person living with HIV experiences negative feelings or thoughts about their HIV status. Almost 8 in 10 HIV patients in the United States report feeling internalized HIV-related stigma.

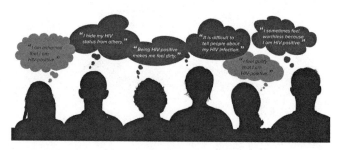

Figure 51.1. *General Statements of People with Internalized HIV-Related Stigma*

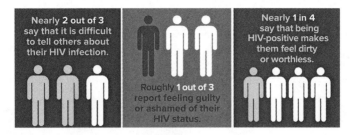

Figure 51.2. *Internalized HIV-Related Stigma—Statistics*

Which Groups Are Most Affected by Internalized HIV-Related Stigma?

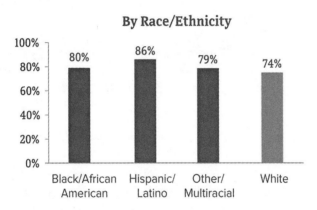

Figure 51.3. *Percentage Reporting Internalized Stigma—By Race/Ethnicity*

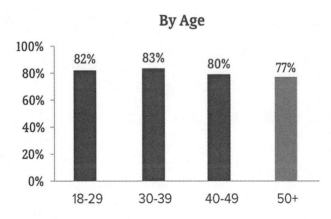

Figure 51.4. *Percentage Reporting Internalized Stigma—By Age*

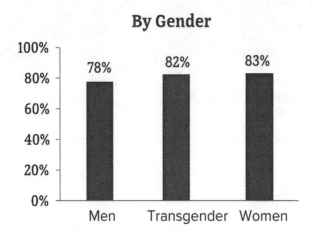

Figure 51.5. *Percentage Reporting Internalized Stigma—By Gender*

How Can People Live with HIV Reduce Internalized Stigma?

• Think about the negative beliefs you may have about yourself. Ask yourself if they are really true.

• Take HIV medicine as prescribed to keep an undetectable viral load—that means the level of HIV in your body is so low that a test can't detect it. Getting and keeping an undetectable viral load can reduce internalized stigma by keeping you healthy and protecting your partner.

• Find a counselor who can help you deal with any negative thoughts and feelings about your HIV status.

• Join support groups and organizations that help people living with HIV. These groups offer a safe environment and can help you overcome the challenges of living with HIV.

How Can People Live Well with HIV?

• Take HIV medicine as prescribed

• Stay in HIV care

• Share your status

• Protect your partners

HIV Treatment Can Keep You Healthy and Protect Others

If you are living with HIV, get in care and start treatment as soon as possible. The sooner you start treatment, the more you benefit. Taking HIV medicine as prescribed can make the level of HIV in your blood very low (called viral suppression) or even undetectable. Getting and keeping an undetectable viral load is the best thing you can do to stay healthy. Also, if you stay undetectable, you have effectively no risk of transmitting HIV to an HIV-negative partner through sex.

Section 51.2

Employment

This section includes text excerpted from "Employment and Health," HIV.gov, U.S. Department of Health and Human Services (HHS), May 15, 2017.

Working with Human Immunodeficiency Virus (HIV)

With proper care and treatment, many people living with human immunodeficiency virus (HIV) lead normal, healthy lives, including having a job. Most people living with HIV can continue working at their current jobs or look for a new job in their chosen field. Your overall well-being and financial health can be more stable when you are gainfully employed.

Getting a New Job or Returning to Work

Working will affect a lot of your life:

- Your medical status
- Your finances
- Your social life
- The way you spend your time
- Your housing or transportation needs

Before taking action on getting a new job or returning to work, you may want to get information and perspectives from:

- Your HIV case manager or counselor, if you have one

- Benefits counselors at an HIV service organization or other community organization

- The Social Security Administrations Work Incentives Planning and Assistance Program (WIPA)

- Other people living with HIV who are working, or have returned to work

- Providers of any of your housing, medical, or financial benefits

- Public and nonprofit employment and training service providers

Here are some questions to discuss with them:

- What are my goals for employment?

- What kind of work do I want to do?

- What are the resources that can help me set and achieve a new career goal?

- Are there state or local laws that further strengthen anti-discrimination protections in the American Disabilities Act (ADA)?

- How do I access training or education that will help me achieve my goals?

- How can I plan to take care of my health if I go to work?

- How will my going to work impact the benefits I am receiving?

Requesting Reasonable Accommodations

Qualified individuals with disabilities, including people living with HIV, have the right to request reasonable accommodations in the workplace. A reasonable accommodation is any modification or adjustment to a job or work environment that enables a qualified person with a disability to apply for or perform a job. An accommodation may be tangible (for example, a certain type of chair) or nontangible (for example, a modified work schedule for someone with a medical condition requiring regular appointments with a healthcare provider). You are qualified if you are able to perform the essential functions of the job, with or without reasonable accommodation.

Your supervisor may not be trained in reasonable accommodations or know how to negotiate them. For that reason, often its best to go directly to the person responsible for human resources at your employer, even if that person works in a different location. In a small business, that person may well be the owner.

When you request an accommodation, state clearly what you need (for example, time off for a clinic visit every third Tuesday of the month, a certain type of chair, or a change in your work hours) and be ready to supply a doctor's note supporting your request. The initial note need not contain your diagnosis, but it should verify that you are under the doctors care and that he/she believes you need the accommodation to maintain your health to be able to fulfill essential functions of your job.

Many people living with HIV do not want to give a lot of details about their health. If you prefer not to provide a lot of information, you may want to limit the medical information you initially give to your employer. However, if your need for accommodation is not obvious, your employer may require that you provide medical documentation to establish that you have a disability as defined by the ADA, to show that the employee needs the requested accommodation, and to help determine effective accommodation options. This can, but often does not, include disclosing your specific medical condition.

Be aware that not all people with HIV or AIDS (acquired immunodeficiency syndrome) will need accommodations to perform their jobs and many others may only need a few or simple accommodations. The U.S. Department of Labor's (DOL) Job Accommodation Network (JAN) provides free, expert, and confidential technical assistance to both employees and employers on workplace accommodations and disability employment issues, which includes resources for employees living with HIV or AIDS.

Section 51.3

Sex and Sexuality and HIV

This section includes text excerpted from "HIV/AIDS—Sex and
Sexuality and HIV: Entire Lesson," U.S. Department of Veterans
Affairs (VA), February 8, 2018.

If you just tested positive for human immunodeficiency virus (HIV),
you may not want to think about having sex. Some people who get HIV
feel guilty or embarrassed. Or they may be afraid of infecting a partner
and decide sex is too risky. These are common reactions, especially if
you got HIV through sex. Chances are, however, that you will want to
have sex again. The good news is that there is no reason why you can't.
People with HIV enjoy sex and fall in love, just like other people. And
there are many ways to have satisfying and safe sexual relationships.

In fact, one of the most effective ways to prevent HIV from passing
to an HIV-negative sex partner is to take your own HIV medications
(antiretroviral therapy, or ART) every day—these not only protect your
health but can prevent transmission of HIV.

If you are having a hard time dealing with negative feelings like
anger or fear, you can get help. Talk to your healthcare provider about
support groups or counseling. Sex is a very tough topic for many people
with HIV—you are not alone.

By reading this section, you are already taking a good first step
toward a healthy sex life. Having good information will help you make
good decisions.

Talking to Your Healthcare Provider

Your doctor or other members of your healthcare team may ask you
about your sexual practices each time you go in for a checkup. It may
feel embarrassing at first, to be honest and open with your doctor. But
he or she is trying to help you stay healthy.

Your clinician and staff will still give you care if you have had sex
with someone of the same sex or someone other than your spouse.
It's OK to tell your providers the truth. It will not affect your medical
benefits. It will help your healthcare team take better care of you.

Make sure you set aside time to ask your doctor questions about
safer sex, sexually transmitted diseases (STDs), re-infection, or any
other questions you might have. If you feel that you need help dealing
with your feelings, ask about support groups or counseling.

Many people with HIV ask their doctor or nurse to talk with them and their partners about HIV and how it is transmitted. They can answer technical questions and address the specifics of your situation. If you live with someone, they may have questions about everyday contact as well as sexual contact.

Telling Your Sex Partners

This may be one of the hardest things you have to do. But you need to tell your sex partner(s) that you are HIV positive, whether you have a primary partner such as a spouse or girlfriend or boyfriend, have more than one partner, or are single or casually dating.

What follows are tips for talking to your main partner, other partners, and former partners.

Talking to Your Main Partner

If you are in a relationship, one of the first things you will probably think about after learning that you have HIV is telling your partner or partners. For some couples, a positive HIV test may have been expected. For others, the news will be a surprise that can bring up difficult issues.

Your partner may not be prepared to offer you support during a time when you need it. Your partner may be worrying about their own HIV status. On the other hand, if you think you may have contracted HIV from your partner, you are probably dealing with your own feelings.

Unless your partner is known to have HIV infection, he or she should get an HIV test right away. Don't assume that the results will come back positive, even if you have been having unprotected sex or sharing needles. Your partner may assume the worst and may blame you for possibly spreading the disease. It is important that you discuss these feelings with each other in an open and honest way, perhaps with a licensed counselor.

Talking to New Partners

Talking about HIV with someone you are dating casually or someone you met recently may be difficult. You might not know this person very well or know what kind of reaction to expect. When telling a casual partner or someone you are dating, each situation is different and you might use a different approach each time. Sometimes you may

603

feel comfortable being direct and saying, "Before we have sex, I want you to know that I have HIV."

Other times, you may want to bring it up by saying something like, "Let's talk about safer sex." Whichever approach you choose, you probably want to tell the person that you have HIV before you have sex the first time. Otherwise, there may be hurt feelings or mistrust later. Also be sure to take your HIV medications every day and to practice safer sex.

Talking to Former Partners

With people you have had sex with in the past or people you have shared needles with, it can be very difficult to explain that you have HIV. However, it is important that they know so that they can get tested.

If you need help telling people that you may have been exposed to HIV, most city or county health departments will tell them for you, without using your name. Ask your doctor about this service.

Remember

Before telling your partner that you have HIV, take some time alone to think about how you want to bring it up.

Decide when and where would be the best time and place to have a conversation. Choose a time when you expect that you will both be comfortable, rested, and as relaxed as possible.

Think about how your partner may react to stressful situations. If there is a history of violence in your relationship, consider your safety first and plan the situation with a case manager or counselor.

Imagine several ways in which your partner might react to the news that you are HIV positive. Write down what she or he might say, and then think about what you might say in response.

Safer Sex

We know a lot about how HIV is transmitted from person to person. Having safer sex means you take this into account and avoid risky practices. There are two reasons to practice safer sex: to protect yourself and to protect others.

Protecting Yourself

If you have HIV, you need to protect your health. When it comes to sex, this means practicing safer sex (like using condoms) to avoid sexually transmitted diseases like herpes and hepatitis. HIV makes it harder for your body to fight off diseases. What might be a small health problem for someone without HIV could be big health problem for you.

Protecting Your Partner

Taking care of others means making sure that you do not pass along HIV to them. If your sex partners already have HIV, you should still avoid infecting them with another sexually transmitted disease you may be carrying.

Most people would agree that you owe it to your sexual partners to tell them that you have HIV. This is being honest with them. Even though it can be very hard to do, in the long run, you will probably feel much better about yourself.

Some people with HIV have found that people who love them think that condomless sex is a sign of greater love or trust. If someone offers to have condomless sex with you, it is still up to you to protect them by being safe.

"Being safe" usually means protecting yourself and others by using condoms for the highest-risk sex activities, specifically for anal and vaginal sex. When done correctly, condom use is very effective at preventing HIV transmission. Over the years, "being safe" has come to include two other important strategies for reducing HIV infections; these are HIV treatment (ART medications) for HIV-positive people and preexposure prophylaxis (PrEP) for HIV negatives. Both of these are very effective at reducing the risk of HIV infection. One or more of them is likely to be appropriate for you—be sure to ask your healthcare provider about them.

What about Antiretroviral Therapy (ART) for HIV Prevention?

One of the most effective ways you can prevent HIV from passing to an HIV-negative sex partner is to take your ART (HIV medications) every day—if they are working well to suppress the HIV in your body they also will prevent transmission of HIV.

What about Preexposure Prophylaxis (PrEP)?

HIV-negative individuals may, under the supervision of their healthcare providers, take an anti-HIV pill every day to prevent themselves from becoming infected. This is called preexposure prophylaxis or PrEP. Usually, these are persons who are at relatively high risk of becoming infected with HIV (for example, because they have a partner with HIV, they have risky sexual exposures, or they share injection drug equipment). The medication used for PrEP is Truvada, a combination tablet containing tenofovir and emtricitabine. PrEP appears to be extremely effective if it is taken every day, and is not effective if it is taken irregularly. Your VA healthcare provider can tell you more about the potential benefits and shortcomings of PrEP for HIV-negative persons.

Risky Sex

Risky sex is sex that may lead to infection of an HIV-negative individual. As indicated earlier, there are many ways to decrease the risk of HIV infection, like (for the HIV-positive partner) taking anti-HIV medications (ART) every day, or (for the HIV-negative partner) using PrEP, or (for partners of any HIV status) using condoms or other latex barriers during sex.

HIV is passed through body fluids such as semen, vaginal, or anal fluid, or blood. The less contact you have with these, the lower the risk. The most sensitive areas where these fluids are risky are in the vagina or anus and rectum (ass). The protective tissue there is thin, and is easily torn, which makes it easier for the virus to enter your body. Saliva (spit) and tears aren't risky.

In general, vaginal or anal sex without a condom is the riskiest.

Here is a list of sexual activities organized by level of risk to help you and your partner make decisions:

High risk

- Anal sex without a condom (penis in the anus)

- Vaginal sex without a condom (penis in the vagina)

Low risk

- Sex with a condom when you use it correctly

- Oral sex, but don't swallow semen (cum)

- Deep kissing (French kissing or tongue kissing)

- Sharing sex toys that have been cleaned or covered with a new condom between uses

No risk

- Hugging, massage

- Masturbation
- Fantasizing
- Dry kissing
- Phone sex
- Cybersex
- Using sex toys that you don't share

Talking about Safer Sex

You and your partners will have to decide what you are comfortable doing sexually. If you aren't used to talking openly about sex, this could be hard to get used to.

Here are some tips:

- Find a time and place outside the bedroom to talk
- Decide what are your boundaries, concerns and desires before you start to talk
- Make sure you clearly state what you want. Use only "I" statements, for example: "I want to use a condom when we have sex."
- Make sure you don't do, or agree to do, anything that you're not 100 percent comfortable with.
- Listen to what your partner is saying. Acknowledge your partner's feelings and opinions. You will need to come up with solutions that work for both of you.
- Be positive. Use reasons for safer sex that are about you, not your partner.

Birth Control and HIV

The only forms of birth control that will protect against HIV are abstinence and using condoms while having sex. Other methods of birth control offer protection against unplanned pregnancy but do not protect against HIV or other sexually transmitted diseases.

Birth control options that DO protect against HIV:

- Abstinence (not having sex)
- Male condom

- Internal or female condom

Birth control options that DO NOT protect against HIV:

- Oral contraceptive ("the pill")
- Injectable contraceptive (shot)
- Contraceptive implant
- IUD (intrauterine device)
- Emergency contraception ("morning-after pill")
- Diaphragm, cap, and shield
- Vasectomy (getting your tubes tied if you are a man)
- Tubal ligation (getting your tubes tied if you are a woman)
- Withdrawal

Considerations for Women with HIV

If you are in a monogamous relationship and your partner also is HIV positive, you may decide to use a birth control method other than condoms.

Safe methods of birth control for an HIV-positive woman with an HIV-positive partner include:

- Using a diaphragm
- Tubal ligation (getting your tubes tied)
- IUD (intrauterine device)

Use only after checking with your provider (these may interact with your anti-HIV medications):

- Birth control pills
- Contraceptive injection (e.g., Depo-Provera)
- Contraceptive implant (e.g., Norplant)

Tips for Using Condoms and Dental Dams

Some people think that using a condom makes sex less fun. Other people have become creative and find condoms sexy. Not having to worry about infecting someone will definitely make sex much more enjoyable.

If you are not used to using condoms: practice, practice, practice.

Condom Dos and Don'ts

Shop around. Use lubricated latex condoms. Always use latex, because lambskin condoms don't block HIV and STDs, and polyurethane condoms break more often than latex (if you are allergic to latex, polyurethane condoms are an option). Shop around and find your favorite brand. Try different sizes and shapes (yes, they come in different sizes and shapes). There are a lot of choices—one will work for you.

Keep it fresh. Store condoms loosely in a cool, dry place (not your wallet). Make sure your condoms are fresh—check the expiration date. Throw away condoms that have expired, been very hot, or been washed in the washer. If you think the condom might not be good, get a new one. You and your partner are worth it.

Take it easy. Open the package carefully, so that you don't rip the condom. Be careful if you use your teeth. Make sure that the condom package has not been punctured (there should be a pocket of air). Check the condom for damaged packaging and signs of aging such as brittleness, stickiness, and discoloration.

Keep it hard. Put on the condom after the penis is erect and before it touches any part of a partner's body. If a penis is uncircumcised (uncut), the foreskin must be pulled back before putting on the condom.

Heads up. Make sure the condom is right-side out. It's like a sock—there's a right side and a wrong side. Before you put it on the penis, unroll the condom about half an inch to see which direction it is unrolling. Then put it on the head of the penis and hold the tip of the condom between your fingers as you roll it all the way down the shaft of the penis from head to base. This keeps out air bubbles that can cause the condom to break. It also leaves a space for semen to collect after ejaculation.

Slippery when wet. If you use a lubricant (lube), it should be a water-soluble lubricant (for example, ID Glide, K-Y Jelly, Slippery Stuff, Foreplay, Wet, Astroglide) in order to prevent breakdown of the condom. Products such as petroleum jelly, massage oils, butter, Crisco, Vaseline, and hand creams are not considered water-soluble lubricants and should not be used.

Put lubricant on after you put on the condom, not before—it could slip off. Add more lube often. Dry condoms break more easily.

Come and go. Withdraw the penis immediately after ejaculation, while the penis is still erect; grasp the rim of the condom between your fingers and slowly withdraw the penis (with the condom still on) so that no semen is spilled.

Clean up. Throw out the used condom right away. Tie it off to prevent spillage or wrap it in bathroom tissue and put it in the garbage. Condoms can clog toilets. Use a condom only once. Never use the same condom for vaginal and anal intercourse. Never use a condom that has been used by someone else.

Do You Have to Use a Condom for Oral Sex?

It is possible for oral sex to transmit HIV, whether the infected partner is performing or receiving oral sex. But the risk is very low compared with unprotected vaginal or anal sex.

If you choose to perform oral sex, you may:

- Use a latex condom on the penis; or

- Use a latex barrier (such as a natural rubber latex sheet, a dental dam, or a cut-open condom that makes a square) between your mouth and the vagina. A latex barrier such as a dental dam reduces the risk of blood or vaginal fluids entering your mouth. Plastic food wrap also can be used as a barrier.

- If either you or your partner are allergic to latex, plastic (polyurethane) condoms can be used.

  If you choose to perform oral sex and this sex includes oral contact with your partner's anus (analingus or rimming),

- Use a latex barrier (such as a natural rubber latex sheet, a dental dam, or a cut-open condom that makes a square) between your mouth and the anus. Plastic food wrap also can be used as a barrier. This barrier is to prevent getting another sexually transmitted disease or parasites, not HIV.

  If you choose to share sex toys, such as dildos or vibrators, with your partner,

- Each partner should use a new condom on the sex toy; and be sure to clean sex toys between each use.

Internal Condom (Also Called Female Condom)

The internal condom is a large condom fitted with larger and smaller rings at each end. The rings help keep it inside the vagina during sex;

for anal sex, the inner ring usually is removed before it is inserted. It is made of nitrile, so any lubricant can be used without damaging it. It may seem a little awkward at first, but can be a useful alternative to the traditional "male" condom. Female condoms generally cost more than male condoms.

- Store the condom in a cool dry place, not in direct heat or sunlight.

- Throw away any condoms that have expired—the date is printed on individual condom wrappers.

- Check the package for damage and check the condom for signs of aging such as brittleness, stickiness, and discoloration. The internal condom is lubricated, so it will be somewhat wet.

- Before inserting the condom, you can squeeze lubricant into the condom pouch and rub the sides together to spread it around.

- Put the condom in before sex play because preejaculatory fluid, which comes from the penis, may contain HIV. The condom can be inserted up to 8 hours before sex.

- The internal condom has a firm ring at each end of it. To insert the condom in the vagina, squeeze the ring at the closed end between the fingers (like a diaphragm), and push it up into the back of the vagina. The open ring must stay outside the vagina at all times, and it will partly cover the lip area. For use in the anus, most people remove the internal ring before insertion.

- Do not use a male condom with the internal condom.

- Do not use an internal condom with a diaphragm.

- If the penis is inserted outside the condom pouch or if the outer ring (open ring) slips into the vagina, stop and take the condom out. Use a new condom before you start sex again.

- Don't tear the condom with fingernails or jewelry.

- Use a condom only once and properly dispose of it in the trash (not the toilet).

Dental Dams and Plastic Wrap

Even though oral sex is a low-risk sexual practice, you may want to use protection when performing oral sex on someone who has HIV.

Dental dams are small squares of latex that were made originally for use in dental procedures. They are now commonly used as barriers when performing oral sex on women, to keep in vaginal fluids or menstrual blood that could transmit HIV or other STDs. Some people use plastic wrap instead of a dental dam. It's thinner.

Here are some things to remember:

- Before using a dental dam, first check it visually for any holes

- If the dental dam has cornstarch on it, rinse that off with water (starch in the vagina can lead to an infection)

- Cover the woman's genital area with the dental dam

- For oral-anal sex, cover the opening of the anus with a new dental dam

- A new dental dam should be used for each act of oral sex; it should never be reused

Section 51.4

Aging with HIV/AIDS

This section includes text excerpted from "Aging with HIV," HIV.gov, U.S. Department of Health and Human Services (HHS), May 15, 2017.

Growing Older with Human Immunodeficiency Virus (HIV)

At the start of the epidemic more than 30 years ago, people who were diagnosed with human immunodeficiency virus (HIV) or acquired immunodeficiency syndrome (AIDS) could expect to live only 1–2 years after that diagnosis. This meant that the issues of aging were not a major focus for people with HIV disease.

But today, thanks to improvements in the effectiveness of antiretroviral therapy (ART), people with HIV who are diagnosed early in their infection, and who get and stay on ART can keep the virus suppressed.

For this reason, a growing number of people living with HIV in the United States are aged 55 and older. Many of them have been living with HIV for years; others are recently infected or diagnosed. According to the Centers for Disease Control and Prevention (CDC), people aged 55 and older accounted for 26 percent of all Americans living with diagnosed or undiagnosed HIV infection in 2013.

Complications Associated with Aging

So the good news is that people with HIV are living longer, healthier lives if they are on treatment and achieve and maintain a suppressed viral load. However, with this longer life expectancy, individuals living with long-term HIV infection exhibit many clinical characteristics commonly observed in aging: multiple chronic diseases or conditions, the use of multiple medications, changes in physical and cognitive abilities, and increased vulnerability to stressors.

Complications Associated with Long-Term HIV Infection

While effective HIV treatments have decreased the likelihood of AIDS-defining illnesses among people aging with HIV, HIV-associated non-AIDS conditions are more common in individuals with long-standing HIV infection. These conditions include cardiovascular disease, lung disease, certain cancers, HIV-Associated Neurocognitive Disorders (HAND), and liver disease (including hepatitis B and hepatitis C), among others.

In addition, HIV appears to increase the risk for several age-associated diseases, as well as to cause chronic inflammation throughout the body. Chronic inflammation is associated with a number of health conditions, including cardiovascular disease, lymphoma, and type 2 diabetes. Researchers are working to better understand what causes chronic inflammation, even when people are being treated with ART for their HIV disease.

HIV and its treatment can also have profound effects on the brain. Although AIDS-related dementia, once relatively common among people with HIV, is now rare, researchers estimate that more than 50 percent of people with HIV have HAND, which may include deficits in attention, language, motor skills, memory, and other aspects of cognitive function that may significantly affect a person's quality of life. People who have HAND may also experience depression or psychological distress. Researchers are studying how HIV and its treatment affect the brain, including the effects on older people living with HIV.

Late HIV Diagnosis

Older Americans are more likely than younger Americans to be diagnosed with HIV infection late in the course of their disease, meaning they get a late start to treatment and possibly more damage to their immune system. This can lead to poorer prognoses and shorter survival after an HIV diagnosis. Late diagnoses can occur because healthcare providers may not always test older people for HIV infection, and older people may mistake HIV symptoms for those of normal aging and don't consider HIV as a cause.

The Importance of Support Services

Living with HIV presents certain challenges, no matter what your age. But older people with HIV may face different issues than their younger counterparts, including greater social isolation and loneliness. Stigma is also a particular concern among older people with HIV. Stigma negatively affects people's quality of life, self-image, and behaviors, and may prevent them disclosing their HIV status or seeking HIV care.

Therefore, it is important for older people with HIV to get linked to HIV care and have access to mental health and other support services to help them stay healthy and remain engaged in HIV care. You can find support services through your healthcare provider, your local community center, or and HIV service organization. Or use HIV.gov's HIV Testing and Care Services Locator to find services near you.

Chapter 52

HIV/AIDS Status Disclosure

Revealing Positive Test Results to Others

It's important to share your status with your sex partner(s) and/or people with whom you inject drugs. Whether you disclose your status to others is your decision.

Partners

It's important to disclose your human immunodeficiency virus (HIV) status to your sex partner(s) and anyone you shared needles with, even if you are not comfortable doing it. Communicating with each other about your HIV status means you can take steps to keep both of you healthy. The more practice you have disclosing your HIV status, the easier it will become. Many resources can help you learn ways to disclose your status to your partners.

If you're nervous about disclosing your test result, or you have been threatened or injured by a partner, you can ask your doctor or the local health department to help you tell your partner(s) that they might have been exposed to HIV. This type of assistance is called partner notification or partner services. Health departments do not reveal your name to your partner(s). They will only tell your partner(s) that they have been exposed to HIV and should get tested.

This chapter includes text excerpted from "Talking about Your HIV Status," HIV.gov, U.S. Department of Health and Human Services (HHS), May 15, 2017.

Many states have laws that require you to tell your sexual partners if you're HIV-positive before you have sex (anal, vaginal, or oral) or tell your drug-using partners before you share drugs or needles to inject drugs. In some states, you can be charged with a crime if you don't tell your partner your HIV status, even if you used a condom or another type of protection and the partner does not become infected.

Healthcare Providers

Your healthcare providers (doctors, clinical workers, dentists, etc.) have to know about your HIV status in order to be able to give you the best possible care. It's also important that healthcare providers know your HIV status so that they don't prescribe medication for you that may be harmful when taken with your HIV medications.

Some states require you to disclose your HIV-positive status before you receive any healthcare services from a physician or dentist. For this reason, it's important to discuss the laws in your state about disclosure in medical settings with the healthcare provider who gave you your HIV test results.

Your HIV test result will become part of your medical records so that your doctor or other healthcare providers can give you the best care possible. All medical information, including HIV test results, falls under strict confidentiality laws such as the Health Insurance Portability and Accountability Act (HIPAA) Privacy Rule and cannot be released without your permission. There are some limited exceptions to confidentiality. These come into play only when not disclosing the information could result in harm to the other person.

Family and Friends

In most cases, your family and friends will not know your test results or HIV status unless you tell them yourself. While telling your family that you have HIV may seem hard, you should know that disclosure actually has many benefits—studies have shown that people who disclose their HIV status respond better to treatment than those who don't. If you are under 18, however, some states allow your healthcare provider to tell your parent(s) that you received services for HIV if they think doing so is in your best interest.

Employers

In most cases, your employer will not know your HIV status unless you tell them. But your employer does have a right to ask if you have any health conditions that would affect your ability to do your job or pose a serious risk to others. (An example might be a healthcare professional, like a surgeon, who does procedures where there is a risk of blood or other body fluids being exchanged.)

If you have health insurance through your employer, the insurance company cannot legally tell your employer that you have HIV. But it is possible that your employer could find out if the insurance company provides detailed information to your employer about the benefits it pays or the costs of insurance. All people with HIV are covered under the Americans with Disabilities Act (ADA). This means that your employer cannot discriminate against you because of your HIV status as long as you can do your job.

Chapter 53

HIV/AIDS Patients and Legal Rights

Chapter Contents

Section 53.1

Your Rights in the Workplace

This section includes text excerpted from "Workplace
Rights," HIV.gov, U.S. Department of Health and Human
Services (HHS), May 15, 2017.

Human Immunodeficiency Virus (HIV), Employment Discrimination, and the Law

The Americans with Disabilities Act (ADA) of 1990 prohibits
employment discrimination on the basis of disability. The ADA, which
covers employers of 15 or more people, applies to employment decisions at all stages. Court decisions have found that an individual with
even asymptomatic human immunodeficiency virus (HIV) is protected
under this law.

The Health Insurance Portability and Accountability Act (HIPAA)
of 1996 addresses some of the barriers to healthcare facing people with
HIV, as well as other vulnerable populations. HIPAA gives people with
group coverage protections from discriminatory treatment, makes it
easier for small groups (such as businesses with a small number of
employees) to obtain and keep health insurance coverage, and gives
those losing/leaving group coverage new options for obtaining individual coverage.

The Family Medical Leave Act (FMLA) of 1993 applies to pri-
vate-sector employers with 50 or more employees within 75 miles of
the work site. Eligible employees may take leave for serious medical
conditions or to provide care for an immediate family member with a
serious medical condition, including HIV/AIDS (acquired immunodeficiency syndrome). Eligible employees are entitled to a total of 12 weeks
of job-protected, unpaid leave during any 12-month period.

The Consolidated Omnibus Budget Reconciliation Act (COBRA) of
1986 allows employees to continue their health insurance coverage at
their own expense for a period of time after their employment ends.
For most employees ceasing work for health reasons, the period of
time to which benefits may be extended ranges from 18–36 months.

Filing a Charge of Employment Discrimination

Any individual who believes that his or her employment rights have
been violated may file a charge of discrimination with the Federal

Equal Employment Opportunity Commission (EEOC). In addition, an individual, an organization, or an agency may file a charge on behalf of another person in order to protect the aggrieved person's identity.

Section 53.2

Laws for Your Welfare

This section contains text excerpted from the following sources: Text under the heading "The Americans with Disabilities Act (ADA) and Persons with Human Immunodeficiency Virus (HIV) / Acquired Immunodeficiency Syndrome (AIDS)" is excerpted from "Questions and Answers: The Americans with Disabilities Act and Persons with HIV/AIDS," ADA.gov, U.S. Department of Justice (DOJ), October 2016; Text under the heading "Family and Medical Leave Act (FMLA)" is excerpted from "Family and Medical Leave Act (FMLA)," U.S. Department of Labor (DOL), February 1, 2002. Reviewed June 2018; Text under the heading "Health Insurance Portability and Accountability (HIPAA)" is excerpted from "Employee Benefits Security Administration—Health Coverage Portability (HIPAA) Compliance FAQs," U.S. Department of Labor (DOL), July 25, 2016; Text under the heading "COBRA—7 Important facts" is excerpted from "COBRA—7 important Facts," Centers for Medicare and Medicaid Services (CMS), February 15, 2018.

The Americans with Disabilities Act (ADA) and Persons with Human Immunodeficiency Virus (HIV) / Acquired Immunodeficiency Syndrome (AIDS)

What Is the ADA?

The Americans with Disabilities Act (ADA) gives federal civil rights protections to individuals with disabilities similar to those provided to individuals on the basis of race, color, sex, national origin, age, and religion. It guarantees equal opportunity for individuals with disabilities in public accommodations, employment, transportation, state and local government services, and telecommunications.

Are People Living with HIV or AIDS Protected by the ADA?

Yes. An individual has a "disability" under the ADA if he or she has a physical or mental impairment that substantially limits one or more major life activities, including major bodily functions such as the functions of the immune system; has a record of such an impairment; or has an actual or perceived mental or physical impairment that is not transitory and minor and is subjected to an action prohibited under the ADA.

Persons with human immunodeficiency virus (HIV), both symptomatic and asymptomatic, have physical impairments that substantially limit one or more major life activities or major bodily functions and are, therefore, protected by the law. Persons who are discriminated against because they are regarded as having HIV are also protected. For example, a person who is fired on the basis of a rumor that he has acquired immunodeficiency syndrome (AIDS), even if he does not, is protected by the law.

Moreover, the ADA protects persons who are discriminated against because they have a known association or relationship with an individual who has HIV. For example, the ADA protects a woman (who does not have HIV) who is denied a job because her roommate has AIDS.

Family and Medical Leave Act (FMLA)

The Family and Medical Leave Act (FMLA) provides certain employees with up to 12 weeks of unpaid, job-protected leave per year. It also requires that their group health benefits be maintained during the leave. FMLA is designed to help employees balance their work and family responsibilities by allowing them to take reasonable unpaid leave for certain family and medical reasons. It also seeks to accommodate the legitimate interests of employers and promote equal employment opportunity for men and women.

FMLA applies to all public agencies, all public and private elementary and secondary schools, and companies with 50 or more employees. These employers must provide an eligible employee with up to 12 weeks of unpaid leave each year for any of the following reasons:

- For the birth and care of the newborn child of an employee

- For placement with the employee of a child for adoption or foster care

- To care for an immediate family member (spouse, child, or parent) with a serious health condition

- To take medical leave when the employee is unable to work because of a serious health condition

Employees are eligible for leave if they have worked for their employer at least 12 months, at least 1,250 hours over the past 12 months, and work at a location where the company employs 50 or more employees within 75 miles. Whether an employee has worked the minimum 1,250 hours of service is determined according to FLSA principles for determining compensable hours or work.

Time taken off work due to pregnancy complications can be counted against the 12 weeks of family and medical leave.

Special rules apply to employees of local education agencies. The Department of Labor (DOL) administers FMLA; however, the Office of Personnel Management (OPM) administers FMLA for most federal employees.

Health Insurance Portability and Accountability (HIPAA)

The Health Insurance Portability and Accountability Act (HIPAA) of 1996 includes provisions of federal law governing health coverage portability, health information privacy, administrative simplification, medical savings accounts, and long-term care insurance.

HIPAA's provisions affect group health plan coverage in the following ways:

- Provide certain individuals special enrollment rights in group health coverage when specific events occur, e.g., birth of a child (regardless of any open season);

- Prohibit discrimination in group health plan eligibility, benefits, and premiums based on specific health factors; and

- While HIPAA previously provided for limits with respect to preexisting condition exclusions, new protections under the Affordable Care Act (ACA) now prohibit preexisting condition exclusions for plan years beginning on or after January 1, 2014. For plan years beginning on or after January 1, 2014, plans are no longer required to issue the general notice of preexisting condition exclusion and individual notice of period of preexisting condition exclusion. Plans are also no longer required to issue certificates of creditable coverage after December 31, 2014. These amendments were made because plans are prohibited from imposing preexisting condition exclusions for plan years beginning on or after January 1, 2014.

COBRA—7 Important Facts

COBRA is a federal law that may let you keep your employer group health plan coverage for a limited time after one of these:

1. Your employment ends:

   - You lose coverage as a dependent of the covered employee

   - This is called "continuation coverage."

2. In general, COBRA only applies to employers with 20 or more employees. However, some states require insurers covering employers with fewer than 20 employees to let you keep your coverage for a limited time.

3. In most situations that give you COBRA rights (other than a divorce), you should get a notice from your employer's benefits administrator or the group health plan. The notice will tell you your coverage is ending and offer you the right to elect COBRA continuation coverage.

4. COBRA coverage generally is offered for 18 months (36 months in some cases). Ask the employer's benefits administrator or group health plan about your COBRA rights if:

   - You find out your coverage has ended and you don't get a notice

   - You get divorced

5. The employer must tell the plan administrator if you qualify for COBRA because of one of these:

   - The covered employee died

   - The covered employee lost his/her job

   - The covered employee became entitled to Medicare

   Once the plan administrator is notified, the plan must let you know you have the right to choose COBRA coverage.

6. You or the covered employee needs to tell the plan administrator if you qualify for COBRA because of one of these:

   - You've become divorced or legally separated (court-issued separation decree) from the covered employee

   - You were a dependent child or dependent adult child who's no longer a dependent

   You'll need to tell the plan administrator about your change in situation within 60 days of the change.

7. Before you elect COBRA, talk with your State Health Insurance Assistance Program (SHIP) about Part B and Medigap.

Chapter 54

Public Benefits and Housing Options for Persons with HIV

Chapter Contents

Section 54.1

Social Security for People Living with HIV/AIDS

This section includes text excerpted from "Social
Security for People Living with HIV/AIDS," U.S. Social
Security Administration (SSA), April 2017.

If you have human immunodeficiency virus (HIV) / acquired immunodeficiency syndrome (AIDS) and cannot work, you may qualify for
disability benefits from the U.S. Social Security Administration (SSA).
Your condition must be expected to last at least a year or end in death,
and must be serious enough to prevent you from doing substantial
gainful work. The amount of earnings that Social Security considers
substantial and gainful changes each year.

If your child has HIV/AIDS, he or she may be able to get Supplemental Security Income (SSI) if your household income is low enough.

Benefits Paid under Two Programs

Social Security pays disability benefits under two programs:

1. The Social Security Disability Insurance (SSDI) program for
    people who paid Social Security taxes; and

2. The Supplemental Security Income (SSI) program for people
    who have little income and few resources.

If your Social Security benefits are very low and you have limited
income and resources, you may qualify for benefits from both programs.

How Do I Qualify for Social Security Disability Benefits?

When you work and pay Social Security taxes, you earn Social Security credits. (Most people earn the maximum of four credits a year.) The
number of years of work needed for disability benefits depends on how
old you are when you become disabled. Generally, you need five years
of work in the 10 years before the year you become disabled. Younger
workers need fewer years of work. If your application is approved,
your first Social Security disability benefit will be paid for the sixth
full month after the date your disability began.

What Will I Get from Social Security?

The amount of your monthly benefit depends on how much you earned while you were working. You'll also qualify for Medicare after you have been getting disability benefits for 24 months. Medicare helps pay for hospital and hospice care, lab tests, home healthcare, and other medical services.

How Do I Qualify for SSI Disability Payments?

If you have not worked long enough to get Social Security or your Social Security benefits are low, you may qualify for SSI payments if your total income and resources are low enough. If you get SSI, you'll most likely be eligible for the Supplemental Nutrition Assistance Program (SNAP) and Medicaid. Medicaid takes care of your medical bills while you're in the hospital or receiving outpatient care. In some states, Medicaid pays for hospice care, a private nurse, and prescription drugs used to fight HIV disease.

How Do I File for Benefits?

You can apply for Social Security disability benefits online at www.socialsecurity.gov, or you can call the toll-free number, 800-772-1213, to make an appointment to file a disability claim at your local Social Security office or to set up an appointment for someone to take your claim over the telephone. The disability claims interview lasts about one hour. If you're deaf or hard of hearing, you may call the toll-free TTY number, 800-325-0778, between 7 a.m. and 7 p.m. on business days.

The Social Security office treats all calls confidentially, and a second Social Security representative monitors some telephone calls to make sure you receive accurate and courteous service.

How Do You Decide My Claim?

All applications received from people with HIV/AIDS are processed as quickly as possible. Social Security works with an agency in each state called the Disability Determination Services (DDS).

The state agency will look at the information you and your doctor provide and decide if you qualify for benefits. Social Security benefits can be paid right away for up to six months before making a final decision on your claim if:

- You're not working;

- You meet the SSI rules about income and resources; and

- Your doctor or other medical source certifies that your HIV infection meets certain criteria based on medical eligibility rules.

How Can I Help Speed up My Claim?

You can help speed up the processing of your claim by having certain information when you apply. This includes:

- Your Social Security number (SSN) and birth certificate and the SSN and birth certificates of any family members who may be applying for benefits; and

- A copy of your most recent W-2 form. (If you're applying for SSI, information about your income and resources will be asked for; for example, bank statements, unemployment records, rent receipts, and car registration.)

The following information is also needed:

- The names and addresses of any doctors, hospitals, or clinics you've been to for treatment;

- How HIV/AIDS has affected your daily activities, such as cleaning, shopping, cooking, taking the bus, etc., and

- The kinds of jobs you've had during the past 15 years.

Additionally, a representative will ask your doctor to complete a form explaining how your HIV infection has affected you. You or your doctor can access form "SSA–4814" for adults or "SSA–4815" for children at www.ssa.gov/forms/index.html or you can call the 800 number to ask for the appropriate form. After your doctor completes and signs the appropriate form, bring or send the form to the Social Security office.

What Happens If I Go Back to Work?

If you return to work, there are special rules that let your benefits continue while you work. These rules are important for people with HIV/AIDS who may be able to go back to work when they are feeling better.

Contacting Social Security

The most convenient way to contact the Social Security anytime, anywhere is to visit www.socialsecurity.gov. There, you can: apply for benefits; open a my Social Security account, which you can use to review your Social Security statement, verify your earnings, print a benefit verification letter, change your direct deposit information, request a replacement Medicare card, and get a replacement 1099/1042S; obtain valuable information; find publications; get answers to frequently asked questions; and much more.

If you don't have access to the Internet, the Social Security offers many automated services by telephone, 24 hours a day, 7 days a week. Call the toll-free at 800-772-1213 or TTY number, 800-325-0778, if you're deaf or hard of hearing.

If you need to speak to a person, your calls can be answered from 7 a.m. to 7 p.m., Monday through Friday.

Section 54.2

Affordable Care Act for People Living with HIV/AIDS

This section includes text excerpted from "HIV/AIDS—The Affordable Care Act Helps People Living with HIV/AIDS," Centers for Disease Control and Prevention (CDC), August 28, 2017.

On March 23, 2010, President Obama signed the Affordable Care Act (ACA) and set into place an effort that will help ensure Americans have secure, stable, affordable health insurance. Historically, people living with human immunodeficiency virus (HIV) and acquired immunodeficiency syndrome (AIDS) have had a difficult time obtaining private health insurance and have been particularly vulnerable to insurance industry abuses. Consistent with the goals of the President's National HIV/AIDS Strategy, the ACA makes considerable strides in addressing these concerns and advancing equality for people living with HIV and AIDS.

Improving Access to Coverage

Currently, fewer than one in five (17%) of people living with HIV has private insurance and nearly 30 percent do not have any coverage. Medicaid, the federal-state program that provides healthcare benefits to people with low incomes and those living with disabilities, is a major source of coverage for people living with HIV/AIDS, as is Medicare, the federal program for seniors and people with disabilities. The Ryan White HIV/AIDS Program is another key source of funding for health and social services for this population.

The ACA is one of the most important pieces of legislation in the fight against HIV/AIDS in our history. As of September 23, 2010, insurers are no longer able to deny coverage to children living with HIV or AIDS. The parents of as many as 17.6 million children with preexisting conditions no longer have to worry that their children will be denied coverage because of a preexisting condition. Insurers also are prohibited from canceling or rescinding coverage to adults or children because of a mistake on an application. And insurers can no longer impose lifetime caps on insurance benefits. Because of the law, 105 million Americans no longer have a lifetime dollar limit on essential health benefits. These changes will begin to improve access to insurance for people living with HIV/AIDS and other disabling conditions and help people with these conditions retain the coverage they have.

For people who have been locked out of the insurance market because of their health status, including those living with HIV/AIDS, the law created the Pre-existing Condition Insurance Plan. More than 90,000 people—some of whom are living with HIV or AIDS—have enrolled in this program, which has helped change lives and, in many cases, save them.

These changes will provide an important bridge to the significant changes in 2014 as the ACA is fully implemented. Beginning in 2014, insurers will not be allowed to deny coverage to anyone or impose annual limits on coverage. People with low and middle incomes will be eligible for tax subsidies that will help them buy coverage from new state health insurance exchanges. The ACA also broadens Medicaid eligibility to generally include individuals with income below 133 percent of the federal poverty line ($14,400 for an individual and $29,300 for a family of 4), including single adults without children who were previously not generally eligible for Medicaid. As a result, in many states, a person living with HIV who meets this income threshold will no longer have to wait for an AIDS diagnosis in order to become eligible for Medicaid.

The ACA also closes, over time, the Medicare Part D prescription drug benefit "donut hole," giving Medicare enrollees living with HIV and AIDS the peace of mind that they will be better able to afford their medications. Beneficiaries receive a 50 percent discount on covered brand-name drugs while they are in the "donut hole," a considerable savings for people taking costly HIV/AIDS drugs. And in the years to come, they can expect additional savings on their prescription drugs while they are in the coverage gap until it is closed in 2020.

In addition, as a result of the healthcare law, AIDS Drug Assistance Program (ADAP) benefits are now considered as contributions toward Medicare Part D's True Out of Pocket Spending Limit ("TrOOP"). This is a huge relief for ADAP clients who are Medicare Part D enrollees, since they will now be able to move through the donut hole more quickly, which was difficult, if not impossible, for ADAP clients to do before this change.

Ensuring Quality Coverage

The ACA also helps people with public or private coverage have access to the information they need to get the best quality care. This includes:

- **Quality, comprehensive care.** The law ensures health plans in the individual and small-group markets beginning in 2014 offer benefits similar to that of a typical employer plan, including prescription drugs, preventive services and chronic disease management, and mental health and substance use disorder services.

- **Preventive care.** Many private health insurance plans must now cover recommended preventive services, like certain cancer screenings, at no additional cost. HIV screening for adults and adolescents at higher risk and HIV screening and counseling for women are also covered without cost-sharing in most private plans. Medicare also covers certain recommended preventive services, including HIV screening for individuals at increased risk, without cost-sharing or deductibles. These services will help people living with HIV and AIDS stay healthy and prevent the spread of HIV as well.

- **Coordinated care.** The law also recognizes the value of patient-centered medical homes (coordinated, integrated, and comprehensive care) as an effective way to strengthen the quality of care, especially for people with complex chronic conditions. The Ryan White HIV/AIDS Program is the pioneer in the development of this model in the HIV healthcare system.

Increasing Opportunities for Health and Well-Being

Despite significant advances in HIV treatment and education, there are an estimated 50,000 new HIV infections annually, and there are significant racial and gender disparities with the majority of new infections among gay men, African Americans, and Latinos. The health of people living with HIV and AIDS is influenced not only by their ability to get coverage but also economic, social, and physical factors.

- **Prevention and wellness.** The law makes critical investments in prevention, wellness, and public health activities to improve public health surveillance, community-based programs, and outreach efforts. This includes increasing coverage for HIV testing.

- **Diversity and cultural competency.** The ACA expands initiatives to strengthen cultural competency training for all healthcare providers and ensure all populations are treated equitably. It also bolsters the federal commitment to reducing health disparities.

- **Healthcare providers for underserved communities.** The ACA expands the healthcare workforce and increases funding for community health centers, an important safety-net for low-income individuals and families. A key recommendation of the National HIV/AIDS Strategy is to increase the number and diversity of available providers of clinical care and related services for people living with HIV. Thanks to the ACA, the National Health Service Corps (NHSC) is providing loans and scholarships to more doctors, nurses, and other healthcare providers that serve approximately 10.4 million patients across the country. The NHSC has nearly tripled since 2008, a critical healthcare workforce expansion to better serve vulnerable populations.

Section 54.3

Housing Options for People with HIV

This section includes text excerpted from "Housing and
Health," HIV.gov, U.S. Department of Health and
Human Services (HHS), May 15, 2017.

Why Is Stable Housing Important for People with Human Immunodeficiency Virus (HIV)?

The conditions in which people with human immunodeficiency virus (HIV) live, work, learn, and play contribute to their ability to live healthy lives. With safe, decent, and affordable housing, people with HIV are better able to access comprehensive healthcare and supportive services, get on HIV treatment, take their HV medication consistently, and see their healthcare provider regularly. However, individuals with HIV who are homeless or lack stable housing are more likely to delay HIV care, have poorer access to regular care, and are less likely to adhere to their HIV treatment.

Throughout many communities, people with HIV risk losing their housing due to factors such as increased medical costs and limited incomes or reduced ability to keep working due to related illnesses. Securing stable housing is a key part of achieving successful HIV outcomes.

Federal Housing Assistance

To help take care of the housing needs of low-income people who are living with HIV/AIDS and their families, the U.S. Department of Housing and Urban Development's (HUD) Office of HIV/AIDS Housing manages the Housing Opportunities for Persons With AIDS (HOPWA) program. The HOPWA program is the only federal program dedicated to addressing the housing needs of people living with HIV/AIDS and their families. Under the HOPWA Program, HUD makes grants to local communities, States, and nonprofit organizations for projects that benefit low-income persons living with HIV/AIDS and their families.

Many local HOPWA programs and projects provide short- and long-term rental assistance, operate community residences, or provide other supportive housing facilities that have been created to address the needs of people who are living with HIV/AIDS and the challenges that come with the disease.

- Statewide HOPWA information. Search HUD's list of HOPWA grantees to find current contact information for grantees in your state.

- Technical Assistance for HOPWA grantees. HOPWA technical assistance is available to assist HOPWA grantees, project sponsors, and communities in identifying and addressing the supportive housing needs of low-income individuals and their families living with HIV. Requests for technical assistance are submitted through the HUD Exchange portal. HOPWA grantees and project sponsors interested in requesting TA should reach out to their local HUD Field Office.

Other HUD Programs for People with HIV

In addition to the HOPWA program, people living with HIV/AIDS are eligible for any HUD program for which they might otherwise qualify (such as by being low-income or homeless). Programs include public housing, the Section 8 Housing Choice Voucher Program (HCVP), housing opportunities supported by Community Development Block Grants (CDBG), the HOME Investment Partnerships Program, and the Continuum of Care (COC) Homeless Assistance Program.

Chapter 55

Caring for Someone with HIV/AIDS

Helping Someone Who Has Been Newly Diagnosed with Human Immunodeficiency Virus (HIV)

There are many things that you can do to help a friend or loved one who has been recently diagnosed with human immunodeficiency virus (HIV):

- **Talk.** Be available to have open, honest conversations about HIV. Follow the lead of the person who is diagnosed with HIV. They may not always want to talk about it, or may not be ready. They may want to connect with you in the same ways they did before being diagnosed. Do things you did together before their diagnosis; talk about things you talked about before their diagnosis. Show them that you see them as the same person and that they are more than their diagnosis.

- **Listen.** Being diagnosed with HIV is life-changing news. Listen to your loved one and offer your support. Reassure them that HIV is a manageable health condition. There are medicines that can treat HIV and help them stay healthy.

This chapter includes text excerpted from "Supporting Someone Living with HIV," HIV.gov, U.S. Department of Health and Human Services (HHS), May 15, 2017.

637

- **Learn.** Educate yourself about HIV—what it is, how it is transmitted, how it is treated, and how people can stay healthy while living with HIV. Having a solid understanding of HIV is a big step forward in supporting your loved one. Have these resources available for your newly diagnosed friend if they want them. Knowledge is empowering, but keep in mind that your friend may not want the information right away.

- **Encourage treatment.** Some people who are recently diagnosed may find it hard to take that first step to HIV treatment. Your support and assistance may be helpful. By getting linked to HIV medical care early, starting treatment with HIV medication (called antiretroviral therapy or ART), adhering to medication, and staying in care, people with HIV can keep the virus under control, and prevent their HIV infection from progressing to AIDS. HIV treatment is recommended for all people with HIV and should be started as soon as possible after diagnosis. Encourage your friend or loved one to see a doctor and start HIV treatment as soon as possible. If they do not have an HIV care provider, you can help them find one. There are programs that can provide HIV medical care or help with paying for HIV medications. Use HIV.gov's HIV Testing Sites and Care Services Locator to find a provider.

- **Support medication adherence.** It is important for people living with HIV to take their HIV medication every day, exactly as prescribed. Ask your loved one what you can do to support them in establishing a medication routine and sticking to it. Also ask what other needs they might have and how you can help them stay healthy.

- **Get support.** Take care of yourself and get support if you need it. Turn to others for any questions, concerns, or anxieties you may have, so that the person who is diagnosed can focus on taking care of their own health.

If you are the sexual partner of someone who has been diagnosed with HIV, you should also get tested so that you know your own HIV status. If you test negative, talk to your healthcare provider about PrEP (preexposure prophylaxis), taking HIV medicine daily to prevent HIV infection. PrEP is recommended for people at high risk of HIV infection, including those who are in a long-term relationship with a partner who has HIV. If you test positive, get connected to HIV treatment and care as soon as possible.

What If a Friend Tells Me That They Have HIV?

More than a million people in the United States are living with HIV, so you may know someone who has the virus. If your friend, family member, or coworker has been HIV-positive for some time and has just told you, here's how you can be supportive:

- **Acknowledge.** If someone has disclosed their HIV status to you, thank them for trusting you with their private health information.

- **Ask.** If appropriate, ask if there's anything that you can do to help them. One reason they may have chosen to disclose their status to you is that they need an ally or advocate, or they may need help with a particular issue or challenge. Some people are public with this information; other people keep it very private. Ask whether other people know this information, and how private they are about their HIV status.

- **Reassure.** Let the person know, through your words or actions, that their HIV status does not change your relationship and that you will keep this information private if they want you to.

- **Learn.** Educate yourself about HIV. Today, lots of people living with HIV are on ART and have the virus under control. Others are at different stages of treatment and care. Don't make assumptions and look to your friend for guidance.

Part Seven

Additional Help and Information

Chapter 56

Glossary of HIV/AIDS-Related Terms

acquired immunodeficiency syndrome (AIDS): A disease of the immune system due to infection with human immunodeficiency virus (HIV). HIV destroys the cluster of differentiation 4 (CD4) T lymphocytes (CD4 cells) of the immune system, leaving the body vulnerable to life-threatening infections and cancers. Acquired immunodeficiency syndrome (AIDS) is the most advanced stage of HIV infection. To be diagnosed with AIDS, a person with HIV must have an AIDS-defining condition or have a CD4 count less than 200 cells/mm^3 (regardless of whether the person has an AIDS-defining condition).

acute HIV infection: Early stage of HIV infection that extends approximately 1–4 weeks from initial infection until the body produces enough HIV antibodies to be detected by an HIV antibody test. During acute HIV infection, HIV is highly infectious because the virus is multiplying rapidly. The rapid increase in HIV viral load can be detected before HIV antibodies are present.

adherence: Taking medications (or other treatment) exactly as instructed by a healthcare provider. The benefits of strict adherence to an HIV regimen include sustained viral suppression, reduced risk of drug resistance, improved overall health and quality of life, and decreased risk of HIV transmission.

This glossary contains terms excerpted from documents produced by several sources deemed reliable.

AIDS-defining condition: Any HIV-related illness included in the Centers for Disease Control and Prevention's (CDC) list of diagnostic criteria for AIDS. AIDS-defining conditions include opportunistic infections and cancers that are life-threatening in a person with HIV.

alanine aminotransferase (ALT): A liver enzyme that plays a role in protein metabolism. Abnormally high blood levels of ALT are a sign of liver inflammation or damage from infection or drugs. A normal level is below approximately 50 IU/L.

amebiasis: An inflammation of the intestines caused by infection with Entamoeba histolytica (a type of ameba) and characterized by frequent, loose stools flecked with blood and mucus.

antiretroviral therapy (ART): The daily use of a combination of HIV medicines (called an HIV regimen) to treat HIV infection. A person's initial HIV regimen generally includes three antiretroviral (ARV) drugs from at least two different HIV drug classes.

assay: A qualitative or quantitative analysis of a substance; a test.

asymptomatic: Without symptoms or not sick. Usually, used in HIV/AIDS literature to describe a person who has a positive reaction to one of several tests for HIV antibodies but who shows no clinical symptoms of the disease and who is not sick. Even though a person is asymptomatic, he or she may still infect another person with HIV.

baseline: An initial measurement used as the basis for future comparison. For people infected with HIV, baseline testing includes CD4 count, viral load (HIV RNA (ribonucleic acid)), and resistance testing. Baseline test results are used to guide HIV treatment choices and monitor effectiveness of antiretroviral therapy (ART).

CD4 cell count: A laboratory test that measures the number of CD4 T lymphocytes (CD4 cells) in a sample of blood. In people with HIV, the CD4 count is the most important laboratory indicator of immune function and the strongest predictor of HIV progression. The CD4 count is one of the factors used to determine when to start antiretroviral therapy (ART). The CD4 count is also used to monitor response to ART.

cervical cancer: Cancer that forms in tissues of the cervix (the organ connecting the uterus and vagina). It is usually a slow-growing cancer that may not have symptoms but can be found with regular Papanicolaou (Pap) tests (a procedure in which cells are scraped from the cervix and looked at under a microscope). Cervical cancer is almost always caused by human papillomavirus (HPV) infection.

chemotherapy: In general, it is the use of medicines to treat any disease. It is more commonly used to describe medicines to treat cancer.

chlamydia: A sexually transmitted disease (STD) caused by Chlamydia trachomatis that infects the genital tract. The infection is frequently asymptomatic (i.e., shows no symptoms), but if left untreated, it can cause sterility in women.

chronic HIV infection: Also known as asymptomatic HIV infection or clinical latency. The stage of HIV infection between acute HIV infection and the onset of AIDS. During chronic HIV infection, HIV levels gradually increase and the number of CD4 cells decrease. Declining CD4 cell levels indicate increasing damage to the immune system. Antiretroviral therapy (ART) can prevent HIV from destroying the immune system and advancing to AIDS.

clinical progression: Advance of disease that can be measured by observable and diagnosable signs or symptoms. For example, HIV progression can be measured by change in CD4 count.

cluster of differentiation 4 (CD4) cell: A type of lymphocyte. CD4 T lymphocytes (CD4 cells) help coordinate the immune response by stimulating other immune cells, such as macrophages, B lymphocytes (B cells), and CD8 T lymphocytes (CD8 cells), to fight infection. HIV weakens the immune system by destroying CD4 cells.

coccidioidomycosis: An infectious fungal disease caused by the breathing in of Coccidioides immitis, which are carried on windblown dust particles.

coinfection: When a person has two or more infections at the same time. For example, a person infected with HIV may be coinfected with hepatitis C virus (HCV) or tuberculosis (TB) or both.

combination therapy: Two or more drugs or treatments used together to obtain the best results against HIV infection and/or AIDS. Combination drug therapy (treatment) has proven more effective than monotherapy (single-drug therapy) in controlling the growth of the virus. An example of combination therapy would be the use of two drugs such as zidovudine and lamivudine together.

computed tomography (CT) scan: A procedure that uses a computer linked to an X-ray machine to make a series of detailed pictures of areas inside the body. The pictures are taken from different angles and are used to create 3-dimensional (3-D) views of tissues and organs. A dye may be injected into a vein or swallowed to help the tissues and organs show up more clearly. A CT scan may be used to help diagnose disease, plan treatment, or find out how well treatment is working. Also called CAT scan, computed tomography scan, computerized axial tomography scan, and computerized tomography.

core biopsy: The removal of a tissue sample with a wide needle for examination under a microscope. Also called core needle biopsy.

drug resistance: When a bacteria, virus, or other microorganism mutates (changes form) and becomes insensitive to (resistant to) a drug that was previously effective. Drug resistance can be a cause of HIV treatment failure.

enzyme-linked immunosorbent assay (ELISA): A laboratory test to detect the presence of HIV antibodies in the blood, oral fluid, or urine. The immune system responds to HIV infection by producing HIV antibodies. A positive result on an ELISA must be confirmed by a second, different antibody test (a positive Western blot (WB)) for a person to be definitively diagnosed with HIV infection.

excisional biopsy: A surgical procedure in which an entire lump or suspicious area is removed for diagnosis. The tissue is then examined under a microscope.

false negative: A negative test result that incorrectly indicates that the condition being tested for is not present when, in fact, the condition is actually present. For example, a false negative HIV test indicates a person does not have HIV when, in fact, the person is infected with HIV.

false positive: A positive test result that incorrectly indicates that the condition being tested for is present when, in fact, the condition is actually not present. For example, a false positive HIV test indicates a person has HIV when, in fact, the person is not infected with HIV.

highly active antiretroviral therapy (HAART): The name given to treatment regimens recommended by HIV experts to aggressively decrease viral multiplication and progress of HIV disease. The usual HAART treatment combines three or more different drugs, such as two nucleoside reverse transcriptase inhibitors (NRTIs) and a protease inhibitor, two NRTIs and a nonnucleoside reverse transcriptase inhibitor (NNRTI), or other combinations. These treatment regimens have been shown to reduce the amount of virus so that it becomes undetectable in a patient's blood.

Hodgkin lymphoma: A cancer of the immune system that is marked by the presence of a type of cell called the Reed-Sternberg cell. The two major types of Hodgkin lymphoma are classical Hodgkin lymphoma and nodular lymphocyte-predominant Hodgkin lymphoma (NLPHL). Symptoms include the painless enlargement of lymph nodes, spleen, or other immune tissue. Other symptoms include fever, weight loss, fatigue, or night sweats. Also called Hodgkin disease.

human herpesvirus 8 (HHV-8): A type of virus that causes Kaposi sarcoma (KS) (a rare cancer in which lesions grow in the skin, lymph nodes, lining of the mouth, nose, and throat, and other tissues of the body). Human herpesvirus 8 also causes certain types of lymphoma (cancer that begins in cells of the immune system). Also called HHV8, Kaposi sarcoma-associated herpesvirus, and KSHV.

human immunodeficiency virus (HIV): The virus that causes AIDS, which is the most advanced stage of HIV infection. HIV is a retrovirus that occurs as two types.

human papillomavirus (HPV): A type of virus that can cause abnormal tissue growth (for example, warts) and other changes to cells. Infection for a long time with certain types of HPV can cause cervical cancer. HPV may also play a role in some other types of cancer, such as anal, vaginal, vulvar, penile, oropharyngeal, and squamous cell skin cancers. Also called HPV.

immune system: A complex network of cells, tissues, organs, and the substances they make that helps the body fight infections and other diseases. The immune system includes white blood cells and organs and tissues of the lymph system, such as the thymus, spleen, tonsils, lymph nodes, lymph vessels, and bone marrow.

immunocompromised: When the body is unable to produce an adequate immune response. A person may be immunocompromised because of a disease or an infection, such as HIV, or as the result of treatment with drugs or radiation.

immunosuppression: A state of the body in which the immune system is damaged and does not perform its normal functions. Immunosuppression may be induced by drugs (e.g., in chemotherapy) or result from certain disease processes, such as HIV infection.

incisional biopsy: A surgical procedure in which a portion of a lump or suspicious area is removed for diagnosis. The tissue is then examined under a microscope to check for signs of disease.

incubation period: The time between infection with a pathogen and the onset of disease symptoms.

Kaposi sarcoma (KS): A type of cancer in which lesions (abnormal areas) grow in the skin, lymph nodes, lining of the mouth, nose, and throat, and other tissues of the body. The lesions are usually purple and are made of cancer cells, new blood vessels, and blood cells. They may begin in more than one place in the body at the same time. Kaposi sarcoma is caused by Kaposi sarcoma-associated herpesvirus (KSHV). In the United States, it usually occurs in people who have a weak immune system caused by AIDS or by drugs used in organ transplants. It is also seen in older men of Jewish or Mediterranean descent, or in young men in Africa.

latency: The period when an infecting organism is in the body but is not producing any clinically noticeable ill effects or symptoms. In HIV disease, clinical latency is an asymptomatic period in the early years of HIV infection. The period of latency is characterized by near-normal cluster of differentiation 4+ (CD4+) T-cell counts. Recent research indicates that HIV remains quite active in the lymph nodes during this period.

lymphocyte: A type of immune cell that is made in the bone marrow and is found in the blood and in lymph tissue. The two main types of lymphocytes are B lymphocytes and T lymphocytes. B lymphocytes make antibodies, and T lymphocytes help kill tumor cells and help control immune responses. A lymphocyte is a type of white blood cell.

lymphoma: Cancer of the lymphoid tissues. Lymphomas are often described as being large-cell or small-cell types, cleaved or noncleaved, or diffuse or nodular. The different types often have different prognoses (i.e., prospect of survival or recovery). Lymphomas can also be referred to by the organs where they are active, such as central nervous system (CNS) lymphomas, which are in the central nervous system, and gastrointestinal (GI) lymphomas, which are in the gastrointestinal tract. The types of lymphomas most commonly associated with HIV infection are called non-Hodgkin lymphomas or B-cell lymphomas. In these types of cancers, certain cells of the lymphatic system grow abnormally. They divide rapidly, growing into tumors.

monotherapy: Using only one drug to treat an infection or disease. Monotherapy for the treatment of HIV is not recommended outside of a clinical trial. The optimal regimen for initial treatment of HIV includes three antiretroviral (ARV) drugs from at least two different HIV drug classes.

non-Hodgkin lymphoma (NHL): Any of a large group of cancers of lymphocytes (white blood cells). Non-Hodgkin lymphomas can occur at any age and are often marked by lymph nodes that are larger than normal, fever, and weight loss. There are many different types of non-Hodgkin lymphoma. These types can be divided into aggressive (fast-growing) and indolent (slow-growing) types, and they can be formed from either B-cells or T-cells. B-cell non-Hodgkin lymphomas include Burkitt lymphoma, chronic lymphocytic leukemia (CLL)/ small lymphocytic lymphoma (SLL), diffuse large B-cell lymphoma, follicular lymphoma, immunoblastic large cell lymphoma, precursor B-lymphoblastic lymphoma, and mantle cell lymphoma. T-cell non-Hodgkin lymphomas include mycosis fungoides, anaplastic large cell lymphoma, and precursor T-lymphoblastic lymphoma. Lymphomas that occur after bone marrow or stem cell transplantation are usually B-cell non-Hodgkin lymphomas. Prognosis and treatment depend on the stage and type of disease. Also called NHL.

nonnucleoside reverse transcriptase inhibitor (NNRTI): Antiretroviral (ARV) HIV drug class. Nonnucleoside reverse transcriptase inhibitors (NNRTIs) bind to and block HIV reverse transcriptase (an HIV enzyme). HIV uses reverse transcriptase to convert its ribonucleic acid (RNA) into deoxyribonucleic acid (DNA) (reverse transcription). Blocking reverse transcriptase and reverse transcription prevents HIV from replicating.

nucleoside reverse transcriptase inhibitor (NRTI): Antiretroviral (ARV) HIV drug class. Nucleoside reverse transcriptase inhibitors (NRTIs) block reverse transcriptase (an HIV enzyme). HIV uses reverse transcriptase to convert its RNA into DNA (reverse transcription). Blocking reverse transcriptase and reverse transcription prevents HIV from replicating.

opportunistic infection (OI): An infection that occurs more frequently or is more severe in people with weakened immune systems, such as people with HIV or people receiving chemotherapy, than in people with healthy immune systems.

positron emission tomography (PET) scan: A procedure in which a small amount of radioactive glucose (sugar) is injected into a vein, and a scanner is used to make detailed, computerized pictures of areas inside the body where the glucose is taken up. Because cancer cells often take up more glucose than normal cells, the pictures can be used to find cancer cells in the body. Also called PET scan.

postexposure prophylaxis (PEP): Short-term treatment started as soon as possible after high-risk exposure to an infectious agent, such as HIV, hepatitis B virus (HBV), or hepatitis C virus (HCV).

The purpose of PEP is to reduce the risk of infection. An example of a high-risk exposure is exposure to an infectious agent as the result of unprotected sex.

protease inhibitor: Antiretroviral (ARV) HIV drug class. Protease inhibitors (PIs) block protease (an HIV enzyme). By blocking protease, PIs prevent new (immature) HIV from becoming a mature virus that can infect other CD4 cells.

rapid HIV test: A screening test for detecting antibody to HIV that produces very quick results, usually in 5–30 minutes. For diagnosis of HIV infection, a positive rapid test is confirmed with a second rapid test made by a different manufacturer.

rapid test: A type of HIV antibody test used to screen for HIV infection. A rapid HIV antibody test can detect HIV antibodies in blood or oral fluid in less than 30 minutes. A positive rapid HIV antibody test must be confirmed by a second, different antibody test (a positive Western blot) for a person to be definitively diagnosed with HIV infection.

reverse transcription: The third of seven steps in the HIV life cycle. Once inside a CD4 cell, HIV releases and uses reverse transcriptase (an HIV enzyme) to convert its genetic material—HIV RNA—into HIV DNA. The conversion of HIV RNA to HIV DNA allows HIV to enter the CD4 cell nucleus and combine with the cell's genetic material—cell DNA.

serologic test: Any number of tests that are performed on the clear fluid portion of blood. Often refers to a test that determines the presence of antibodies to antigens such as viruses.

superinfection: When a person who is already infected with HIV becomes infected with a second, different strain of HIV. Superinfection may cause HIV to advance more rapidly. Superinfection can also complicate treatment if the newly acquired strain of HIV is resistant to antiretroviral (ARV) drugs in the person's current HIV treatment regimen.

syphilis: A primarily sexually transmitted disease (STD) resulting from infection with the spirochete (a bacterium) *Treponema pallidum*. Syphilis can also be acquired in the uterus during pregnancy.

T cell: A type of lymphocyte. There are two major types of T lymphocytes

treatment failure: When an antiretroviral (ARV) regimen is unable to control HIV infection. Treatment failure can be clinical failure, immunologic failure, virologic failure, or any combination of the three. Factors that can contribute to treatment failure include drug resistance, drug toxicity, or poor treatment adherence.

tuberculosis (TB): Infection with the bacteria Mycobacterium tuberculosis, as evidenced by a positive tuberculin skin test (TST) that screens for infection with this organism. Sometimes, TST is called a purified protein derivative (PPD) or Mantoux test. A positive skin test might or might not indicate active TB disease. Thus, any person with a positive TST should be screened for active TB and, once active TB is excluded, evaluated for treatment to prevent the development of TB disease. TB infection alone is not considered an opportunistic infection indicating possible immune deficiency.

undetectable viral load: When the amount of HIV in the blood is too low to be detected with a viral load (HIV RNA) test. Antiretroviral (ARV) drugs may reduce a person's viral load to an undetectable level; however, that does not mean the person is cured. Some HIV, in the form of latent HIV reservoirs, remain inside cells and in body tissues.

viral load: The amount of HIV in a sample of blood. Viral load is reported as the number of HIV RNA copies per milliliter of blood. An important goal of antiretroviral therapy (ART) is to suppress a person's VL to an undetectable level—a level too low for the virus to be detected by a VL test.

viral set point: The viral load (HIV RNA) that the body settles at within a few weeks to months after infection with HIV. Immediately after infection, HIV multiplies rapidly and a person's viral load is typically very high. After a few weeks to months, this rapid replication of HIV declines and the person's viral load drops to its set point.

Western blot (WB): A type of antibody test used to confirm a positive result on an HIV screening test. (The initial screening test is usually a different type of antibody test or, less often, a viral load test). The immune system responds to HIV infection by producing HIV antibodies. A WB for confirmatory HIV testing is done using a blood sample.

window period: The time period from infection with HIV until the body produces enough HIV antibodies to be detected by standard HIV antibody tests. The length of the window period varies depending on the antibody test used. During the window period, a person can have a negative result on an HIV antibody test despite being infected with HIV.

X-ray: A type of high-energy radiation. In low doses, X-rays are used to diagnose diseases by making pictures of the inside of the body.

yoga: A mind and body practice with origins in ancient Indian philosophy. The various styles of yoga typically combine physical postures, breathing techniques, and meditation or relaxation.

Chapter 57

Directory of Organizations for People with HIV/AIDS and Their Families and Friends

Government Agencies That Provide Information about HIV/AIDS

AIDSinfo
P.O. Box 4780
Rockville, MD 20849-6303
Toll-Free: 800-HIV-0440
(800-448-0440)
Phone: 301-315-2816
Toll-Free TTY: 888-480-3739
Fax: 301-315-2818
Website: www.aidsinfo.nih.gov
E-mail: ContactUs@aidsinfo.nih.gov

Centers for Disease Control and Prevention (CDC)
1600 Clifton Rd.
Atlanta, GA 30329-4027
Toll-Free: 800-CDC-INFO
(800-232-4636)
Phone: 404-639-3311
Toll-Free TTY: 888-232-6348
Website: www.cdc.gov
E-mail: cdcinfo@cdc.gov

Resources in this chapter were compiled from several sources deemed reliable; all contact information was verified and updated in June 2018.

Effective Interventions

Centers for Disease Control and Prevention (CDC)
Toll-Free: 866-532-9565
Phone: 240-645-1756
Website: effectiveinterventions.cdc.gov
E-mail: interventions@danya.com

HIV Testing and Care Services Locator

Website: locator.aids.gov

National Cancer Institute (NCI)

9609 Medical Center Dr.
BG 9609 MSC 9760
Bethesda, MD 20892-9760
Toll-Free: 800-4-CANCER (800-422-6237)
Website: www.cancer.gov
E-mail: cancergovstaff@mail.nih.gov

National Institute of Allergy and Infectious Diseases (NIAID)

Office of Communications and Government Relations (OCGR)
5601 Fishers Ln.
MSC 9806
Bethesda, MD 20892-9806
Toll-Free: 866-284-4107
Phone: 301-496-5717
Toll-Free TDD: 800-877-8339
Fax: 301-402-3573
Website: www.niaid.nih.gov
E-mail: ocpostoffice@niaid.nih.gov

National Institute on Aging (NIA)

Bldg. 31 Rm. 5C27
31 Center Dr. MSC 2292
Bethesda, MD 20892
Toll-Free: 800-222-2225
Toll-Free TTY: 800-222-4225
Website: www.nia.nih.gov
E-mail: niaic@nia.nih.gov

National Prevention Information Network (NPIN)

Centers for Disease Control and Prevention (CDC)
Website: npin.cdc.gov
E-mail: NPIN-info@cdc.gov

Office of AIDS Research (OAR)

National Institutes of Health (NIH)
5601 Fishers Ln.
MSC 9840
Bethesda, MD 20892-9310
Phone: 301-496-0357
Website: www.oar.nih.gov
E-mail: oartemp1@od31em1.od.nih.gov

Positive Spin

U.S. Department of Health and Human Services (HHS)
Website: positivespin.hiv.gov

U.S. Department of Health and Human Services (HHS)

200 Independence Ave. S.W.
Washington, DC 20201
Toll-Free: 877-696-6775
Website: www.hhs.gov

U.S. Department of Veterans Affairs (VA)
810 Vermont Ave. N.W.
Washington, DC 20420
Toll-Free: 877-222-VETS
(877-222-8387)
Website: www.va.gov

U.S. Food and Drug Administration (FDA)
10903 New Hampshire Ave.
Silver Spring, MD 20993
Toll-Free: 888-INFO-FDA
(888-463-6332)
Website: www.fda.gov

Private Agencies That Provide Information about HIV/AIDS

AIDS InfoNet
2200 Pennsylvania Ave. N.W.
Fourth Fl. E.
Washington, DC 20037
Website: www.aidsinfonet.org
E-mail: webmaster@aidsinfonet.org

AIDS Vaccine Advocacy Coalition (AVAC)
423 W. 127th St.
Fourth Fl.
New York, NY 10027
Phone: 212-796-6423
Fax: 646-365-3452
Website: www.avac.org
E-mail: avac@avac.org

AIDSmeds.com
Website: www.aidsmeds.com

AIDSVu
Phone: 202-854-0480
Website: www.aidsvu.org
E-mail: info@aidsvu.org

American Academy of Family Physicians (AAFP)
P.O. Box 11210
Shawnee Mission, KS 66207-1210
Toll-Free: 800-274-2237
Phone: 913-906-6000
Fax: 913-906-6075
Website: www.nf.aafp.org
E-mail: aafp@aafp.org

American Academy of HIV Medicine (AAHIVM)
AAHIVM National Office
1705 DeSales St. N.W., Ste. 700
Washington, DC 20036
Phone: 202-659-0699
Fax: 202-659-0976
Website: www.aahivm.org

American Sexual Health Association (ASHA)
P.O. Box 13827
Research Triangle Park, NC 27709
Phone: 919-361-8400
Fax: 919-361-8425
Website: www.ashasexualhealth.org
E-mail: info@ashasexualhealth.org

Antiretroviral Pregnancy Registry (APR)
1011 Ashes Dr.
Wilmington, NC 28405
Toll-Free: 800-258-4263
Toll-Free Fax: 800-800-1052
Website: www.apregistry.com
E-mail: SM_APR@INCResearch.com

The Body.com
The Complete HIV/AIDS Resource
750 Third Ave.
Sixth Fl.
New York, NY 10017
Phone: 212-541-8500
Website: www.thebody.com

Center for AIDS (CFA)
Information and Advocacy
P.O. Box 66308
Houston, TX 77266-6308
Toll-Free: 888-341-1788
Phone: 713-527-8219
Fax: 713-521-3679
Website: www.centerforaids.org
E-mail: info@centerforaids.org

Elizabeth Glaser Pediatric AIDS Foundation (EGPAF)
1140 Connecticut Ave. N.W.
Ste. 200
Washington, DC 20036
Toll-Free: 888-499-HOPE
(888-499-4673)
Phone: 202-296-9165
Fax: 202-296-9185
Website: www.pedaids.org
E-mail: info@pedaids.org

Elton John AIDS Foundation (EJAF)
584 Bdwy.
Ste. 906
New York, NY 10012
Phone: 212-219-0670
Website: www.newyork.ejaf.org
E-mail: info@ejaf.org

The Foundation for AIDS Research (amfAR)
120 Wall St.
13th Fl.
New York, NY 10005-3908
Toll-Free: 800-39-amfAR
(800-392-6327)
Phone: 212-806-1600
Fax: 212-806-1601
Website: www.amfar.org
E-mail: E-mail: info@amfar.org

HIV Medicine Association (HIVMA)
1300 Wilson Blvd.
Ste. 300
Arlington, VA 22209
Phone: 703-299-1215
Fax: 703-299-8766
Website: www.hivma.org
E-mail: info@hivma.org

HIV Vaccine Trials Network (HVTN)
1100 Eastlake Ave. E.
Seattle, WA 98109
Phone: 206-667-6300
Fax: 206-667-6366
Website: www.hvtn.org
E-mail: info@hvtn.org

International AIDS Vaccine Initiative (IAVI)
Website: www.iavi.org
E-mail: info@iavi.org

National Clinician Consultation Center (NCCC)
University of California, San Francisco (UCSF), Zuckerberg San Francisco General Hospital
1001 Potrero Ave.
Bldg. 20, Ward 2203
San Francisco, CA 94110
Toll-Free: 800-933-3413
Phone: 415-206-5792
Fax: 415-476-3454
Website: aidsetc.org/aetc-program/national-clinician-consultation-center

National Minority AIDS Council (NMAC)
1000 Vermont Ave. N.W.
Ste. 200
Washington, DC 20005-4903
Phone: 202-853-0021
Website: www.nmac.org
E-mail: info@nmac.org

National NeuroAIDS Tissue Consortium (NNTC)
NNTC Data Coordinating Center (DCC)
401 N. Washington St.
Ste. 700
Rockville, MD 20850
Toll-Free: 866-NNTC-BRAIN (866-668-2272)
Phone: 301-251-1161 ext. 244
Fax: 301-576-4597
Website: www.nntc.org
E-mail: nntc@emmes.com

North American Syringe Exchange Network (NASEN)
535 Dock St.
Ste. 113
Tacoma, WA 98402
Phone: 253-272-4857
Fax: 253-272-8415
Website: www.nasen.org
E-mail: info@nasen.org

NYU School of Medicine
550 First Ave.
New York, NY 10016
Website: www.med.nyu.edu

Pacific AIDS Education and Training Center (PAETC)
Pacific AIDS Education and Training Program, University of California, San Francisco (UCSF)
550 16th St.
Third Fl. UCSF MC 0661
San Francisco, CA 94158-2549
Phone: 415-476-6153
Website: www.paetc.org
E-mail: paetcmail@ucsf.edu

Project Inform
273 Ninth St.
San Francisco, CA 94103
Toll-Free: 877-HELP-4-HEP (877-435-7443)
Phone: 415-558-8669
Fax: 415-558-0684
Website: www.projectinform.org

Services & Advocacy for Gay, Lesbian, Bisexual and Transgender Elders (SAGE)
305 Seventh Ave.
15th Fl.
New York, NY 10001
Phone: 646-576-8669
Website: www.sageusa.org
E-mail: info@sageusa.org

U.S. Military HIV Research Program (MHRP)
6720A Rockledge Dr.
Ste. 400
Bethesda, MD 20817
Phone: 301-500-3600
Fax: 301-500-3666
Website: www.hivresearch.org
E-mail: info@hivresearch.org

The Well Project
P.O. Box 220410
Brooklyn, NY 11222
Toll-Free: 888-616-WELL
(888-616-9355)
Website: www.thewellproject.org
E-mail: info@thewellproject.org

Index

Index